Healthy Medicine:
A Guide to the Emergence of Sensible, Comprehensive Care

© in 2005

(a 2nd book 2006)

Book envisioned changes to org2d medical syst —

Robert J. Zieve, MD

(created?
Zieve went into a alt cancer care network

seems to be overflow — mat'l left for prev bk, no further work specific to dr—cooperative — a network vision

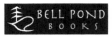
BELL POND
B O O K S

Published by Bell Pond Books
Great Barrington, Massachusetts 01230
www.bellpondbooks.com

ISBN: 0-88010-560-7

Library of Congress Cataloging-in-Publication Data is available.

10 9 8 7 6 5 4 3 2 1

Printed in the United States of America

TABLE OF CONTENTS

interesting sections

Part III: Why We Become Ill and How We Can Heal

Part IV: Illness and the Psyche

Part V: Comprehensive Medicine: Health Care that Works

IMAGINE

Imagine you are living some time in the near future. You have concerns about an illness in your life. You call the health association to which you belong and to which you make regular payments. These payments may vary depending on your income. You make an appointment to see a comprehensive medicine practitioner, who is part of a team at the clinic. In the meantime, you go on the Internet and download the freely available material that describes the nature of your illness. The association encourages you to do this, and your practitioner, who is your partner in healing, will be glad about the research you do. You may also go to any one of the educative meetings at the association facility.

When you go to your appointment with the practitioner you have chosen, the visit is paid for partly by you and partly by the association to which you belong. You receive a thorough evaluation, which includes a battery of tests. Many of these are comprehensive medicine tests that have become commonly accepted as often more valuable than the conventional laboratory tests and X rays that used to be the only testing done. Before this visit, you have been coming to the Association clinic regularly for evaluations, with appointments that last much longer than the ten-minute visits to which you used to be limited.

Whereas ten years earlier you feared that there would not be enough money or good facilities to care for you and help you heal, you know now that there are both. You understand that you have to play a more active role in your care and make necessary lifestyle changes. But you can now see the strong support you receive and can relax in the knowledge of this, which also helps your health.

The health association established a comprehensive medicine clinic several years before your current visit. It has practitioners of many backgrounds and training who work together as teams. These teams include conventional medical doctors, herbalists, and shamans. The old control that medical boards wielded over practitioners has been uprooted and replaced with certification requirements and evidence-based research that has shown results. Because health care is no longer primarily pharmaceutically or surgically based, there are no special interests behind the scenes that benefit from your remaining ill and needing their products. So you can relax and wait for good care from people who like what they do and receive appropriate compensation for reasonable work hours.

As you wait to see your practitioner, you think back a number of years and remember what it was like then. At that time you went to a crowded and impersonal doctor's office, saw the doctor for five or ten minutes at the most, and received a prescription, which you filled at a drugstore, filled with chemical products that contributed to your body's toxic buildup.

A few years back, faced with a crisis in health care, both in quality and financing, a number of individuals and groups in public and private care called for complete overhaul of the health care system. A small group of physicians who were practicing what was then called alternative, complementary, or integrative medicine began to push for changes. Their efforts were backed by a growing volume of evidence-based research on the value of practicing health care in this integrative way. Many so-called "fringe" healers and practitioners were invited to partake in these changes.

Before the new health association, you used to go to your local hospital for drug-based therapy, surgery, and radiation diagnostics and therapies. The hospital had a large billing department where clerks worked with stacks of files making sure that the hospital was paid for its services by insurance companies whose employees were rewarded for minimizing such payments. Although the hospital still does some of the same surgeries, surgery is now performed much less frequently because there is less need for it. The integration of various energy medicine therapies into the care provided by your hospital and local clinic has greatly decreased the need for the tremendously expensive surgeries that were common before. Payment is now made directly to the association and the amount of your bill is based on both your income and your compliance with the association's healthy lifestyle guidelines.

You have become acquainted with and have experienced many new therapies, such as microcurrent and infrared technologies, color and light therapies, homeopathy, IV infusions, oxygen-based therapies, and heavy metal chelation and detoxification. It is still amazing to you that these are now more of the norm than the exception. It was not too many years back that the medical establishment derided these methods as quackery, and medical boards revoked the licenses of good physicians for providing them to their patients. And the eye movement and color therapies that helped you heal much of your stored emotional traumas are now part of most people's care.

Your name was just called. Time to go and get some healthy medicine, and then to head home to your loved ones and to the work you enjoy.

ABOUT THIS BOOK

Healthy Medicine: A Guide to the Emergence of Sensible, Comprehensive Care is written for both health care professionals and laypeople.

PART I begins with a picture of our health care system today. It then explores how we arrived at the current position and how we can create a new and effective health care system.

PART II looks at the model of comprehensive medicine, describes how it offers the solution to effective and financially affordable health care, and discusses how allopathic practitioners can make changes in their practices in order to become more integrative. This details some integrative medicine diagnostic and treatment modalities.

PART III provides an explanation of illness and its underlying causes and an introduction to lifestyle changes to transform our lives from illness-driven, to embarking on and maintaining a therapeutic path.

PART IV explores the psychology of illness as a road to transformation. Through images from myth, fairy tales, and the creative arts, this section provides the reader with a template for this journey of healing through illness. Many of the illnesses from which we physically suffer have their origins in stored conflicts and trauma experienced many years before the onset of illness. This section brings attention to that part of ourselves that, if we make deep changes, will improve our therapeutic process.

Books are guides, a way for us to become more aware and reflective on the human condition. Reading is not about getting through a book as fast as you can in order to glean as much information as possible. It is about pausing and reflecting. Reading is like breathing in, pausing, and then breathing out. It is in life's pauses, the twilight and dawn times of transition between day and night, inspiration and expiration, that insight and intuition develop. I urge you, as the reader, to permit them to develop within you as you read this book.

INTRODUCTION

Healthy Medicine: A Guide to the Emergence of Sensible, Comprehensive Care provides an in-depth explanation of the model of effective and affordable health care that we need to establish if we are to have a health care system that works.

In the book, I call the model I present "Comprehensive Medicine" because it goes beyond terms such as "integrative medicine" and enables us to achieve a unity of all the realms of healing in an intelligent, inclusive way. Through Comprehensive Medicine, we can achieve the goal of healthy medicine, which is a system of medicine that clearly promotes health and healing for all.

Comprehensive Medicine integrates areas that were previously kept separate, or which are sometimes put together haphazardly, but which we now know are interconnected. The term "integrative medicine," as it is currently used, refers to a medical approach that combines allopathic/conventional medicine and alternative/complementary medicine. There are as many ways of combining these disciplines as there are practitioners, however. For some practitioners, combining the conventional and the alternative translates into primarily prescribing pharmaceuticals while slowly integrating nutritional supplements and herbal medicine as the practitioner gains knowledge and experience in their use. For others, it means relying on pharmaceuticals, while recommending acupuncture and Chinese herbs. Still others primarily use the more alternative/complementary therapies and rely on conventional medicine with only a small number of patients.

While being willing to employ a range of therapies is the first step in going beyond the conventional medical approach, practicing comprehensive medicine requires integrating these areas of medicine into a comprehensive whole. When we comprehend something, we see the whole picture, or a greater picture than we saw before. We see how the parts work together. This is intelligence, as opposed to the intellectual over-analysis of information that is characteristic of medicine as it is practiced conventionally today.

The use of the word "medicine" is deliberate in the title. In its essence, the word reflects something sacred. It used to be that medicine was from the earth, or that good medicine was the essence of a loving relationship. Unfortunately, the word today refers to a large bureaucratized institution. We need now to reclaim the original realms encompassed by the word "medicine," and restore them to a comprehensive medical model.

In this book, you will find other terms that may be new to you, such as energy medicine. These will be explained as we go along. But as an example of the comprehensive nature of the new medicine, let me say here that in the category of energy medicine are the MRI's and EKG's of conventional medicine as well as the traditional therapies acupuncture and homeopathy. The category also includes newer forms of older experience in light and sound therapies, infrared treatments, and treatments based on the deeper understandings of physics in medicine and healing.

In our modern approach to education, we learn to compartmentalize. Notice the "mentalize" of the "part" in this word. This book endeavors to integrate such compartmentalized areas as medicine, psychology, economics, myth, fairy tale, and spiritual principles into a wider, yet more practical view of what we need to be developing as Medicine for Healing.

Over the past 25 years as a practicing physician, I have watched a progressive disintegration of our health care system. On the surface, it may not seem that way to everyone. Television advertising and specials make it appear that things are improving. Yet the rate and severity of chronic illness are increasing, as is the cost of chronic care. We are slipping into an abyss even if we don't realize it. I worked for many years as an emergency room physician. In this work, I saw how conventional medical technology could be of great use when it comes to emergencies, surgery, and certain diagnostics. And this is where the money is in health care—not in caring for sick people. Most people who visit the emergency room actually do so for chronic illness care, or care for an acute illness, rather than for emergencies. As an emergency physician, I so often witnessed how lost, fearful, and isolated my patients felt. They were often thankful for receiving care, but I knew the care was woefully inadequate for their problems. And I knew that five minutes in their doctor's office would be almost totally ineffective. I felt deep sadness at these realities, and they have only become progressively worse.

While integrative medicine provides an opportunity to help people in a deeper way, it is still insufficient when it is practiced in the context of today's medicine. Some patients need a half-hour session; some need four hours. I know through my practice of comprehensive medicine that to do it right, to get to the core of why a person is ill, and to craft an effective treatment program, requires time and money, neither of which is available to many patients in the medical care system today.

Alternative/complementary therapies are unaffordable in the current model, where most people feel forced to determine their care based on insurance and government financial support. Most integrative practitioners with busy practices can scarcely afford the time and money required to do deep healing work with patients.

Of course, the patient also must be ready for this deep healing work. Most are not—even most of those who see integrative physicians. It is this deep healing work that our illnesses now call upon us to do, both individually and collectively, so that our lives can become more meaningful. To do the deep healing work in the early 21st century requires fundamental life changes on the part of both patients and practitioners. And it requires us to rethink our approach to the social and institutional fabric of health care.

We need an infusion of new energies into health care. This is beginning to happen. Some city hospitals, notably Jefferson Hospital in Philadelphia and

Beth Israel in New York City, are developing departments of integrative medicine. In many other areas of the country, practitioners of non-allopathic medicine are greatly increasing in numbers. But the change is coming slowly.

This book is about the deep and fundamental changes we need to make now in our health care system and how we, both the public and health practitioners, can begin taking on this challenge. We need changes in our attitudes, our understanding of illness, our acceptance of non-allopathic practitioners, the economics of how we pay for health care, and our entire professional medical-legal system in which medical boards often act within the law to protect and defend the guild of conventional medicine under the guise of "scientific proof." The book explores a wide range of topics, integrating areas that have too often been kept separate. To aid in bringing these areas together, I present a template that combines economics, psychology, medicine, physiology, and mythology. It can serve as support and guidance for making the changes necessary for a new model of medicine in the 21st century.

I am reminded of the words spoken by the U.S. president, played by Michael Douglas, in the movie *The American President*: "America isn't easy. America is advanced citizenship. We have serious problems to solve, and we need serious people to solve them."

Together we can create a health care system that works, that makes healing affordable to everyone. This is a big task. Health care is now neither effective nor affordable for most, and it is becoming less effective and more expensive.

Consider what is in these pages and consider beginning to make the recommended changes in your own life, in your relationships, communities, and in your approach to politics and economics. Our health and well-being depend on it.

The reader can gain much from this book in depth of understanding and in guidance to life-changing and health-supporting activities. If each of us can begin to make changes, however small they may be at the beginning, we will engender a movement toward the health care system we so greatly need.

ACKNOWLEDGEMENTS

This book is the culmination of almost two decades of study and experience. Increasingly, it is obvious how much we learn from each other. I have been blessed with being able to learn from and observe many good teachers and practitioners. In what follows, I would like to thank each and every one of these individuals for the time and energy they offered me. The cumulative effort of my relationships with these people has helped me to increasingly fulfill the endeavor given to me in this life: to work in the healing profession.

Dietrich Klinghardt, M.D., Ph.D., Director
American Academy of Neural Therapy, Bellevue, Washington

Thomas Rau, M.D., Medical Director
Paracelsus Klinik, Lustmuhle, Switzerland

Gerard Gueniot, M.D, Homeopathic Physician
La Medeleine-Lez-Lille, France

Larry Wilson, M.D., Prescott, Arizona

Joseph Mercola, D.O., Optimal Wellness Center
Schaumburg, Illinois

Karl Maret, M.D.,
Dove Health Alliance and Heart Mind Communications
Aptos, California

Tony Cocilovo, Lightforms, Inc.,
Prescott, Arizona

Dickson Thom, N.D. Portland, Oregon

Garry Gordon, M.D., Gordon Research Inc.
Payson, Arizona

Ross Rentea, M.D. and Andrea Rentea, M.D
Paulina Medical Clinic, Chicago, Illinois

Ann Szaur, N.D., R.N., Nevada City, California

Patricia Kane, Ph.D.
Haverford, Pennsylvania, and Millville, New Jersey

Dane Rutledge, Esq., Attorney at Law
New York City

Frank George, D.O., Scottsdale, Arizona

Scott Moyer, BioEclectic Research Institute,
Santa Rosa, California

Rob Robb, Personal Advisor

Gillian Schoemaker, Therapeutic Eurythmist
Kimberton, Pennsylvania

Bruce Shelton, M.D.
President, Arizona Homeopathic Medical Board, Phoenix, Arizona

Frank Shallenberger, M.D.,
The Nevada Center of Alternative and Anti-Aging Medicine
Carson City, Nevada

Steven Johnson, D.O., Foxhollow Clinic
Crestwood, Kentucky

Donald Gill, Albuquerque, New Mexico

Henry Williams, M.D., Lancaster, Pennsylvania

My deep thanks to Eve Greenberg, MA, without whose assistance this book
would not have been prepared and published.

Also special thanks to my friends: Lana Strouse; Sharon McFeely; Wayne
Lehrer; Brian Stern, D.C., L.Ac.; Bill Westendorff, D.D.S.; Ulrich Bold; Will
LeStrange; Diane Del Chiaro; Clare Helfrich; Chrystyne Jackson; Kim Levin;
Vickie Ragsdell; Peter Moscow; Tish Mosvold; Jacqueline Small; Valerie
Schultz; and Joy Wallen; all of whom helped me in this process.

And to Stephanie Marohn, whose excellence in editing has helped shape the
final form of this material.

And to the late John Foster, M.D., whom I hardly knew, but to whom I felt
very close and whose loss I felt deeply.

FOREWORD

By Dietrich Klinghardt, MD, Ph.D.

In the last 200 years humans have solved the most haunting problems we have faced for millennia: we have developed systems of government and conduct with each other that have given us a reasonable amount of personal safety, peace and some freedom. We have figured out how to secure a reliable and lasting food supply and how to provide shelter for most of us. We have also created a health care system and medical technologies that improve our chances of survival in life threatening situations and offer us a scientific understanding of our physical and emotional sufferings.

There were always cultures which had achieved these basics for a while – however against the backdrop of less evolved starving and often angry neighbors. Instead of sharing their wealth and knowledge in a brotherly way, the more evolved cultures defended their progress with military might, until another culture emerged with better weapons or more skillful warriors. In the constant turmoil ideas about health and wellness came and went -- without a chance for a universal body of knowledge and truth about medicine emerging that was complete, effective, gentle and accessible to everybody. Whenever there was starvation and war, beyond the care for the injured warrior there was little interest in health, longevity, caring for the elderly and infants, no interest in poetry and love or relationship. Whenever there was peace and abundance, medical knowledge and systems of healing and caring evolved that included preventative measures (such as acupuncture or the Kosher diet), caring for pregnant women and infants and for those who were disadvantaged.

Our current young medical system developed over the last 200 years parallel to the industrial revolution and against the backdrop of major wars, revolutions and the threat of total extinction of life on the planet. It is medicine for acute problems and has never really evolved beyond the field of emergency medicine. We know how to treat gunshot wounds, fractures and skin lacerations. But our current medical model does not address the issues effectively that most people really suffer from: the lack of zest and interest, chronic fatigue and depression, chronic pain syndromes, feelings of loneliness and lack of belonging - and the ever increasing presence of neurological illness and cancer. This is a time of relative peace and safety and therefore a time and an opportunity to address those issues and create a healing and health care system that can successfully guide people towards more fulfilling and joyful lives.

This is a time to use the global contemporary and historical knowledge from all healing traditions and rediscover solutions that are already here. It is also time to attend to those struggling with chronic rather then acute problems. Why do so many children have asthma? Why do so many grown-ups not feel well? There are so many questions conventional medicine has no answers for.

Many of these questions have long been answered by alternative practitioners. Many of the new discoveries in Medicine lead to treatments that are 2500 years old: Acupuncture can up-regulate the infection and cancer fighting cytokines instantly and often lastingly. A compassionate conversation with a client can often free up that portion of the immune system that has been asleep for years. Science often provides the understanding for traditional methods of healing - which have often been ridiculed by those intentionally misinterpreting true science in order to cater to special interests.

True science fully embraces many traditional, alternative and conventional approaches in healing and can create a meaningful synergy between them. It can provide the proof and respect wherever it is due. It can also reject some of the approaches in each of these categories. A true scientist cannot be limited by the dogma of his or her time. Buddha once said: "Truth is what works". In Medicine it is up to science to prove why certain methods work. It is not up to science to declare certain methods as "unscientific" because currently science does not understand it. Science is currently still blind in many areas and cannot and should not be the gatekeeper of medical methodologies. It is up to the practitioner to make wise choices for his or her clients against this backdrop.

Dr. Robert Zieve has been my colleague and personal friend for many years. He is the only medical doctor and physician who could have written this book. Life has prepared him well: in his early upbringing he was deeply steeped and connected to the philosophical and practical teachings of Europe's 20th century mystic and enlightened master, Rudolph Steiner. By working in the emergency room for many years he stayed solidly grounded in the current technology and methods used in good western medicine. But he knew from his contact with anthroposophical thinking in medicine that there is a whole other world out there. Dr. Zieve explored that world carefully. He sought out the best teachers and scientists of this time and did his due diligence. By also working for many years in private practice he explored what worked and what did not.

I know that he has practiced most of the methods he introduces in this book. It sets him aside from most other authors in our field. Many of them create philosophical models that were never tested and are too theoretical to be implemented. Many of them have stopped practicing medicine long before they started writing their books. Many of them do not have the solid background in science that is required to move our field forward. Beyond that, I have known Dr. Zieve not only as a broad minded thinker and philosopher, but also as a pragmatic scientist and equally as a compassionate and very gifted healer. These ingredients make this book unique.

In the early part of the book, Dr Zieve introduces us to the ***context*** of modern western medicine – the political, social, economical and psychological backdrop against which medicine has evolved so far. It also exposes the many ways in which modern medicine is stuck and is resisting change. He makes the point painfully clear why we need a freer and encompassing body of knowledge and applied methodology in healing.

In the following parts of the book he takes us onto a journey into the ***content*** of healing and to deeper and deeper levels of understanding of the human condition in regards to health -- and the specific treatment strategies and paths of healing that are currently available. Dr. Zieve uncovers the hidden order behind health problems, the deepest causes -- and always points towards targeted and practical solutions. I consider this book a vision of a future that is already here. Many of us are aware of the hidden health care system already available to many who search for it, a system which is compassionate, dependable, highly effective and gentle. Many scientists, creative and intuitive minds, gifted and connected individuals have co-created it in the last twenty years.

This is the first book reaching the depth of understanding of complementary and alternative Medicine that reveals its inherent principles and honors it with Dr. Zieve's intelligence and sensitivity.

This book will leave the reader more intelligent, wiser and able to make far better choices in health care. It will give the health care provider an understanding of where she or he is right now in their personal and medical development - and give a map of meaningful future learnings and courses to take. It will give the current powers-to-be a valuable map outlining the necessary and unavoidable steps to create a new health care system.

The current system in its alignment with corporate interests will eventually lead us into death and extinction through environmental pollution, misguided and shortsighted manipulation of our food supply, contamination of our air and water and ever-increasing and severe damage to the most precious gift of all times: our children. The health care system this book leads us to is life affirmative on all levels and will lead us into a sustainable future. May it shorten the often painful transition phase from the rigid past to a liberated future!

Thank you Robert!

FOREWORD

By James Oschman, Ph.D.

Medicine and health care are changing rapidly in many countries around the world. The cost and ineffectiveness of virtually all health care systems has placed an unbearable financial and spiritual burden on the governments and the people in many nations, including the U.S.

During this transitional time, when many of the old systems are self-destructing, it is critical that the creative minds of our world contemplate what a new medicine might look like. Robert Zieve has contributed an important perspective on this puzzle in his book on Healthy Medicine.

The importance of this book goes beyond imagining a new health system. Dr. Zieve challenges us to pay attention to the many dimensions in which our health is being subtly and not so subtly influenced by the health care business as it is presently carried out. For example, television and advertising and world affairs subconsciously feed our fears. We are increasingly tense and worried, and this creates chaos in our lives and in our social fabric. To survive and remove this turbulence, we all need to pay closer attention to the subtle forces that are being exerted on our lives. Only through awareness can we heal the fractures and disharmonies being generated within and around us.

For example, we have a system that profits financially from our dependence and trust in it. We do not expect our health care system to take advantage of us when we are most vulnerable, but this is what has happened. Moreover, cash does not flow until we become ill, so there is little real motivation for prevention. Our best options for taking care of ourselves are rarely discussed, except in the context of some product we can purchase. What is left out of this equation is a simple reminder that our bodies and our spirits are remarkably resilient, and capable of efficient self-repair.

Dr. Zieve's book contains information that is vital to everyone involved in the evolutionary process that is upon us. From my perspective, this book is essential reading for all who will soon become key components of the comprehensive medical practices Zieve is envisioning and that are actually being created right now.

For all of this to work, we must be aware of the mistakes that have taken place in the past, so we do not repeat them. One of these mistakes is to focus on symptoms and fixing parts that have problems. The body in fact contains no isolated systems; injuries are not localized; eliminating pain is not healing. A change in emphasis is essential, for we rely on our medicine to maintain and strengthen our vitality, our joy, and our ability to participate in the world around us. Dr. Zieve's prescription is to bring together the best of all therapies, and to offer exactly what each patient needs. This is a formula for a much brighter future for all of us.

Dr. Oschman is the author of Energy Medicine: The Scientific Basis.

PART I:

FAILING HEALTH CARE
VERSUS
AN ECONOMY OF HEALING

CHAPTER 1

HEALTH CARE USA

The American health care system is ill. Although conventional medical breakthroughs are reported regularly on the evening news, and cures for cancer, heart disease, and many other diseases, are touted as just around the corner, the reality is quite different from this optimistic picture. The culture-wide disintegration and decay of family structure, schools, child-care, transportation infrastructure, politics, and our food and water supplies, is occurring in the way we provide health care as well. Health care availability differs depending on ability to pay and geographical location. Even for those who have money to purchase health care, which makes health care a commodity, the over-mechanized and specialized approach of conventional medicine ensures its ineffectiveness in treating most chronic illness beyond the short-term benefits it may provide.

Health care has become an industry. It has strayed from its true vocation, which is to serve as a vehicle for personal growth and development. Health, along with education and the arts in this country, has become subservient to economic forces. Our culture has become rigid, narrow-minded, protective of its self-interests, obsessed with mechanistic thinking, and reliant on pharmaceuticals and technology as its almost exclusionary form of fixing people. In our refusal to take responsibility for our own health, observing the conditions of our illnesses, and addressing them actively in our daily lives, we are collectively responsible for the development of a highly paternalistic medical profession.

There is a growing lack of trust in and respect for the medical profession as a whole. This is true even though there are many in its ranks that mean well. The problem is in the structure of the health care model we have created. The doctor-patient relationship as a vehicle for personal growth and development has all but disappeared. Patients are whisked in and out of the office, given a prescription, and another appointment in the near future. There is little, if any, appreciation of the real purpose of illness—to act as a vehicle for change. Through healing illness, a person has the opportunity to develop into a more self-directed human being. We too often perceive illness as a curse to be feared rather than as a blessing to be trusted. The trust between two people, doctor and patient, has fragmented, which has contributed to the current malpractice climate.

The American medical system is going bankrupt, obsessively driven by more expensive technology and drugs that are less affordable to many people, to the government, and to private insurers.

M.D.: MUTUAL DENIAL

A negative agreement exists between doctor and patient today. This works in the following manner: The doctor agrees to use his or her narrowly intellectual and mechanistic understanding of the human body and its diseases to decide on a drug to prescribe, or an operation. The doctor holds out the promise of protocols to eliminate a patient's unpleasant symptoms.

The symptoms are treated as if they are the illness. This is a big mistake in conventional medicine (and also, and unfortunately, often in what we call alternative medicine). The symptoms are not the illness. Yet when the symptoms are made to go away with drugs or surgery, then both doctor and patient think that the disease is gone. When the symptoms do not go away after a treatment, then stronger suppressive therapy is applied.

In return, the patient agrees to arrange payment either through government or third-party insurance, or through out-of-pocket payments that often take large chunks out of a weekly paycheck.

In this arrangement, neither party acts responsibly. The doctor does not spend much time or pursue depth of relationship in trying to understand the patient's illness. Likewise, the patient is not required to assume any responsibility for lifestyle conditions that led to the illness. These negative agreements are built-in defects in the medical system.

This system of mutual denial is bankrupting us for a number of reasons:

- It fosters continued dependence on professionals.

- It permits us to avoid looking at the seeds of illness in our lives and then making necessary changes—until incapacitating accidents or illnesses occur.

- It keeps us frozen in a mechanistic approach to life. Health care is equated with automobile care. Diseases are treated part-by-part, organ by organ. If a part is not working, then it needs to be replaced or cleaned out and overhauled. The image of the whole is fractured, like the fairytale mirror cracked into a thousand pieces.

- Because we are addicted to perfection, many of us demand ever-more expensive technology to treat a disease, are intolerant of mistakes, and are quick to sue if something goes wrong.

Most people are trapped in insurance and government plans that support these imbalances. As long as this system of mutual denial continues, it matters not whether we have a single-payer insurance system, or continue the present system of financing health care.

GOOD INTENTIONS ARE NOT ENOUGH

These mutual denial collusions are sometimes difficult to perceive. Many people in medicine have good intentions and want the best for their patients. A health care provider may have good intentions and sincerely want to help others, and still unwittingly do harm. Treating only symptoms can cause a patient's illness to worsen or to go more deeply into the patient's body, manifesting years later in another illness, and the connection between the two illnesses pass unnoticed.

Real healing requires more than having good intentions. It requires attention to basic principles. People may intend to do well, yet still do harm if they are unwilling to perceive how they have been subtly influenced to think and act in a certain way. The education of health professionals is designed to promote certain values and mechanistic intellectual approaches to illness. When the entire health care system economically and professionally rewards these values and approaches, then it becomes more difficult to penetrate the veils of illusion and respond to what people really need.

DENIAL: THE ILLNESS OF AMERICA

When I was an intern, I made rounds with the other physicians on my team. We visited each patient, and at the end of the rounds returned to the nurse's station for lively discussions about the diseases we had seen and the laboratory tests we would order. I remember feeling disconnected in this way of practicing medicine. We were expressing enthusiasm about diseases and not talking at all about the patient's life, the effects of the illness, or why the illness developed. To me, this was denial, staying in the comfortable and financially rewarding area of treating symptoms and not looking deeper.

Most physicians play it safe, offering medical care by formula, prescribing drugs as treatment, and seeing too many patients per day. This is denial, a denial of the heart, and the denial of being willing to feel the depth of suffering in another. It was much easier then, and still is for most in medicine to stay at the surface and fix the symptoms. While I practiced that way for a while, my need to look deeper eventually led me to comprehensive medicine, as it has led many others.

When you look deeper, you discover that the seeds of illness are in our lifestyles, our lack of awareness and consciousness, and our denials. Our daily

lives are too often consumed with denial. There is denial of real feelings, denial of what our true motives are in a relationship or at work, and denial of the
degree to which we are driven. Many people deny that they have problems at
all. Patients who are under extreme stress often deny to their doctor that they
have stress. Or they deny that their thoughts, words, and deeds could have
anything to do with why their relationships have turned sour. It has become
easier to blame others. We have a health care crisis because we are well practiced in denial. We refuse to do what is necessary in our daily lives. Instead,
we procrastinate, deny, and blame.

There is corporate denial on a massive scale. Our businesses and corporations have become adept at denying how the toxic by-products of industry are
making us ill.

Our health care institutions support this collective denial because they
benefit from it. We deny that our symptoms mean that something is out of
balance in our lives. We have evolved a medical system that supports this denial. It promises to fix our symptoms, as if these symptoms are really our
illness. The current mechanistic view has us believe that a pill can alter our
biochemistry, rid us of a symptom, and heal our illness.

Symptoms do not originate in our physical body chemistry, as we would
like to believe. Symptoms develop or precipitate out of our imbalanced lifestyles. This is true for contagious diseases as well as chronic diseases of the
internal organs. The illness is in the way we live.

Denial blinds us. We are unable to think clearly, to see the obvious, to as-
sess our imbalances, and then to make decisions on courses of action. This is
as true in our daily lives as it is in our health care system.

Many people blame malpractice as the reason for the increase in health
care costs. There is a partially correct perception here. The fear of being sued
does lead physicians to order more tests than may be necessary. Diagnostic
tests also enhance the diagnostics industry, however. Increasingly, those who
make the decisions about expensive diagnostic evaluation benefit financially
by doing such tests. For example, many patients with upper abdominal distress, which is often functional in nature, rather than being a disease, are
advised to have upper GI and gall bladder x-rays, or patients with headaches
are given CT scans and MRI's, which most often than not are unnecessary.
These are reimbursed by insurance companies. Yet tests to determine if such
headaches are secondary to food allergies, which is a far more common cause
of headaches than brain tumors, are not often reimbursed. Further, consumers
bear some of the responsibility for rising health care costs. Many of the same
people who blame malpractice costs also demand that other people fix them,
and are willing to blame others, doctors included, for the results (illnesses) of
their own denials.

Many elderly people blame drug companies for the high cost of drugs; for
many, prescription drugs are their single largest monthly expenditure. They

have become attached to being mechanistically fixed by their doctors. Yet many of the elderly choose to deny that years of imbalanced lifestyles have led to the diseases that keep them dependent on drugs. They demand that someone else pay the high costs of the miracle drugs that they have spent a lifetime worshiping.

Much of the public refuses to confront other explanations for rising costs, especially aging and technology, believing that health insurance should pay for any treatment that will save their lives, no matter the cost. This collective attitude is a major problem. There is no agreement today as to what is appropriate health care.

Instead, there is denial. We want one side of the coin without the other. We want health without honestly evaluating our illness-generating lifestyles. We want to see ourselves as good without acknowledging our undesirable traits. We want the warmth of family without being honest and observant about how families often become adept at collusively denying and keeping hidden many of our shortcomings. We demand to be fixed by others and deny recognition that part of healing involves making changes in our own lives. We want to enjoy the fruits of a materialistic culture without taking into account how we are suffering from the toxic by-products that permeate our daily lives.

Our health care system is ill because our society is ill. Almost everyone in our culture is ill. This is not a condemnation or a judgment. Illness is not bad. Acknowledging illness does not mean we use it as an excuse for all of our problems, or that we become dependent on medical treatment. It simply means that we need to change our perception, as in the following two points:

- Acknowledging the reality of illness is an opportunity to become more conscious and creative human beings

- We have to leave the womb. We need to stop demanding to be taken care of—by government, insurance company, job, doctor, or family.

In the 20th century we have seen two polar opposite approaches in the United States. Before 1932, there was no social welfare support net. We were on our own. Business was largely unregulated. There was no health care insurance. Beginning in 1965 with Medicare, a multifaceted program of what have come to be called entitlements has gradually been introduced into our social fabric.

Today we have taken this approach too far. Now people expect care regardless of the cost. The technology that has in some respects made our lives more comfortable has been put on a pedestal. People are denying that their lifestyles may be generating illness and are not being told otherwise. This is prolonged adolescence, coupled with a refusal to mature.

The health care crisis that is now in sharp focus gives us the opportunity to bring things into balance. Denial destroys balance, and balance is the key to healing. Denial leaves us open to being driven by what we are denying. It drives us to one extreme of behavior or the other.

Times of crisis require actions to change the complacent way we have been living for years. The illness of denial is deeply ingrained in our lifestyles at this time, and it must be met and gradually changed on a daily basis, with vision and purpose. This includes encouraging support groups, honest meetings between people in local communities and workplaces, and between physicians and other health practitioners whose primary focus and source of joy in life is in helping people heal. People will then be able to emerge from their protected and isolated states of unfulfilled wants and desires, and support each other in breaking through the web of denial.

Forums for living social dialogues between people need to become as important as learning principles from textbooks. Something new will then be given an opportunity to develop. Instead of a top-down, highly controlled and regulated health care system, either private or governmental, a system will develop that grows upward from a new living soil. Imagine a plant that grows upward in the light and heat of the sun to support and nourish our growth. In human life, the sun represents clear thinking (light) and enthusiasm (heat) in cooperative efforts. Illness is the reminder of our denials. Healing involves a change in consciousness.

DECAYING HIERARCHIES

Old hierarchical social agreements, old lines of authority that extend from the top down are breaking apart today. We must mature and no longer rely on paying a professional to be responsible for our health and well-being. These relationships need to become partnerships in responsibility.

This principle of maturation applies to all professional situations. In law, the legalese terminology and manipulation that characterizes our present legal system needs to be replaced with a system of common law based on common sense and right relationship. In medicine, the regality of professionals who tell their patients what to do based on a mechanistic and intellectual understanding of human illness and who become intolerant when their directions are not followed needs to be replaced with the model of physician as facilitator or guide for our development through the journey of illness.

The American and French Revolutions over two centuries ago were fought to break with old forms of social contracts. Yet these old forms of doing business are still strongly rooted in our economic system and extend into most professional fields, especially medicine. The word professional derives from "profess," which is what one professes to be, as opposed to who one really is.

Professional status has become a rigid and separate way of maintaining positions of economic privilege and social recognition. As a result of specialized intellectual training, the professional medical doctor finds his niche, his formula for success. Everyone else in the health care system, from nurses to hospital administrators, attend to the doctor because the doctor is the source of income. Physicians and other professionals are rewarded for what they know rather than who they are. Equating intellectualism with status is a central problem in Western civilization. It has become very difficult to bring light and clarity to the professional so that he can see the deficiencies of this system. This is the case because he has too much invested in its continuance.

The self-help movement and support groups in the United States, including those in alternative and complementary medicine, are a positive response to the negative agreements between doctor and patient, doctor and hospital, and hospital and insurance company. Unfortunately, orthodox professionals often deride the worth of support groups. Sometimes the support groups themselves become extensions of the medical model, as has happened with societies that raise funds for multiple sclerosis research, for example. Other self-help groups, such as Defeat Autism Now, are doing significant research in many important aspects of autistic spectrum disorder that is largely ignored by conventional medicine.

Medical doctors often feel threatened by informed patients, responding by speaking to them in a patronizing manner, putting them down, or even refusing to work with them. Many patients have reported to me how doctors have dismissed their questions. This especially happens with female patients going to male doctors. Quite a few patients I've seen have reported being dismissed by their doctor for not following the doctor's advice. Others have told stories of their doctor literally getting up and walking out of the room when they, the patient, started to show the doctor some literature on their illness, even if the literature was from mainstream medical journals.

Almost all physical illnesses have a psychological component. Conventional medicine ignores this fact. Doctor visits for lifestyle consultations are almost never covered by insurance or governmental health care. The situation is worse for thousands with depression, anxiety, and other psychological imbalances. Most people are not able to afford expensive psychotherapy. Funds for mental health programs are drying up across the country, leaving only private insurance that enables the few who can afford it to check into hospital programs. With the closing of many mental hospitals, patients end up on the streets, often homeless, and from there are sent to prison where no adequate treatment is available, and they further deteriorate. An estimated 35 to 40 percent of inmates are mentally ill. It is unfortunate that many programs for people with addictive behavior and other psychological imbalances do not draw on the wealth of practical experience of health workers in alternative and complementary medicine. This is another example of the restrictiveness and exclusivity that characterizes the medical profession today, which is strangling both itself and our health care system.

The mindset in this country is that if a patient's insurance company does not cover the treatment, then that treatment is unavailable to the patient. Insurance is allowed to dictate the level of care. Patients are in collusion with the insurance companies, allowing an impersonal, unavailable insurance company to make even life-or-death health care decisions for them.

LOOKING FOR SCAPEGOATS

Unfortunately, many in the medical field are quick to place the blame for their problems on a source outside themselves—government, insurance companies, lawyers, "quack" holistic doctors, to name four common scapegoats. Actually, the core of the crisis is in the model itself.

As we have seen, physician-professionals are at the apex of the pyramid of an old, rigid, decaying hierarchical structure. It is our collective responsibility today to ensure the reformation of this system into one that is:

1. More tolerant and inclusive of other approaches to healing, and which permits people to see the practitioner of their choice, licensed or unlicensed

2. More life-sustaining in support of human development through illness, and focused on discovering the functional imbalances that occur well before physical disease manifests

3. More economically affordable and available to all, which will occur as the first two reforms are implemented.

By placing blame on others, the medical profession has become possessed by a Scapegoat Complex. In reality, the inherent weaknesses of professionalism are the real problem. Narrow intellectual perceptions, a limited mechanistic understanding of illness, and a paternalistic approach to patients are some of these weaknesses. Old-boy types of relationships have developed between doctors and other main players in medical economics. An example is the continued willingness by many physicians to accept gifts from drug and medical technology companies. This interrelationship goes deep. Most conventional MD's update their medical knowledge primarily through magazines and seminars often funded by pharmaceutical companies.

CODEPENDENT AND ENABLER

The doctor-patient relationship today is one of codependent and enabler. The profession, for its own narcissistic gratification and rewards, needs to

8

have sick people who are dependent on it in order to maintain its position of authority and its economic benefits. This applies to the economic institutions of pharmaceuticals, medical technology, and insurance companies that provide rewards to the doctor for being allowed to be the front person in this relationship. This structure is increasingly fostered and supported by the volume of technical information that is published weekly. The information is so technical that the public must rely on the professional for interpretation.

In truth, the health professional needs to serve as a mediator between patient and technology. When the professional is too allied with technical experts, then true service to the patient is more difficult. The doctor-patient relationship needs to be based on trust. Yet this trust becomes more difficult when the doctor is tied to economic incentives. When trust is not there, health costs rise due to malpractice insurance and an increase in unnecessary diagnostic procedures in an attempt to reduce the risk of malpractice suits. As long as physicians permit this system to continue and as long as patients demand the latest drug or technique to "heal" them, then these collusive denials will continue to worsen the state of health care.

TWIN ILLUSIONS

Twin illusions: "Time is money" and "Knowledge is power."

These partners in crime against the soul are like Romulus and Remus, the twins who were suckled by the she-wolf in the myth of the founding of ancient Rome. Rome was a hardened and masculine culture. Roman law was based on property, as are our legal codes. Roman medicine was developed around the ideas of the physician Galen, who focused on human anatomical changes as the sources of disease, as allopathic medicine does today. This repudiated the earlier Greek teachings of Hippocrates that emphasized the interrelationship of bodily functioning and human behavior in the form of four humors, or what today are called the four temperaments: melancholic, choleric, sanguine, and phlegmatic.

Our major institutions of today, medicine included, are driven by mechanistic approaches to disease. What supports these institutions economically are the two sacred twins: time is money, and knowledge is power. These twin pillars hold up the temple of professionalism. The average physician perceives that he must severely limit his time with each patient in order to maintain the economic standard of living he has come to expect. This dependence on intellectually focused information as the primary means of making a living is increasing dramatically, which is why many physicians want to specialize.

In the emerging field of integrative alternative medicine, which is a step toward change in health care, practitioners can be effective and comfortable in a general practice. They know that by initially spending time going to the source of their patients' illnesses, they will save time and money in the long run. And while intellectual information is required, this information is bal-

9

anced by the dynamic and holistic way that integrative alternative practitioners perceive illness and healing.

To transform health care in this country, the separation of professionalism from the wider expanse of the realms of healing must be bridged. The twin illusions—time is money and knowledge is power—must be cast aside so that those in the healing professions can fulfill their vocation, which is to guide people through illness to health and a life of renewed purpose. Eliminating professionalism will liberate physicians and patients from their present codependent-enabler relationship based on collusion and denial. Addiction to intellectual and mechanistic information traps everyone in roles that engender mistrust, and veils us from becoming consciously aware of our potential.

It is imperative that health professionals, especially physicians, focus on how these shadow forces are at work in their own lives, in the institution of medicine, and in the lives of their patients. Physicians resist doing this necessary work of healing because they fear losing control. Those in the medical profession who are sincere in their desire to help others, and there are many, will find a greater opportunity to help when they stop blaming others, let go of the fear of losing control, and face their own shadows. The medical profession is presently walled behind mistrust. How can it do anything but radiate this mistrust to all with whom it interacts? Most illness exists because we have lost our capacity to trust our own instincts and intuition. We too often do not trust ourselves, or each other. Instead we give our trust to the physician who hides behind intellect and professionalism, who cannot help but disappoint us because he, too, is coming from a place of mistrust.

MEDICOLEGAL CLIMATE

Let us focus on the current medico-legal climate as an example of these walls of mistrust. When doctors give advice and treatment to their patients, they are conscious of the invisible presence of a lawyer who may threaten their livelihood. They worry about making a mistake. Physicians, patients, and the legal system are all responsible for the current climate of mistrust in health care. We refer again to the codependent-enabler relationship that exists in many families, and between physicians and patients.

While intolerance, judgment and breakdown of trust have been increasing in society as a whole, the medical profession needs to be honest in acknowledging its role in fracturing trust in the medical field. Dependence on intellectual professionalism with its mechanistic approach to illness has made the practice of medicine too abstract and too limited in the promotion of healing because it excludes patient participation in the process of self-healing. It also excludes other diagnostic methods and therapies that can complement the healing process, such as those of integrative alternative medicine. This exclusion has been a great error of conventional medicine, one that has created too much unnecessary suffering.

THE INFORMATION GOD

Of course, we need information to guide us in our decision-making processes. But what has happened in the medical profession is the elevation of statistical and quantifiable information to a height of absolute authority. If a study has not shown certain data, the effectiveness of a treatment is dismissed. Information is the vehicle of communication, but worshiping the Information God prevents communication. The misuse of information to justify a point of view and position of authority that a particular person or institution has an interest in maintaining is the situation in the medical profession today. It is no different from what the Catholic Church did with Galileo in maintaining that their information on the structure of the Universe was the truth and was not to be questioned.

Many books today preach that knowledge and information are keys to success. This addiction to information creates a certain position of power and control for those who have it. In our culture, our attachment to acquiring great volumes of intellectual data without deeper integration and wisdom interferes with the human imaginative and creative process, and the capacity of people to work together. Rationalizations support the rule of the Information God, as more information is necessary so that physicians can be more competent in their specialized fields. Unfortunately, this is increasingly so in alternative medicine as well.

What became lost in this overemphasis on information is the image of the whole, and the relationship of biographical events and social life to illness. Conventional medicine does not integrate approaches such as traditional Chinese medicine or homeopathy, which teach us to perceive the relationship of symptoms in one part of the body to imbalances in other parts. These relationships are understood intuitively, that is, with our deeper level intelligence, rather than through linear intellect.

Addiction to intellectual information and mechanistic approaches to medical care engender euphoria in many physicians. The intricate biochemistry and physiology of an illness is understood. Therefore, the correct drug to manipulate these values can be applied and predictable results observed. Physicians feel good when this occurs. They believe that they are doing their job, which they may be doing on a cellular level, but often not on a personal and social level because they have not related the disease to the human condition. The same sometimes holds true in alternative medicine, where this same information-based approach is applied in alleviating symptoms with an herb or supplement, without investigating the patient's lifestyle. Herbs and supplements, like pharmaceuticals, may also suppress healing.

11

Thus the craving for both information and control is satisfied. How often do we hear that any approach to healing has not been proven effective if there have not been controlled studies? This is a rigid mindset, a raising of technology to the level of a God. Interestingly, most of the drugs and procedures used in conventional medicine today do not have controlled studies to back them up. Mercury dental fillings are an example. Though they have never been tested by the FDA, and there are no studies that document their safety, they are approved as "the standard of practice" in dentistry.

The capacity of physicians and researchers to manipulate study results for a desired end demonstrates a cleverness that could be seen as the trickster in medicine. The trickster archetype is common to many indigenous cultures, including that of the Native Americans. The trickster deceives us into substituting the part for the whole, and in this case affects the thinking of the public. Many people do not believe that their physician is doing a complete job unless laboratory tests and X rays are performed. Often these tests reveal little. Many internal imbalances take years to develop, during which time most commonly used objective laboratory tests are normal. If they are abnormal, then many people feel relieved at getting a diagnosis, even though they have no idea what caused their illness and how to eliminate the cause. Most people have no real intent to do anything besides depend on the physician's prescribed drugs, surgery, or both. If the tests are normal, they either believe there is no reason to be concerned, or they spend even more money using the same type of tests to continue to look for abnormalities.

Integrative alternative medicine has developed objective testing of blood, hair, urine, saliva, and body temperature that can provide insights into internal imbalances before they become disease. These tests give insight into the whole, into the relationships between body parts. They are a constructive addition to health care. Yet conventional medicine still looks condescendingly on many of these approaches, because they are less mechanistic and analytical. These tests give us a picture of how the whole is functioning, and why a problem in one part of our body may be related to something going on in another body part.

The entire emphasis on information in education in the United States is based on becoming a material success in the world. We measure success by position and the accompanying financial benefits. This attitude creates a climate of illness and of mistrust. There is nothing evil about money. However, when money becomes a commodity rather than a medium of relationship and exchange between people that enhances their lives of spirit, then social order and conscience has entered a decaying process. We are well into this decay at the start of the 21st century. The confidence that needs to be present in all healing relationships has been dissipated.

Many problems and illusions exist because we as a whole have come to rely on our physical sense perceptions as the only reality. Subjective feelings and intuitions are discounted as unreal. This is the price we pay and the way we suffer for being such a head-centered society. The faculties necessary for observation and imagination are not encouraged in education, especially in medical education. We come to trust only what the physical senses can perceive, and what can be quantifiably measured. We measure the level of bacteria in a specimen or the numerical values of our blood pressure and perceive these as the illness, much in the same way that we count our money and perceive the amount we possess as the measure of our security and value.

Many people are deficient in the positive sense of self that develops out of observation, imagination, and trust. Deficient in this sense of self and distrusting of our capacity to sense and respond to imbalance, we then tend to rely on objective tests, the results of which require professionals to interpret. The success of the professionals too often depends on patients continuing their patterns of denials, illusions, and lack of sense of self. All of this creates a climate for more illness, in spite of the promise of conventional medicine that great cures are just around the corner. This climate that encourages illness will continue to add stress to our lives and increase the cost of health care. The climate will only change when we understand and take steps to end our growing dependence on, and worshiping of, an information- and position-oriented professional society.

One of the major areas illuminated by Rudolf Steiner, the founder of anthroposophy, was that too much intellectual information early in life could lead to chronic illnesses later in life. This idea is a foundation of the Waldorf approach to education. In these schools, the arts and imagination are the primary focus of teaching, and the intellectual information of spelling and mathematics are not taught in the abstract way they are in most other schools. Math is taught through stories and games and colors, not just with a pencil and numbers on a blackboard. In this way, learning the information of mathematics becomes part of a child's whole being. Children don't just learn mathematics with their heads, but also with their feelings of joy and laughter, with fairy tales and colors, and with movements and games.

In our culture, most people are fragmented. Thinking goes one way, emotions pull us another way, and our movements become habitual and not purposeful. This creates the internal biological terrain for illness. I constantly have to battle the information-orientation model in myself. I frequently feel uncomfortable at the thought of the volumes of information on integrative medicine that I am not keeping up with and feel I should be—the latest on what vitamin works with what illness, what hormone test is most accurate. All of this is important. But I also notice when I am in these states, my internal milieu, my physiology, shifts. I am less relaxed, and slightly fearful that I do not know enough information to help my patients.

When I step away from this battle, I realize the faulty thinking in it. I play the flute or take a short walk in nature to break the cycle of imbalanced addiction to information that characterizes most of us. Many of my patients come into the office with reams of information off the Internet about their illnesses.

What they do not have, what they are deficient in, is an internal process of organizing this information. This means thinking in terms of connectedness, patterns, and inter-relationships. It also means looking at illness in the context of one's life, asking: What is this illness teaching me about my imbalances?

In my practice, I see a number of women with interstitial cystitis, a chronic bladder inflammation without an associated infectious organism. Chronic urogenital problems, when viewed from a homeopathic perspective, are the working through on a physical level of a difficulty in assimilating one's past. A part of the person has stayed in the past and has difficulty integrating an experience, and so it is internalized as a conflict. Dr. Gerard Gueniot, a French homeopathic physician, teaches these ideas.

There are an increasing number of herbs and supplements with application to this illness, and always more information to learn about the latest treatment. But without also seeing the illness from the homeopathic perspective, for example, and getting caught up in accumulating more quantifiable data, a healing impulse will never be discovered and activated. Both patient and doctor stay in a maze and never find the way out.

NARROW THINKING

Two people called into a radio talk show to speak with the doctor host. One was having a sensation of burning in her feet that was worse at night. The doctor was somewhat stumped. He did not have a good mechanistic and pathological disease into which this symptom would fit. He advised her to see a neurologist to make sure this was not a disease of the peripheral nerves, as would occur with diabetes. What the doctor did not know is that there could have been a toxic buildup in the woman's body that was concentrating in the peripheral nerves. This buildup might not as yet have produced pathologic changes detectable in a laboratory. Many acupuncturists and natural medicine practitioners are familiar with this type of story. It can often be successfully treated before it manifests into overt pathological disease.

The other person who called in had been experiencing intermittent pains along the left side of her body since having root canal work on the left side of her mouth. The host physician dismissed the notion of her symptoms having anything to do with her root canal work. By his tone of voice, it was clear that he regarded any suggestion of an interrelationship as ridiculous. As many integrative physicians know, however, such a connection is a reality. (For more insight into this oral-systemic relationship, refer to the book by George E. Meinig, *The Root Canal Cover-Up*, and to later parts of this book.)

The intolerance in the medical profession today is based on a narrow, intellectual, and mechanical understanding of illness. There are many people who have similar complaints that cannot be explained by conventional medicine because they do not fit into the standard model. There is often a good reason for these symptoms, and, more ever, seemingly unrelated symptoms are often connected. Yet too often the patient is dismissed as crazy, or given a prescription for an antidepressant, especially if the patient is a woman. This most definitely needs to change if the health care system is to become effective.

PHARMACEUTICAL OBSESSIONS

In 1998, it was reported in an article in the Journal of the American Medical Association that the fourth leading cause of death in the United States is adverse reactions from drugs taken in the amounts prescribed. This is still true today. The "medical-pharmaceutical complex" is a new term coined by Jay Cohen, M.D., associate clinical professor at the University of California, San Diego, School of Medicine. In his book *Over Dose*, Dr. Cohen describes how physicians generally prescribe drugs. Rather than using the least amount to do the job, they often prescribe much higher amounts because of the information they receive from the drug companies.

Dr. Cohen describes how the media is a big public relations organ for the pharmaceutical companies, and how the need to control information dictates how well physicians are informed about prescribed doses of drugs. This need to be in control applies not only to the drug companies, but also to physicians, insurance companies, and hospitals.

There is a huge gap between official American Medical Association (AMA) policy, which states "the patient's right to self-decision can be effectively exercised only if the patient possesses enough information to enable an intelligent choice," and the way drugs are commonly prescribed in higher than necessary doses, and by physicians who often feel threatened by a patient who asks any questions.

There is rising public concern over the high cost of prescription drugs, and there are growing demands that the government put caps on prices, or help senior citizens. The pharmaceutical industry is the most profitable industry in the United States. It spends more than five billion dollars on marketing alone; this figure includes parties, paid vacations, symposia, and other gifts to doctors. Pharmaceutical companies are increasingly appealing directly to the public, encouraging people, via television and magazines, to ask their doctor for the latest drug for particular diseases. It has been a seller's market, with the companies raising prices at will because the demand is so high for their products.

Both conventional medicine and the public are obsessed with using pharmaceutical drugs at the exclusion of most other approaches to healing. Many of these drugs bring quick symptomatic relief and short-term results. Morphine, antibiotics, anti-hypertensives, aspirin, and calcium channel blockers, to name a few, offer results that are biochemically measurable and provide short-term improvement in symptoms. Yet in the long term we are weakened by this exclusively drug-oriented medical approach because of the effects these drugs have on our immune systems and our internal biological terrain.

This pharmaceutical trend parallels what has manifested in the country as a whole, especially over the last two decades of the twentieth century: an emphasis on short-term results, quick turnover of profits, instant food or cash. Collectively, these trends are the picture of illness. They run counter to the stream of life, which requires development, time, and patience to unfold fully. There is no separation between the condition of the economy and the condition of our individual and collective lives. The increase we are experiencing in the incidence of chronic illness is an important signal that, although we may opt for short-term results and quick turnover of profit, our bodies are not responding favorably.

In what ways are we weakened by this cultural addiction to prescription and nonprescription drugs? Many of these drugs take the work of healing away from us. In some instances, drugs are necessary. However, the attitude behind the medical administration of drug therapy and people's willingness to take them is the belief that these drugs will make us better and promote healing with little effort from us. When an infection is suddenly made to disappear with an antibiotic, for example, we believe that bacteria must have been the cause. It is far easier to accept that conclusion than to acknowledge that the cause arose from our lifestyles. Without helping the inner terrain, the drugs cover up underlying problems, and, ultimately, we are the worse for this. People improve in the short term, but decay inwardly. This decay will show up years later in disease that may be different from the one initially treated with pharmaceuticals.

Too often, medication is the protective barrier that stands between our obsession with living a life of pleasure and convenience and the many perceived threats to this lifestyle. Those who seek help in dealing with unpleasant symptoms of illness are rarely required to change their lifestyles as part of treatment. In the institution of conventional medicine and for the millions of people who take prescription drugs, there is very little willingness today to perceive illness, not with fear, but in its true light: as a process that reveals how our current imbalances in life may guide us toward renewal and regeneration This lack of insight is a great tragedy and it is what we are being called upon to address.

Our dependence on drugs has intensified in the past 25 years. An intimate relationship exists between the pervasive dependence on prescription and nonprescription drugs that supposedly heal all the ills to which flesh is heir and the pervasive use of illegal drugs that help many to forget these ills. Both are forms of escape. The former is institutionally sanctioned. The destructive nature of illegal drugs is much more obvious, due to both the rapidity with which they unravel a person's life as well as the criminal and destructive nature that society is keen to recognize and punish.

The similarly destructive nature of many prescription drugs is not so obvious or recognized. This is because the nature of their destructiveness is subtler. Illness has come to mean something wrong that has no place in life and must be eliminated as quickly as possible. The illusion of today is that someone can take away our ills by giving us a drug, or even a vitamin or an herb, so that we may return to our illness-generating lifestyles. And so we go on hiding from life. We are paying a heavy price, both personally and culturally, to continue these illusions.

It is helpful to step back and look at the bigger picture in relation to pharmaceuticals. These drugs, the toxic chemicals that permeate all aspects of our lives, and the plastics on which we are heavily dependent in our throw-away economy are all connected. The same companies often produce both the drugs and the toxic chemicals, and now the genetically modified foods. While these three products—drugs, chemicals, and plastics—have brought conveniences of modern life, our overdependence on them has brought us to a point of national crisis. Our reliance on them for energy, health, and convenience has eroded local economies, polluted the environment, and weakened people's health.

Chemicals, plastics, and drugs have given us a so-called freedom. We can get in our cars and travel wherever we want to go. We can buy any consumer product we can afford and ignore the waste of the packaging and manufacturing by-products if we choose. We can make the symptoms of illness disappear quickly. Yet symptoms of illness do not disappear. They only go deeper into the body or the psyche to appear years later as chronic diseases. Likewise, the massive accumulation of plastics in garbage is destroying the environment. This so-called freedom is really license to indulge and then deny the devastating results and blame others. This license and denial are characteristic of the United States today.

The crises facing us today were created by us. Our energy crisis exists solely because of our dependence on fossil fuels and an abundance of consumer goods that need to be trucked to us at great expense from distant places. Our environmental crises from global warming to estrogen-stimulating chemicals, exists because of our disconnection from nature. Similarly, there is no health care crisis except what we have created out of our addiction to a "quick cure" with pharmaceutical drugs.

CHAPTER 2

THE HEALTH INSURANCE CRISIS

The foundation of conventional health care in the past 50 years has been health insurance. People have come to expect that they will be financially protected from the increasing costs of treating their illnesses and accidents. In the previous chapter we looked at major reasons why health care costs are rising dramatically. The focus of this chapter is health insurance and what brought it to its current crisis state. This discussion is important because effective health care reform will only come about by making major changes in our definition and approach to health insurance.

THE CURRENT SITUATION: OUR SICKNESS CARE SYSTEM

Over 40 million people in the United States do not have health insurance. Many of them have jobs and pay taxes. Many young people today, from infants to young adults, are uninsured. We have collectively decided to prop up the past by stealing from the future. This is identical to what has occurred in the national economy.

Divorced people are often no longer able to purchase health insurance at the affordable premiums they obtained while married to someone who was insured through work. For some people with significant health care needs, this is a factor in their remaining in relationships that are not working. Others become vulnerable to high health care costs as they make lifestyle changes.

Elderly people fear not having enough money for health care as they age. Many working people do not seek help for illness because they know they cannot afford it, and in the current medical system they are often correct. A visit to the emergency department for a broken bone could cost up to one-fourth of a person's monthly salary.

Among American children who do not have health insurance, 80 percent have at least one parent working. These working parents are increasingly caught in the gray area between making too much money to qualify for Medicaid for their children's health care, and making too little money to afford private health insurance. Women without health insurance have almost a one-third increase in the probability of a bad pregnancy outcome, such as infant illness or death. It costs much less for nine months of prenatal care than for care of a premature infant in the neonatal intensive care unit.

Because the Sickness Care System is so controlled, and most people still believe that drugs are the only way to treat illness, it is becoming increasingly difficult for parents to afford treatment for common pediatric problems. A course of an expensive antibiotic for a child with recurrent ear infections may cost up to $100. Asthma medicine for a child may cost $500 to $1,000 per year. When people are unable to afford health care, they often do not seek health care or they wait until their health has deteriorated and then show up in an emergency department.

There are people who remain in jobs they do not like only because of the health insurance benefits. The results of this are often not considered. They include:

- Decrease in immune system function because of a decrease in enthusiasm and the lack of a sense of self in the work environment

- Increase in the use of drugs and other forms of escape from an inwardly difficult but outwardly necessary situation

- Increase in work-related injuries and worker's compensation liabilities, both acute and chronic, which are related to lack of attentiveness by those who are physically at a job but otherwise not mentally focused

- Decrease in the quality of products and work by those who feel trapped in jobs they do not like.

The entire system is riddled with deception, as illustrated in the following examples:

- Insurance companies attempt to enroll individuals and businesses, and then make things so complex that it is difficult to determine what one is paying for. Furthermore, insurance companies increasingly refuse coverage for certain treatments and make it difficult for anyone with a previously diagnosed illness to become insured. Essentially, these companies want to insure so-called healthy people to protect their investment.

- Medical specialists seek to keep their positions and rewards. They lead the fight against meaningful changes in the system by feeding the hysterical fear that people will no longer be able to get their needs met if changes are made.

- Everyone participates in this deception by believing that if they pay an insurance premium, they will be taken care of and need not change their illness-generating lifestyles. This way of doing things rewards people for being irresponsible with themselves and toward those with whom they work. They continue to expect to be entitled to health care at whatever the cost, while someone else pays.

The underlying premise is: Pay a premium to a third party and receive protection against expensive health care bills. The concept of insurance, aside from catastrophic, is based on perpetuating the fear and denial of illness, and the illusion that someone else can fix it. There are hundreds of insurance companies that spend thousands of bureaucratic hours on paperwork and regulations. It is odd that people rant against the bureaucracy of government yet ignore the wasteful bureaucracy of big health care conglomerates.

In the present system, health insurance companies collect premiums and pay a certain amount for health care expenditures; most of the health care they cover is biotechnological in nature and provides only short-term relief at best. Each family and each employer gives over to an agency the responsibility for health care. We allow this to continue because it permits us to live in denial about our addictive and habitual lifestyles, as someone else pays for the illnesses and accidents that result from our lifestyles. Much of this behavior is subconscious, but it is nevertheless present.

MISDIRECTED PRIORITIES

The reality is that we do not invest in health education and preventive medicine. We do not teach people how to observe and become more aware of the patterns of illness in their daily lives. Instead, we wait until they are on their backs and then rifle their wallets and mortgage their future with the high costs of conventional medicine. And most people and businesses permit this folly to continue. When people are insured they often give up control to statistics. Insurance companies decide the level at which they are going to reimburse patients and other health care players by terms such as "usual," or "reasonable," or "common." These are vague terms that permit companies to escape their commitments. Health insurers develop complex formulas for reimbursement. These force employers, hospitals, and doctors to hire more people to interpret these complexities so everyone can maximize their own profits. Billions of dollars in wasted administrative costs appear in our national health care budget.

In now common scenarios, an employee at a hospital or physician's office calls someone who is often on the other side of the country employed by a managed health care company. The call is made in order to get approval for a particular treatment. In other words, the health care provider wants to make sure that it gets paid. Employees at these companies do not know the patient. They make their decisions using computers, based on the complaints and diagnosis given to them by the health provider. Using complex financial and procedural formulas, they decide whether to give approval. The patient's health and well-being are not a consideration. Only statistically significant and quantifiably measurable diseases are economically reimbursable.

I could continue endlessly with these illustrations, many all too familiar to the reader, that reveal our current health insurance situation. By understanding where we are and how we have gotten into this predicament, imaginative and innovative remedies will begin to emerge.

THE EVOLUTION OF HEALTH INSURANCE

In the past 50 years, health insurance has evolved in a three-fold way. Understanding this three-fold aspect is the key to gaining insight into our current dilemma and finding our way out of the maze of often deliberate and deceptive complexities, so we can develop remedies to the current crisis.

There have been three major participants in the evolution of health care insurance:

- Government
- Private nonprofit companies
- Commercial and investor-owned insurance companies.

At one pole is the government. In the 20 years after Medicare was passed, the federal government permitted hospitals and doctors to bill the government for whatever they deemed necessary. The government paid whatever it was billed. This is called a cost-plus basis. It is a fundamental reason why we have a health care crisis today. It is exactly what occurred with the Savings and Loan crisis: The government gave free reign to the private sector and paid for what it was billed.

With the increase in the percentage of people older than 65, the proliferation of chronic disease, and the explosion in expensive medical technology to treat these diseases, the government's bill in this massive entitlement program has skyrocketed. The bill is now a significant percentage of the yearly federal budget and is well defended by strong interest groups who want to continue things as they are. Hospitals and doctors have become cleverly adept at getting around recent federal efforts to limit these costs, while at the same time blaming government, insurance companies, and others for their current problems.

At the opposite pole has been the explosion of both private commercial and investor-owned health insurance companies. Their primary goal is profit, not service.

Buying health insurance is like putting money in the bank. The supposed agreement is that we will receive a service later for money we save now. The problem with this relationship is that it is based on mutual selfishness. This arrangement is another of the fundamental sources of the decay of our current system.

In this back-to-back relationship, each party—insurance company and patient (or family or business)—is interested primarily in gaining its own advantage. Consumers are primarily interested in how little they can pay into the insurance fund and still have someone else pay for their health care, regardless of their lifestyles. The insurance company is interested in how high a rate it can charge and still get away with not having to pay for services. This becomes mutual selfishness and distrust instead of mutual support and trust.

Secretive lifestyles proliferate. There is the secretive lifestyle of the person who purchases health insurance, and then demands that the illness consequent of a lifestyle of denial and habitual living be paid for. And there are the secretive business motives and dealings of insurance companies that permit large amounts of money to be circulated in incestuous-like currents of collusion between hospitals, doctors, insurance companies, and biotechnology firms.

After World War II, private nonprofit companies originally were a strong middle force in health care. The best example is Blue Cross/Blue Shield. This company used to be the conscience of medicine. It provided health insurance at a small cost to all who enrolled, whether they were healthy or incapacitated.

The intention of insurance companies was to act as representatives for those they insured, exacting substantial discounts from hospitals in return for contractual agreements. Significantly, they planned to use money saved to subsidize care for the sick and elderly. This is in sharp contrast to major commercial health insurance companies whose profits go toward investors or diversification.

In 1965, Congress passed Medicare. What initially was believed to be a positive advance in health care soon gave rise to the split in health care that has reached crisis proportions. This split was a polarization of extremes with a weakening of the middle.

There used to be inclusiveness in health care insurance. All people were insured and the money was pooled to pay for this. Today, commercial and investor-owned private insurance companies increasingly and very competitively go after the so-called "healthy" people. In this way they collect higher premiums each year while paying out little for health care. If a "healthy" person becomes ill and requires expensive treatment, then that person's next premium will increase by a large amount. He or she will likely join the growing numbers of uninsured. Or the group rates for that person's business may skyrocket. To guarantee their economic survival, many Blue Cross companies today have become essentially the same as private commercial companies.

The soil on which Blue Cross was built was destined to erode because of the forces unleashed in America during the past half-century. These forces of clever and ruthless economics have not only largely taken over health care, but have also taken over the federal government.

Insurance companies were destined to fail once our health began to be insured by distant and impersonal companies that do not have our best interests at heart. Insurance works as long as the person enrolled in a plan shares the risk and the responsibility involved in illness and health. This means that enrollees in an insurance plan have a responsibility to their own health care and to the viability of the plan. This responsibility is to change their illness-generating lifestyle habits in order to continue to be enrolled. Yet all insurance plans, including Blue Cross/Blue Shield and the government-sponsored plans of Medicare and Medicaid, embrace the distant approach and discard the model of shared responsibility.

NEW ENTITIES

Efforts to control health care costs over the past few decades have spawned new entities such as health maintenance organizations (HMOs). HMOs grew out of attempts on the part of corporate America to curb rising health care costs by ensuring large numbers of people, especially businesses. For a fixed amount of money paid each month by individuals or partly by a major employer or small business employer, each person receives whatever health care they need. Groups of health "consumers" contract for services with groups of health "providers." Why isn't this working as planned?

Many have pointed to such factors as: the rise in costs of medical care, especially drugs and technology; the general public's increasing demand for perfect health; the aging of the population; and medico-legal entanglements. These are indeed obvious contributing reasons as to why HMOs and other similar attempts have been doomed to failure. However, all of these factors, aside from the aging population, are not the cause of the failure, but rather the results of our Sickness Care System.

The reason these and other so-called innovative approaches such as "managed care" are will continue to fail is that their focus is strictly mechanistic. With general public agreement, they perceive Sickness Care in mechanistic terms and then try to control costs by limiting services and patients' choice of doctors. These mechanical solutions can only worsen the problem because they are trying to fix a system that, as presently constituted, cannot be effective.

HMOs, in their current form, are profitable if they keep prices down. They do so primarily in two ways: by keeping health "consumers" out of the hospital and by limiting what they pay to "health providers." The focus of such attempts is still on cost control and other business terms.

THEFT OF THE CENTER

The idea behind managed care—that a third party needs to be involved with the first party (doctor) and the second party (patient) in making decisions about expensive diagnostic and therapeutic procedures—is a sound idea. The problem is in the way it is being carried out.

The decisions are being made on monetary grounds. This keeps our health care materialistic and mechanistic, since the two are wed in health care today. This approach disregards that there are other factors to consider, such as the prognosis of the patient, how the patient has lived his or her life, what the value of a procedure is to the well-being of the patient, and whether there are other effective ways of approaching the problem, such as those in complementary/ alternative medicine.

The decisions are made by someone at a computer terminal in a distant city. The third party involved in this process needs to be accountable, not to the hospital or insurance company or utilization-review company, but to the community.

All participants, both "consumers" and "providers", need to develop agreements that place real value on human development rather than on money and mechanistic improvement at the expense of inner enrichment and purposeful living. Without these agreements, health care insurance reforms will not succeed. They may appear to succeed, as perceived from the mechanistic view of fixing body parts, killing microorganisms, or altering genes. Yet people will become more ill until new principles are invoked and integrated into contractual agreements in health care.

There have never been any agreed-on principles of individual and mutual responsibility and accountability. There has never been a clear definition of health. And there has been very little in the way of education that is necessary if people are to become responsible for directing their lives. The health insurance industry focuses on keeping people scared, unaware, and dependent.

As long as chronic diseases did not proliferate with an aging population, and people did not become addicted to expensive health care technology and demand to be fixed instead of changing their lives, the weaknesses of such a health care system could be hidden. Health insurance has been the great hidden medium between us, and those who "fix" us—doctors, hospitals, pharmaceutical companies, and medical technology companies. Due to the polarization of this system and the theft of the middle, this system is in trouble. Whether people exercise clear thinking and perceive the situation, or whether they retreat in further denial remains to be seen. We are now being forced to deal with and confront what we have created through our denials and rationalizations.

THE NEED FOR REFORM

We need to find a new way to have health insurance. There is no turning back the clock. We have developed technology as a useful aide in health care. For example, the value of CT (computed tomography) scans for acute head injuries cannot be underestimated. Thus catastrophic insurance makes sense for everyone, because of the expensive nature of diagnostic tests and surgeries, which we still rely on too much but which are a reality.

We need to recognize and be honest about the hidden driving forces in the economics of health care, and acknowledge our collective responsibility in permitting these to predominate.

Current specialty-oriented reimbursement procedures encourage physicians to continue ordering and performing them, which helps physicians maintain a high standard of living. Such procedures to look for physical tissue changes that have occurred, often after decades of denial on the part of patients regarding their illness-engendering lifestyles, are reimbursed far more frequently than are biographical consultations that form the basis of preventative medicine and self-educative healing.

Most Americans carry health insurance that has many loopholes. Those without insurance, unless they are wealthy, live in fear of illness and its financial costs. Most health insurance companies try to recruit people whom they determine will not need major moneys to pay for health care. And most of these companies confine their coverage to the prevailing (and largely ineffective) conventional medical approach to chronic illness. Until we break this pattern and become more creative and supportive of healing, our health insurance crisis will worsen.

CHAPTER 3

CULTURAL DECAY AND ILLNESS

O ur culture is in the process of social and economic decay. The old order is breaking down and giving way. This decay extends not only to health care, but to traditional institutions such as the family, schools, religious organizations, and the criminal justice system.

The fuel for a consumer-driven economy is based on informational learning that prepares us for technological jobs to compete as a nation with other nations and maintain our illusion of technological superiority. According to the conventional ways that successful education is measured, our system is failing and getting worse all the time. Traditional religious institutions are failing to provide a living image for a spiritual life that goes beyond religious dogma and sectarianism. The nuclear family is breaking down. With rising divorce rates, the number of single-parent families is increasing. "Sandwich" families, where adults have the responsibility of caring for both their children and their parents, are also on the rise. Our present economic structure makes success in handling both of these family responsibilities very difficult. The process of decay is also apparent in the environment. We are witnessing a dramatic increase in environmental toxins and public concern over food safety, among other environmental issues.

Most people have been psychologically veiled from the consequences of this decay because the consequences develop slowly and cumulatively. For example, the economy of the United States is built around the automobile. Yet the automobile is a major contributor to air pollution and congestion in cities. Today continued economic growth depends on people buying cars often. Thousands of jobs and family livelihoods depend on this. It is not difficult to see the situation we have collectively created. Fewer cars sold leads to worker layoffs with a resultant decrease in consumer spending and an adverse effect on the economy. To halt environmental decay, we must make the transition to automobiles that are more fuel-efficient and less polluting. This will cost more money that people do not have. Despite the fact that the gasoline that fuels cars creates problems with pollution and entails scarcity issues as an energy source, manufacturers have for years fought attempts to develop solar hydrogen-powered cars, which utilize the sun as the energy source and produce water as the by-product.

The advertising industry has been tremendously successful in stimulating artificial wants in a consumer-driven society. We have a cultural obsession with buying and wanting more material goods without understanding how

27

these material goods are not allowing our inner inadequacies to surface. Our cultural obsession has contributed significantly not only to environmental pollution, but also to an increase in individual psychological imbalance. We have painted ourselves into a corner where we fear that what we need to do in order to have a healthier environment will bring an economic downturn.

On a personal level, many people ignore or deny the significance of illness-generating habits such as smoking, not sleeping enough, eating poorly, and inactivity in their daily lives and the lives of their children. For example, people do not want to hear about the effects that foods with hydrogenated fat and high sugar content have on their children's health and capacity to learn. If they did, there would be a big uproar about the soft drinks and sugar-laden foods that greet the consumer on entering most grocery stores.

People's habitual behaviors typically continue until an incapacitating illness or accident puts them on their backs. They often ignore warning signs of the illness or deal with them in a superficial manner. They do not recognize the need for inner transformation or acknowledge the need for change in the aspects of their lives that are not providing positive and constructive energy. So illness enters in as a teacher and as a rectifying force.

If we step back and look at illness today, several points become obvious:

- There is widespread illness in society as a whole.

- Because of greater communications and interrelationship in the economic sphere, every person on this planet is connected to every other person

- Illness has become not just a personal matter. Much illness derives from social problems such as chemical and heavy metal toxicity

- Illness often involves a refusal to let go of old habits and ways of thinking

- Illness is a reality today because of the breakdown in contemporary culture and the chemical, heavy metal, electromagnetic, and the psycho-emotional toxicities that this breakdown generates. Everyone is affected. In the context of these realities, life is more about maintaining a dynamic ongoing process of healing and regeneration than it is about achieving a static state of perfect health.

The decaying elements of a dying culture are the contributing factors to illness today. We individually and collectively resist recognizing how these elements pervade our lives in multiple ways. Our refusal to take steps to transform these elements leads to the growth of chronic and unnecessarily incapacitating illnesses. Our present economic structure of "health" care delivery in this country does not support a process of understanding. Rather, it supports a pattern of collective denial by both doctors and patients of the deeper causes of illness.

An example of this denial is the focus on cholesterol. Cholesterol has become a virtual obsession. In order to keep the heart and blood vessels healthy so that we may live healthier physical lives as we age, we must supposedly reduce our consumption of foods that supposedly raise blood cholesterol levels and take drugs that lower high blood cholesterol. This sells drugs that lower blood cholesterol. But it ignores the deeper causes of high cholesterol: liver dysfunction, intestinal imbalances in absorption, and toxic microorganisms and chronic inflammation in the gastrointestinal tract and blood vessels.

The medical profession backs this effort. Major food chains have "no cholesterol" signs in front of many foods. To be sure, this movement is a positive step toward taking responsibility for nutritional intake and the role of foods in illness. What often occurs, however, is that one element of this equation, in this case cholesterol, becomes magnified into an obsession. While grocery stores, drug companies, and the medical profession may contribute or benefit from this obsession, cholesterol is a collective cultural obsession that arises from our fears and denials, in particular our fear of death and of aging. Obsession with one element is also a reflection of the desire to find the magic pill that will make illness go away. The obsessive search for the magic pill is actually the illness. Obsessions are patterns of illness that are widespread in our culture, and are not limited to the small select group of people who are labeled as ill. The denial of this reality is a problem facing us today.

With obsession, there is a loss of perspective. In the case of the cholesterol and other health obsessions, it is as if one part of the body has become much larger than normal, at the expense of atrophy in other parts. In reality, we are not either healthy or ill. It is not black and white. Rather, illness and health are two ends of a continuum. Our lives are in constant flux. Illness enters our lives on a daily basis, and we live somewhere along the spectrum of illness, and healing in a living dynamic field of experience. When people become possessed with their own subconscious forces, such as the fear of death, as happens with obsessions, they lose the perspective of the greater whole. Advertising plays on and manipulates these subconscious forces in order to sell products.

The character traits that act as shadowy figures and emerge in destructive habits are hidden parts of us, of which we are often unaware or ignore. Yet shadowy forces are the major contributors to illness today. They function on an individual and collective level and can be personal, family-related, and even national and racial. We need to take account of these forces and create an economic structure in medicine that does not relegate our shadow to the

29

fields of psychology and mental health but facilitates family practitioners exploring it with patients for a greater understanding of and willingness to work with illness.

The threshold between our conscious and subconscious lives is dissolving. The increase in the frequency and severity of drug addiction, psychopathic behavior, and other major illnesses today, bears witness to this reality. The increase in illnesses related to diet and nutrition is a manifestation of the growing effects of continuing to ignore the subconscious as it affects our lives and health. The ignoring occurs on an individual level, as in the continued popularity of fast foods, and on a collective level, as in the poisoning of the food supply. Through the veil of an excessively material culture, we continue to harbor the illusion that the negative effects do not exist, or if they exist, they may affect others, but they won't affect us.

PROMETHEAN GIFTS

The liver is the major organ where cholesterol is synthesized in the body. In Greek mythology, Prometheus stole fire from Zeus on Mount Olympus and brought it down to humanity. The fire had the potential to bring warmth and light. It would transform and give humanity the opportunity to achieve consciousness through the warmth of the heart and the light of intelligence. Prometheus was caught and punished for this. He was chained to a rock in the Caucasus Mountains where a vulture clawed at his liver every day. Each night his liver would regenerate, and each day, the vulture would destroy it again.

What does this myth signify for our present culture and in the context of understanding illness? The liver in the myth is destroyed during the day, the time when we are awake and strive to become more conscious individuals. This process of awakening involves a general breakdown of body organs as the substance of the body is metabolized in activity and thought. When we sleep, body organs have an opportunity to regenerate.

What occurs when we do not use the gifts that have been provided by higher and guiding forces, such as the gift of fire, in conscious and constructive ways? Poisoned and devitalized food eats away at our livers just as the vulture did to Prometheus. Our imbalanced and often obsessive emotional lives do the same. We refuse to become conscious and responsible for our gifts and talents, and instead continue to live primarily out of the forces of heritage, unconscious patterns of family behavior, religious sectarianism, national exclusiveness, and racial bias. We are actually refusing to die to the past. So the dying elements of the past prey on us like the vulture in the myth. Prometheus represents all humanity. The forces of heritage continue to play dominant roles in our personal, social, and economic lives. We see this in the food we consume, our emotional drives, and in the structure of our economy.

30

The liver is the seat of our metabolism. It is the body's oven, the warmest internal organ. Heat is generated by movement. The activity of the liver provides fuel for this movement so that we can carry out our will in activities.

As we refuse to recognize how the dying elements of the past prey on our livers, our will is weakened through our imbalanced lifestyles and indulgent habits. This same will, both individual and collective, is necessary for transformation and for entering into a new, more enriching life. We have the potential to roll the stone away from the sepulcher of death and enter into a new and more expanded life. The word liver signifies life, to live. The fire that Prometheus brought to humanity has been turned over to technology in order to fuel all the material desires of a consumer society. Many of these technologies do play a positive role. But many cause us to die small deaths over and over again.

This same fire has waned from our inner lives. The fire of enthusiasm is needed to provide an impetus for a renewal of civilization, in the same way that Prometheus stimulated this renewal with the fire he brought. Now, humanity must do the work and not rely on the gods. In the same way, when it comes to health, each person must do the work of self-research and self-evaluation, and not depend solely on the health professional.

CHAPTER 4

THE ILLNESS OF THE
MEDICAL PROFESSION

For more than 20 years I led three tracks of experience. One life was as a homeopathic and nutritional practitioner. The second was as the president of a nonprofit educational foundation that sought to create a bridge between the healing arts and the creative arts. And the third was as a board-certified emergency physician in a major city hospital.

Early in my emergency department career, I was fired twice. Not for incompetence, but for my arrogance and difficulty in working with the nursing staff. I was defensive, acted superior, and behaved like a tyrant, verbally mistreating my coworkers. I experienced firsthand these traits that are present in many allopathic physicians, and even in some integrative physicians. The firings forced me to face up to my attitude and learn how to work with and treat others respectfully. It took me a long time to unlearn the superior, narcissistic attitude that likely was there before I ever went to medical school, but which was reinforced during medical training as the accepted stance for our profession.

Unless we are very strong, most of us will compromise our values to maintain a degree of comfort in what we do. (I discuss this in more detail in Part II.) To remain a part of emergency department life, I too participated in the "us versus them" attitude. I became annoyed with patients' questions. I became annoyed if the patient's diagnosis and therapy were not obvious to me, or their symptoms did not fit into one of the neat categories I had learned.

Many of the people with whom I worked did not like their job. They could not wait to get off work and go home or on vacation. Most were what I would consider good and caring people. For years I watched doctors in various specialties swing into the emergency department and, either through their posture or their voice, demand that their needs be met right then and that their patient be ready to be seen. It was rare to see a staff physician be really present with a patient or the staff. The stop to see a patient in the ER was to be done quickly. This behavior was not limited to the ER, however. I witnessed it in physicians' offices as well. Most of the allopathic doctors, in their heart of hearts, were not happy with or deeply fulfilled by their work. They had little humility, little tolerance for anything not going their way or anyone questioning their decisions, and little grace in working with nurses and other staff. For years, I was like this. Medicine is a paternalistic profession. This means that medical professionals have the attitude, "We know what's best for you; leave it to us. We will tell you what to do and we expect you to do it." This is a prime example of the immature masculine attitudes of arrogance and domination that still pervade our culture. Those who strive to bring a spirit of renewal to health care's over-mechanized approach need to understand the elements of this immaturity in order to initiate the necessary changes. The use of "masculine" here does not mean that only men carry these attitudes. Both men and women have a masculine part and it can be immature in either sex.

People want to feel better. They believe that the medical profession and the health care industry have what they want. People will pay to buy what they need, or someone else, like an insurance company, will pay for them to purchase it. The role of the health care professional is to become technically proficient in a special area of diagnosis and treatment, fix people, and live a financially comfortable life. This way of doing business in health care requires neither the physician nor others who work in health care to change inwardly and to invoke the principles of healing in their own lives.

In the United States, the doctor and many others in various professional pursuits have been elevated to godlike status, with people coming to receive what the doctor has been technically trained to dispense. Just like priests in churches of earlier times, the present immature masculine structure of medical institutions continues to permit both physicians and the general public to hide in the shadows of denial rather than do the necessary and often difficult work to become mature human beings who approach illness as teamwork and a journey of transformation.

The Jungian psychologist Robert Moore has described four basic archetypes of the masculine in both their immature and mature aspects. An archetype is an elemental image that we all share in our collective unconscious. Four masculine archetypes—king, warrior, magician, and lover—are directly related to our health care crisis and provide guidance in what can be done to bring about change.

KING

For health care to represent the king, it would, as an institution, encourage and support people to creatively order their lives and become more integrated and centered. People would learn through their illnesses to become stewards of the realm in their own lives. Until people define their own creative ordering principles to live by every day, the chaos of illness-generating lifestyles will continue to consume millions of people and drive health care costs upward.

Currently, physicians and others in positions of authority in health care are acting out the immature masculine qualities of the king. The inflated ego attitude that is full of what the Greeks call *hubris* is commonplace. With pride and arrogance, doctors presume like gods to know what is best for others—namely the mechanistic and technical approach to medicine. No other approach to healing is considered unless it can be proven mechanistically and technically through double-blind studies in a laboratory. This ensures the continuity of medicine exactly as it is practiced today.

This limiting and controlling attitude is fostered by the narcissism endemic to the socially sanctioned status of doctors. The immature masculine archetype applies to both men and women who act out the role. Instead of the benevolent king, we have in health care today the usurper king who protects his position and resists change if it threatens both position and the intellectual concepts held sacred in conventional medicine. For a transformed health care system to be effective, this has to change.

WARRIOR

The warrior has courage, decisiveness, perseverance, and motivation. There are many people in medicine who have these attributes. Indeed, physicians are often driven by warrior qualities. The problem is that they become loners who fix others while not taking care of themselves. Performance stress in health care is high among those who hold higher professional positions. How can anyone who is so driven be able to perceive clearly what a patient requires for healing? The illness of being a professional and the denial of this illness blind the person to clarity of perception. While a physician may be a proficient technician, being a healer is something quite different. The immature warrior tries to maintain his position as hero, with the adulation and control that goes with this hero position.

The warrior in his positive and socially supportive state has a transpersonal commitment. This commitment is often lacking in the present narcissistic medical profession. Without a transpersonal commitment, the spirit of service, the attributes of the warrior that enable the professional to succeed mechanistically and materially turn against him. This results in the shadow warrior who is comfortable with the material success of mechanical medicine and its superficial therapeutic results. No real healing is brought about.

MAGICIAN

The magician is thoughtful and aware, with the capacity for insight into any situation. He is the detached observer. Yet without the right motive he becomes the detached manipulator. This is someone who feigns innocence of hidden power motives. With its secretiveness and superior attitudes, the medical profession looks down on others, such as those who practice alternative medicine, and also looks down on patients who want to know "too much" about their illness. The immature magician uses his learned information primarily for his own benefit and only secondarily for the healing of others. He manipulates the practice of medicine by supporting laws and regulatory agencies that prosecute skilled practitioners in other areas of healing and that reimburse specialists far more than generalists.

Many sincere health professionals have ignored this obvious destructiveness in health care. By doing so, they passively support the consequences. As long as those in positions of responsibility in health care continue to live in the shadow of the magician (when the immature magician is in control) they will be unable to create a sacred space for healing. This is true whether the sacred space is the physical space of an office, the relationship between professional and client, or the internal space of a person's physical body. Neither professional nor patient will be able to access the magician's depth of awareness and insight into illness and healing. And the collusive mutual denial will continue to create problems.

LOVER

The masculine archetype of the lover in his positive expression is sensitive, imaginative, and appreciative of individual differences. Through these qualities, he feels a sense of connectedness to others. Yet as many have observed, these qualities are often missing among many health professionals in the industry, or are overshadowed by a narrow mechanistic mind. Health care corporations are run by people who perceive their clinics as "patient feeder systems," in Wall Street terminology. Such a therapeutic environment will never support real healing because there is no feeling of connectedness. Nor is there much appreciation of individual differences, except to the extent that these affect short-term profit margins.

As with other masculine archetypes, when the positive attributes of the lover are not expressed, either in an individual's life or in the health care institution as a whole, then the shadow of the lover is in control. One aspect of this shadow is an over-attachment to the body. In other words, our health care system overemphasizes relief of physical symptoms even if this means the illness is driven deeper (for example, by drugs that suppress symptoms) into the body and shows up later in a different form.

The immature lover lusts for the physical and material and will compromise his principles in order to have greater material comfort.

If we are going to reform health care, we must recognize that the crisis has been created by tunnel-vision attention on the form, the physical body, while we have avoided life within the form. This life within the form consists of the energetic, emotional, mental, and spiritual components of life, and how these more subtle but real qualities interface and interpenetrate with the physical body. Collectively, we are the picture of one of the lover's shadows, the restless addict, as we compulsively try to rid ourselves of every imperfection in the body and view illness as getting in the way of having fun and being happy.

The lover in his positive state is an expression of artfulness in everyday life. This artfulness enables us to be attentive to real human needs. People who work in the health care field need to integrate the qualities of the lover into their lives and work.

To be able to meet real human needs in times of illness, the medical profession and the entire health care industry need to undergo transformation. Both need to emerge out of the shadows of the immature masculine with its negative qualities of paternalism and control. The positive attributes of the mature masculine, put into daily practice, will encourage health care practitioners to grow personally and professionally and actively encourage their patients to do the same.

THE ILLNESS OF PROFESSIONALISM IN MEDICINE

One of the manifestations of the immature magician archetypes in our society is in our addiction to experts. We seek out a specialist for the part of our body where we believe disease exists, not considering that other parts of our body may also contribute to the disease. We raise our children to believe that if they develop an area of expertise, the chances are much greater for material success and position. The message is that knowledge is power. Schools become vehicles for perpetuation of this message. Today even kindergartners and first-graders undergo aptitude tests. The stress on their nervous systems and digestion often goes unnoticed.

The doctor of today goes to work, intellectually determines how to succeed by having learned the necessary facts. He gives orders, and collects money. This is called formula living. He is often set apart and excused from living and working like other people. As long as he is technically proficient and produces measurable results, everyone is satisfied. He has done his job, and is financially rewarded. The economy has supported this arrangement because everyone is believed to benefit.

However, this professionalism generates illness in professionals and clients because the primary emphasis is placed on the intellect at the expense of the simultaneous development of feeling and conscious will. This imbalance begins in early school years and often continues throughout life, unless one is fortunate enough to become ill and receive the message illness offers. The head-centered and narcissistic existence of the professional world supports our comfortable material way of living. It does so at the expense of pushing aside our dreams or callings.

Physicians, and other professionals as well, are often protected from having to look at their character weaknesses and from having to make changes. When the walls of social protection become too limiting and rigid, and an inner life and sense of self that always seeks expression does not develop, then a severe illness or accident may occur. Even in situations of illness, however, the professional and others may be shielded from becoming more self-aware by that wonderful mechanism and ancient archetypal force that we have built into our legal structure: the scapegoat, someone or something to blame.

FOURTEEN ATTRIBUTES OF THE PHYSICIAN AS PROFESSIONAL EXPERT

The following are the central attributes and behaviors of a physician that shield him from seeing beyond the confines of his professional role.

1. Over-education:

Many professionals are overeducated. They do not know how to live life as a common man. Consequently, they are unable to perceive the reality of the crisis in health care from a common sense perspective. Farmers can see how the weather affects their crops. Plumbers notice how water pressure in one area affects flow in another. Yet the over-analytical physician sees a cancer and operates on it or radiates it, without wondering if something elsewhere in the body is related to the development of the cancer. This inability to perceive connections keeps physicians unable to see clearly the real causes of illness in patients. The professional way of life blocks real change in our approach to healing.

2. Desire for control:

A key part of professional life is the desire to control people and events. This control is usually focused on maintaining a certain economically successful lifestyle and social position of power at the expense of other health care workers and the general public. Medical school education fosters the ability to control. It is why professionals hide in their narrow fields of practice.

3. Separation between the inner and outer selves:

To be a professional means to profess to be something or someone that is often different from who you really are. This results in a divided person cut off from this inner source. Energy goes toward maintaining a mask of an outwardly successful professional personality, while the inner self withers. Many professionals experience this division in their late thirties and early forties. By this time they are so entrenched in position and family and the desire to retire at 50 that they are hesitant to look at their own inner emptiness. The world supports them in continuing to hide. People who seek professional assistance are often ill due to what they are denying. If the professional is also blinded by denial, then nothing substantial can happen in the doctor-patient relationship.

4. Human doing:

Being professional means being able to perform at a high level of excellence and being rewarded for this. People often become human doings, rather than human beings. Our families and our school system reward human doings.

5. Trapped in the head:

Professionally based training and work keeps professional people trapped in intellectually abstract and mechanistically conceptual thinking as the primary way of relating to the world. Many medical doctors view health and illness through a lens of intellectually abstract and mechanistically conceptual thinking. This makes it difficult to look at the whole picture of illness in a patient's life. The physician is also blocked from being able to acknowledge the effectiveness of approaches such as acupuncture and homeopathy that view illness and healing from a perspective of the whole and not just isolated parts.

6. Lack of listening:

Professionals spend little time really listening. The physician of today in most practices allows five to ten minutes per patient in a busy office. After asking questions and giving directions, this leaves very little time for listening. This is how the professional protects himself from being in relationship with another person, and keeps in control.

7. Analysis, not synthesis:

The physician examines parts of the body in isolation. Laboratory tests and sophisticated X rays isolate disease in a particular organ that is then treated with a drug or surgery. The perspective of the whole is lost. Thus there is no real healing.

8. Continuing a heritage:

The head-centered professional lifestyle is most often solidified in the early twenties during professional training, after years of our educational system's emphasis on intellect. The successful professional works for financial and material success. He is part of the problem that permits the illness-engendering climate to continue. The public has faith that the doctor is working to heal patients. Neither the public nor the professional believe that the professional is part of the problem. While a doctor may have good intentions to heal, the results are often the opposite because of the framework and thinking in medicine.

9. Intolerance for other approaches to healing:

The growing attractiveness of alternative therapies to many people is a threat to the financial and controlling position of the conventional medical profession and all those who reap great economic benefits from continuing the allopathic approach to health care. Alternative therapies are offensive to the physician's rational mind because they cannot be proven in double-blind laboratory conditions. Our obsession with this standard of judgment has blinded us to the benefits of incorporating many successful alternative approaches to healing that work on different principles than double-blind laboratory studies may test. The economics of medicine has also permitted us to forget that healing does not take place because of a bottle of pills, but rather because of the living relationship between two people.

10. Aloofness:

Many professionals would like to remain in the ivory tower that is supported by intellectual prowess, position, and arrogance.

11. Hiding:

The physician hides behind the veneer of being a professional, which keeps him from having a real relationship with others. Thus the professional may hide from himself and not have to make real changes in his character, which inner life calls us to make.

12. Cleverness:

The education of professionals is based on the recycling of information from others in the field—learning by formula. The learned formulas give the illusion of people getting better. These formulas ensure material success and are protected by legal codes. These formulas are tombs for the creative spirit and imaginative faculty.

13. Laziness:

Many professionals work long hours. Yet these are often long hours of formula work, whether in diagnostic and surgical procedures, or treating sore throats. The laziness comes in being able to hide in this type of work, rather than extending oneself in a healing relationship with another.

14. Arrogance:

Many professionals assume and demand that all others serve them. This is slowly beginning to change as the public becomes more assertive. The physician's intolerance to patient questions is one way that this arrogance manifests.

These fourteen attributes describe what has been called the Illness of Professionalism. This illness is at the core of our collective resistance to change. It forms the center of problems in our present specialized phase of medicine.

Our intellectual lifestyle has grown to prominence in the past half-century and has blinded us to the causes of many illnesses by focusing on formulas, specialization, and symptoms. The physician, to help people heal, needs to be honest, observant, discriminative, and imaginative.

Society in general and many professionals in particular need to change from a life based on intellect, which is a life of illness, to a life focused on consciousness, which is a life of healing. The process of emerging from an exclusively intellectual lifestyle that eclipses the light of conscious awareness is the requisite of all healing.

As a guide to evolving practitioners, I would paraphrase one of my teachers, the French homeopath Dr. Gerard Gueniot:

> Your power is in your internal authority.
> Practice with love and serenity.
> Have a connectedness with what you are doing.
> You do not need to be respected by conventional medicine, which is really all about the commercial exploitation of disease.

Our current health care crisis allows us to observe in the open what has lain hidden in the shadows. Fear of disease and death has reached epidemic proportions, and is draining both our creative reserves and our economy. Widespread professional narcissism feeds this problem. Not only does this enable many professionals to hide from themselves, but the entire system that is geared to and run by health care professionals, including insurance companies, hospitals, and pharmaceutical companies, gives license to others in society to live in the same manner. The opportunity is now upon us to deal with this state of crisis. The bridge between the Illness of Professionalism and the individual life of purpose and living one's dreams can now consciously be built. It is this process that will give sustenance to the future.

THE WORKPLACE, ILLNESS, AND HEALING

Our interactions in the workplace are indicative of our strengths and weaknesses. The dynamic relationship between illness and work creates an opportunity to transform weaknesses in our temperament and character. If left imbalanced, these imbalances will eventually and often unnecessarily precipitate physical disease in a person.

My experience as a conventional physician sheds light on the relationship between illness and work. While I was hiding behind my position, behaving arrogantly, and reaping the financial rewards of my work, my life was falling apart, from abuse of alcohol and marijuana, overeating and weight gain, and relationships that lacked heart.

Due to the influence of some key people who entered my life when I was choosing a medical specialty, I went into emergency medicine. Several positive developments arose from this. First, I learned how to work with other people. Unlike being a doctor in private practice with his own office, hiring and firing at whim, emergency medicine required me to respect others, or get fired myself. As I mentioned previously, I was fired twice early in my emergency years for my treatment of hospital staff.

Second, working in emergency departments taught me how to act spontaneously and respond to what was needed in the moment. After spending most of my life in my head, with both abstract intellectual thinking and fantasy, emergency work became an antidote. I learned how to observe first and read afterwards, which is the reality of the present moment. And I had to deal with whatever the day presented, instead of being able to control my circumstances and dictating whom I wanted to see.

Third, emergency department work brought me into direct contact with people of different heritages. I began to observe the constitutional, temperament, and character imbalances that are peculiar to each heritage. I also noticed how most people do not begin to emerge from the influence of their heritage and become more free-thinking until something major occurs in their lives, such as an illness or an accident.

The workplace is an excellent environment for developing relationships with people one might never choose to be with. Yet this rarely occurs. I worked for six years in one emergency department and realized on leaving that I hardly knew anyone beneath the surface.

Most work situations deaden our individual creative natures. We too often see work as a necessary evil to tolerate in order to make money and return home to the family, and to save money for vacation and retirement. Work becomes the means to an end rather than an end in itself. When we view work this way, our focus is not on the present. The workplace has the potential to become a place of healing. If all our workplaces were places that supported healing, our economy would be much better.

For many people, work is increasingly consumed by mindless and repetitious work with low pay. The so-called and ironically named "service" jobs are becoming the fastest growing type of work in our economy. The jobs of higher pay are the professional jobs, and those in the computer/ technological fields, and even these are diminishing in compensation.

Mindless repetition or working for excessive material gratification deadens the soul. These polarities of work tear apart our social fabric. The workplace needs to become a place of individual growth and the development of relationships that take us beyond the sometimes-narrow confines of heritage. When this occurs, we can return home to family and bring the healing principles of connectedness into family life. The workplace needs to become a living community in the true sense. This means that we can trust in the heart of those with whom we work, we can hold and be held by others, and we can bring deeper meaningfulness to work.

Then the day again will become whole and people will recover their enthusiasm for life. Chaos in the world, greed in the marketplace, and abstract intellectual teaching in schools all undermine our ability to live artful lives. As a result, more people's lives are breaking down and chronic illness is growing. All the promise of genetic research will not alter this unless we change our lifestyles. To think otherwise is delusional.

More anger is surfacing today. Anger without understanding often degenerates into chaos. This chaos manifests not only outwardly in ways that are seen on the nightly news, but also in the chaos of internal organ function. The incidence of chronic illnesses of the internal organs has dramatically increased, and this epidemic is draining our economic capacities.

More people are becoming ill. Why? The subconscious parts of our selves seek an outlet of expression. When they are denied a healthy outlet, these forces turn against us as illness or accidents. Repetitive work often puts people to sleep while they are awake. As a result, accidents are becoming more frequent. Accidents and uncomfortable symptoms of illness often bring us immediately into the present, which is where we need to focus.

In the crisis orientation of the emergency department, many people become so consumed with their own life situations that they are either unaware of or do not care about the life of another person. This applies to patients, their families, and also many emergency department personnel. Though many try, it becomes difficult for overworked personnel to care deeply about sick people. This environment becomes remarkably similar to any other assembly-line workplace. Both workers and patients have come to perceive medical care in mechanistic ways, fixing the parts.

Witnessing the limitations of this work led me into a deeper phase of work as an integrative alternative physician. I spend time getting to know my patients. Being an emergency physician led me to overcome and transform tendencies in myself that would have created problems in this new life.

We need to create different types of work that do not limit our creativity, imagination, and capacity to live flexible lives. Workplaces need to become places where we may more consciously learn about working with others and healing our own weaknesses and imbalances. Then work becomes a part of life, and preventive medicine becomes more than having blood pressure and cholesterol levels checked periodically. Work and healing become interwoven. This can happen only if we confront and change the current materially driven environment in the health care workplace.

CHAPTER 5

THE THREE PHASES OF THE MEDICAL INSTITUTION

In order to understand the institution of medicine where it is now, where it is headed, and where it needs to go if it is to be renewed, it is important to understand the growth cycle of economic institutions, of which medicine is a part. The growth of most economic institutions, including hospitals, can be described as occurring in three phases. These three phases are called pioneer, organizational or bureaucratic, and integrated. They correspond respectively to past, present, and future. The following are the nature of these phases in institutional medicine.

PIONEER PHASE: THE PAST

Photo displays of history from conception to the present are typically found in hospital lobbies. At conception the small initial building often looked like a one-room schoolhouse. Next to these photos are photographs of the initiators of the hospital, many of who served in multiple capacities. An old surgeon from that time will talk about performing operations, delivering babies, and setting bones. Often these doctors have a gleam of longing in their eyes when they talk of those times.

They were part of the first phase of medicine, the pioneer phase. Small teams of people who in many cases knew each other well worked together in multiple and often changing capacities to begin a project. Camaraderie and a familial kind of bond developed among these people. Even though the earlier work required much effort, there was often simplicity to the work that many people long for when the institution has progressed to another phase.

ORGANIZATIONAL PHASE: THE PRESENT

Following the progression of the photo exhibit, the small hospital gradually develops into a large institution, now called a medical center. This is the organizational or bureaucratic phase, which characterizes most of our major

medical institutions today. During this phase there is development of a bureaucracy with rules and regulations, division of labor, and the development
of specializations and sub-specializations.

During this phase, there is tremendous growth in specialization among
medical doctors and other health professionals, which has occurred in our current medical system. Each becomes competent in a narrow area and takes
steps not to cross into the domain of another specialist. This is perceived as
necessary because of:

- the volume of technical information in each field

- public demand that the doctor be perfect, with litigation the
  consequence of imperfection

- financial rewards for the surgical and diagnostic procedures
  of specialties

In most instances, the financial reward aspect leads to an increasing
cultural dependence on special procedures with highly expensive technology used because it is there. Diagnostic procedures permit physicians to
view directly physical changes inside the body. We have come to believe
that these physical changes are the disease. All sectors of health care—
doctor, insurance company, government agency, and patient—demand
these diagnostic proofs.

These physically observed changes are then treated with pharmaceutical drugs or surgery. The changes seen under a microscope or in a
laboratory are treated, not the person. If a blockage is seen in the heart
blood vessels, for example, then a drug is given to remove this blockage.
What becomes of paramount importance, and what is financially rewarding to physician, hospital, pharmaceutical company, and medical supply
firm, is the pathology of the body tissue. The nature of specialization today is such that the relationship of the part to the whole is lost or only
given lip service. Specialization is the obsession in medicine, a result of a
general public that does not care to educate themselves about the nature of
illness.

Furthermore, the organizational form is a bureaucratic hierarchy with orders coming from the top down. Most people who work in hospitals have little
direct role in decisions about the whole hospital or even about their own particular department. Barring a crisis, there is no sense of community and
shared responsibility among people in a large medical institution, as there was
during the earlier pioneer phase. Each department has its own rules and regulations that often take volumes of notebooks to categorize.

The present trend in health care is bureaucratic centrist thinking, a classic
pyramidal organization with management at the top and many intermediate

layers with differentiated levels of work. Authority moves from above to below. It is ironic and mystifying that many Americans are aware of the pitfalls of governmental bureaucracy and yet are blinded to the destructiveness and wastefulness of the bloated bureaucracy of health care and the private health insurance industry.

The holy concept of efficiency is worshipped at this phase. Efficiency is not measured in human terms but in statistical numbers. For example, the number of nursing personnel assigned to an emergency room is determined by the number of patients seen, not by the hours a nurse may need to spend with a complex problem. The mid-level bureaucrat cares not whether patients have simple problems that take little time to help, or whether the same numbers of patients have complex medical and surgical problems that require hours of treatment and reevaluation. The longer a nurse spends with a patient, the fewer number of nurses will be assigned to the emergency department. The god is efficiency. The goals are to reduce costs and make more profits, at the expense of patient well-being.

This centrally oriented bureaucracy, be it public or private, controls people and stifles creativity. Keeping profit margins high and labor costs low leaves no time for creativity and human initiative. Most people, both in the general public and in health professions, perceive health care in mechanistic terms with material objectives. The public has accepted these limitations, and demands that someone else, that is, the insurance company, pay for the expensive care that has resulted.

We have reached the point in our societal evolution where mechanism no longer works as the modus operandi. It is clear that the organizational or bureaucratic phase is overripe for change. Health care is rapidly becoming unaffordable. More important, in its current fragmented and chaotic form, medicine has no opportunity to contribute to the spiritual and cultural development of most people. This is because we have permitted health care to become subservient to the forces of the marketplace.

The gap between human and machine is closing. In the world of machines, it is correct to strive for efficiency, emphasizing mechanization and automation. In the world of human beings, the striving for creativity is paramount. The potential exists to change our organizational forms in health care. We need to change our image of health care from one that is primarily mechanistic and economic, to one that serves individual growth through appreciating the positive and transformative role of illness in healing.

Hospitals and other health care institutions have tried to humanize the bureaucracy. There are "employees of the month" and other perks for incentive. Yet the system remains largely the same. We are unable to breathe new life and new creativity into health care reforms because it is too invested in mechanistic thinking and materialistic results. The major players have too much invested in keeping things the way they are.

47

Health care has become an industry, where hospitals, insurance companies, and doctors battle for money and become highly possessive of patients. Many doctors are so fearful of losing a patient that they will prescribe a drug when one is not needed, because the patient expects it. The same holds true for expensive diagnostic procedures that the physician is aware having little value in determining treatment for the patient's illness.

The current medical model is now in decay. As we continue to hold on to economics and our mechanistic ideas about disease, more and more people will become incapacitated with physical or psychological illness for which they will be less able to afford care. Many millions of Americans are without any health insurance and millions more have Medicaid that is accepted by fewer and fewer doctors and are less able to be financed by state governments. More and more doctors refuse to accept Medicare patients. The institution of medicine in its bloated organizational phase is in need of critical attention.

INTEGRATION PHASE: THE FUTURE

The third phase, integration, is an opportunity to reawaken the enthusiasm that was felt during the pioneering phase. This enthusiasm must be incorporated in a different way than it had been earlier, because the organizational phase does have a great deal to contribute. We need to be able to combine enthusiasm with creative new approaches that enable the people in bureaucracies to work together in more effective ways for patient care. What are the main principles of this third phase, the phase of integration? Broadly speaking, there are four. The phase of integration involves:

- equality of responsibility
- group process
- interchangeability
- redefinition of values

Equality Of Responsibility

The emphasis on professionalism that characterizes the present-day second phase has created great inequalities and a general lack of authentic relationship among people in a hospital workplace. Progressing to the integration phase requires forming a community based on equality of responsibility. In such a community, a nurse's aide or a kitchen worker holds no less value than a doctor. The vertical hierarchy of the organizational phase, which is based on knowledge and specialization, becomes a horizontal hierarchy in which value to the whole is determined by factors other than technical know-how. These other determinants are defined in terms of principles such as commitment, responsibility, and readiness to do what is needed in the moment.

The guiding organizational principle in hospitals, clinics, long-term care, and other health care facilities needs to be changed from one that is driven by bottom-line efficiency to one that balances the efficiency of machines with the creativity of human beings. We can say that efficiency proceeds from the physical whereas creativity proceeds from the spiritual. We need to create a living bridge between the spiritual and the physical in health care. There is nothing wrong with efficiency if it is guided by human principles and not by principles that govern machines.

Our present vertical hierarchy is ruled by the adage "Knowledge is power." Pharmaceutical drugs and surgery seen as the models for medical treatment is a result from mechanical and abstract models of disease. Most patients and health care workers remain compliant with this medical approach. In this approach, healing is only the illusion of wellness, determined by absence of symptoms. In the phase of integration, the sleeping will is awakened. Rather than the present pyramidal form of organization in corporate health care, what we need to develop is a geometry of interlocking policy-making groups. The two forms of organization are illustrated in the accompanying diagram.

Present Pyramidal Hierarchy:

Medical Doctors

Nurses

Psychologists/
Social Workers

Financial

Maintenance

Future:

Medical Doctors

Psychologists/
Social Workers

Nurses

Financial

Administration
and Maintenance

In the integrated system, there would be no managerial intermediary levels dictated by an arbitrary top-level management. Each point on the star is a group with a particular mandate for certain tasks. All groups are of equal rank. From these groups, representatives to a central policy-making group are chosen. In these ways, we reconnect the value of human labor to the value of health.

Group Process

In the present system, physicians have control because of their knowledge and position. Surgical procedures are more profitable than psychological counseling or art therapy, according to current reimbursement standards. This needs to change. Each person in a therapeutic environment must recognize the value of each participant in a group process that is guided by the spirit of service and focuses on the illness in the life of a particular patient.

Professionals need this new phase, the integrated phase, perhaps more than patients do. Physicians and other health professionals have a difficult time today. This is not often visible because an abundance of money allows the physician to hide his problems with professional and family relationships. Most professionals are overeducated and over-trained. As a result, many do not know how to live life as a common man with common sense. Many have lost their sense of compassion.

Slanderous, though supposedly humorous, statements about patients include calling patients "gomers," an acronym for "get out of my emergency room." Another favorite phrase is "There goes another one of those health nuts." Alcoholics are derided. A woman with lower abdominal pain will be dismissed with a moralistic tone as a "PID" (pelvic inflammatory disease, often caused by sexually-transmitted microorganisms).

The impulse of respect for the common person used to be what the United States stood for and a principle on which it was founded. Yet the spell of specialization and bureaucratic organization separates people and promotes a superior attitude in some toward others. Physicians and other health professionals need to recognize the need for a new phase, not only for the health of the nation but also for their own health and well-being. It will be difficult to transform the health care system by changing laws and methods of financing without addressing these underlying principles.

What we need today are socially organized people who can carry or support each other when that is needed. This idea of being held is very important in group work so that the whole life struggle is not on an individual's shoulders alone.

Often, people stick together in families in their attempt to be carried and held during their lives. But there is also another way to live with, work with, or be in community with people with whom you are not blood related. This can be with a spouse or intimate partner, or with others. The idea is to receive help in going through life's difficult times. This help is given out of kindness, not out of materialism.

Interchangeability

A third principle in the phase of integration is that of interchangeability. The goal is to break down the division of labor of the organizational phase that keeps people isolated and protected from the vulnerability of relationship. Today many of us believe that division of labor has given us a high quality health care system that functions efficiently and makes people well. This is not true. In spite of great publicity about technological advances in conventional medicine, people on the whole are becoming more ill and are not being provided with educational tools for self-healing.

The present division of labor enables the physician to remain in a position of control and authority. The growth in malpractice insurance and in medico-legal claims is the public's mostly unconscious response to this control and fractioning of the human being. Medical professionals should not be surprised that: fractured people without any sense of the whole; and lacking professionals who offer the principles of self-educative healing; become possessed by the same scapegoat complex that obsesses the medical profession.

Imagine walking into a clinic and observing the doctor assisting the nurse in removing the used sheets from an examining table or helping to unpack supplies. Most of us would be flabbergasted. This is not the physician's defined responsibility. His time is much too valuable. This attitude is the problem. Too much value is placed on intellect and knowledge at the expense of relationship and respect.

This attitude of separatism does not support human growth and development gained through the process of coming to terms with illness. Physicians put themselves in the situation of being trapped by the demands of time, hurrying from one patient to another in order to maintain their income status. Physicians place blame for the failing system on health insurance companies, as in "If control was returned to the doctors like it used to be, we would all get better." This is a dangerous illusion. As long as the medical profession is heavily invested in control and in an elitist way of thinking about illness and healing, the same problems will haunt us.

What if a physician spent five minutes helping to make a bed or doing another task outside of his or her habitual professional pattern? Or what if a physician spent several hours working in the garden to learn about the herbs he or she uses with patients? Such physicians would be helping to break down the old decaying system of values. In so doing, they would lessen their own addiction to information and to a certain lifestyle. They would gradually come to understand that value is not defined by one's knowledge, but rather by one's willingness to respond to what is needed in the moment. They would come down off the thrones upon which they are trapped, and begin to live as they really want to live.

On a larger scale, people working in a clinical setting that embraced the principle of interchangeability would engage in regular meetings in which tasks and responsibilities would be agreed on. The needs of the whole would guide the agreement. Such meetings could be called circles of responsibility. To become effective, those who participate in caring for the ill would redefine the purpose of their work. Clocking in and out, doing assigned tasks, and picking up a paycheck every two weeks would not be the norm.

The present way of doing things is merely an extension of the womb. It is the protected environment in which we are not encouraged to change our character, but rather remain hidden in roles such as doctor, nurse, technician, or billing clerk. Is not this act of hiding in our jobs and collusively agreeing to let each other hide merely an extension of the way we hide in families and in society? We need to be accountable to ourselves and to each other.

There are certain areas of work in a hospital, clinic, or any complex modern enterprise that are best performed with training. However, there are many other opportunities where interchangeability is a positive approach. People could experientially learn other labors. Working in a clinic garden and pulling the weeds around herbs used in the clinic is one example. Direct experience is especially necessary for head-trapped professionals. When a business owner began as a worker who rose through the ranks of a business, learning through direct experience along the way, he or she gained a perspective that is lacking in today's climate of protecting one's turf. It would be a valuable experience for a physician or administrator to occasionally help unload delivery trucks or serve dinner in the cafeteria.

REDEFINITION OF VALUES

The phase of integration requires new approaches to economics. Currently, wages for people in clinical environments are set by market values. Yet, as we have seen in other areas such as the environment, market values often run counter to the valuation of human development. How can we bring about a rapport between these two seeming opposites?

Human spiritual development is the purpose of the cultural sphere of life. Medicine and many other institutions are really part of the cultural sphere, and over the centuries have been taken over by and driven by the forces of the economic sphere.

In the phase of integration, professional people would voluntarily agree to accept lower wages in order to be an active part of a community. Most health professionals are in definite need of this type of arrangement to heal their often narcissistic and mechanistic lifestyles. The implications of this reorganization are far-reaching and significant, requiring redefinition of values and reevaluation of the economic structure of medicine.

Such a change would obviously need to be phased in over time. A community of health workers would need to recognize the realities of medicolegal responsibility that society currently places on physicians, and allow for this financially. (Books such as *Money Is Love: Reconnecting to the Sacred Origins of Money,* by Barbara Wilder, may be of great help.) Furthermore, such arrangements will require that the people involved in these arrangements strive to redefine their relationship to money, value, and trust. Changes such as those described herein may generate turmoil in the psyches of participants, as old subconscious patterns and fears make their presence felt. Such changes are not merely mechanical or financial. They require us to make fundamental changes on psychological and spiritual levels.

TIME TO RENEW OUR HEALTH CARE SYSTEM

It is time to make the transition from the organizational phase to the integration phase. Just as many people in their late thirties and early forties yearn to re-enliven the dream of their lives that has been squashed in the organizational phase of life and work, many health professionals yearn to have more meaning in their work. We cannot return to the pioneer phase of anything, just as we cannot return to our childhood. However, we can reawaken the feeling of the pioneer time of life—the awe and wonder, the innocence, the camaraderie—in order to deepen our understanding of illness and enhance our capacity to serve.

For a renewed health care system to be effective, everything must become different, from economic structure, to the way people work together, to the type of health care services offered. The idea is to build more conscious relationships between human beings who share a common striving. In these ways, we will fashion living social structures enlivened by human warmth.

It is no accident that the words integration and integrity have the same root. Restructuring health care and transforming it from the organizational phase into the phase of integration will enhance the feeling of integrity and purpose in all who participate. Those who seek help in dealing with illness will understand and be willing to accept the need to assume more individual responsibility. Medicine will have moved much closer to its true vocation: providing the soil for self-educative healing to grow and flower. In this way, a new, more beneficent culture will emerge in the United States.

CHAPTER 6

THE SOUL AND MEDICINE

M edicine has lost its soul. Wholeness has been fractured by an industry that measures health by cost-effectiveness, and promotes a rigid and exclusive mechanistic understanding of human illness. The three aspects of the human soul as described in anthroposophy—thinking, feeling, and willing—are from the narrow point of view of conventional mechanistic medicine merely abstractions that are relegated to the fields of psychology and religion, and are not seen as having any practical relationship to disease. The moods and temperaments that bridge the soul to the body are discounted because they do not easily fit into diagnosis-related categories for hospital billing purposes. Moods and temperaments cannot be seen under the microscope of cellular pathology.

Present attitudes about organ transplants reveal how conventional medicine has lost its soul. As we rush into this era of organ transplants, most people view the replacing of a human heart with one that is mechanical or with the heart from another as a positive development. Yet whether or not the transplant is done, the central question is always avoided. What is the relationship of the diseased organ to the whole life of the person? Are we really so deluded to think that replacing one organ with another addresses the depth of human illness and the reason the organ needed to be replaced?

Futurists hold out the promise that one day soon all organs will be replaceable. Yet this is already financially unaffordable. When the State of Oregon transferred funds from organ transplants for the poor and redistributed the funds to provide health care for many people, the state was accused of rationing. The Canadian health care system is denounced because some people have to wait years for a heart transplant. These criticisms are driven by fear. They accentuate the illusion that one can continue to live one's same lifestyle, and when this lifestyle destroys an organ, that organ can be replaced with limited changes required in one's lifestyle.

This is a collective denial of the reality of the human soul. This denial is built into our economic system of medical care. It is indeed a denial of death, and an attempt to live forever as a rigidly imbalanced personality with many points of view but little in the way of principles.

The organs we were born with decay so that our inner life of soul and spirit will be born. This is an example of anthroposophical understanding.

55

When we learn to invoke these inner impulses in daily life through family, work, education, creativity, and other areas of endeavor, our organs are given the opportunity to regenerate. Then organ transplants will become rare and unnecessary. What is leading these organs toward continuing decay without regeneration is our denial that our driven wants and desires are obsessive/compulsive and addictive in nature.

All of our major institutions further this unnecessary decay by supporting cultural denial. Medicine denies the process of psychosocial development in its model of health care. Education is just beginning to move away from a primarily head-oriented system of education, which taxes the internal organs early in life and leads to disease years later. (The growing popularity of Waldorf and other arts-based approaches to education are examples of this trend.) Popular entertainment primarily stimulates the physical senses without providing people with the opportunity to experience themselves as beings of soul and spirit through the arts. Religion is obsessed with fanaticism, doctrines, and dogma. The list goes on.

Illness is often a time of death to our old ways, encouraging us to become more aware of ourselves as beings of soul and spirit. This death births regeneration. Without a fundamental change in attitude toward the diseases of internal organs, people will be further possessed by their own as well as society's forces of decay even as they receive new organs.

The soul is far from an abstract phenomenon that has no relationship to our daily lives. Our souls communicate and live in our physical bodies through our organs. In reality there is no separation between the way we live our lives and the function and vitality of our internal organs. All deeper traditions of healing, such as Chinese, Ayurvedic (Indian), and Anthroposophical (German) Medicine understand this deep inner connectedness.

The soul's image is wholeness and connectedness. The growth of the environmental movement worldwide attests to this growing awareness in the collective mind and heart of humanity. We are finally more willing to be responsible for the decay and death that our lives of denial have produced. This principle of connectedness also applies to the internal organs.

The principle of interconnectedness is vital to our redesigned health care system. With interconnectedness, which is the nature of soul relationships, the soul will reenter mainstream medicine. This principle needs to be built into the structure and function of health care. Then we will have the strength to transform the narrow mechanistic medical model that currently dominates health care today.

The key is to look at diseases of the internal organs with the light of interconnectedness to guide us. At the present time, cultural attitudes in most areas of medicine are driven by material incentives, intellectual pursuits, and a public fear of death and disease. It is becoming obvious that we are performing too many heart surgeries on people who do not benefit either physically or spiritually. We are investing millions of dollars in multi-organ transplants and

are not giving attention to weaknesses in people's constitutions, temperaments, and characters, which appeared in the internal organs years before the
crisis occurred. Giving this attention is practicing soul-oriented medicine.

As discussed repeatedly, many people seek lifestyles that are comfortable,
convenient, and financially rewarding. Following such a lifestyle is often the
path of least resistance, and it is where many lose sight of their soul's memory
of their life's dream.

Our cherished cultural institutions, including medicine, encourage us to
continue with these illusory lifestyles. Family members may deny that there
are relationship problems within the family while the teenage drug user is
blamed for being antisocial. A woman who drinks and overeats may deny that
her physical symptoms have any relationship to her lifestyle. In denials and
illusory lifestyles, in escape through holidays or addictions, our personalities
become hardened. We expend energy to defend our supposedly self-chosen
activities. We may also become more attached to our particular opinions and
points of view in order to keep control of these lifestyles and fantasies. Intolerance of others often follows.

More often than not our conversations are based on points of view rather
than principles. How then can our souls communicate to our rigidly controlled
and intolerant personalities that this is not the life of wholeness, development,
and creative individuality that is our destiny? The result is that the soul is relegated to the abstract non-real entity to which we give lip service in religious
services. Or its existence is denied altogether, as in science, which also denies
the relationship of the soul to the body and mind because science cannot prove
the existence of the soul in a laboratory.

One way that our souls communicate with us is through crisis and illness.
Crises happen in people's lives in order to awaken the conscious human will.
These crises are often unnecessary accidents or incapacitating illnesses.
Through these situations we are given opportunities to wake up.

We are born with the potential to become human, though for years we live
primarily out of the animal part of ourselves through wants rather than needs.
Becoming fully human is the work of life. To do this work requires the activity of the conscious human will. All illness needs to be seen in this light.
There are too many potent forces in the world that tear apart the often delicate
and subtle fabric of the soul.

How does one awaken the conscious human will? Exercises and disciplines, such as meditation, mindfulness, and others described by many world
teachers from the Dalai Lama to Rudolf Steiner, when done on a regular basis,
support the awakening of the conscious human will. It requires effort. It involves going beyond what comes easy to us, beyond the supposedly safe
confines of old associations, which include family, religion, or school. It is
not that these associations are bad. However, many of the groups in which we
participate in the first 21 to 28 years of life are based on collective agreements
to hide from life, to hide family dysfunctional patterns, and/or to hide in intellectual pursuits in order to escape from feelings.

The agreements of these groups—family of origin, religious institutions, schools—also dominate our present institutions and are obstacles to real change. Groups such as those that control medicine are based on the will of strong personalities whose activities are often not guided by soul-infused principles. Patients who enter such a health care system seeking help are not enlivened by soul principles. In other words, their unresolved and illness-generating power issues from family or work are not worked with. In this context, all therapy becomes palliative.

When we are able to associate with people who are more focused on needs rather than wants, principles rather than points of view, the soul has found a home. We then enter into a process that takes years, in which we are supported to contact and maintain a relationship with our soul's purpose. With time this purpose is felt more consistently in daily life and in relationship with others. The active group process involves those with whom one recognizes an inner bond. There is a mutually felt purpose and commitment that holds people together.

Through having a living connection with our soul we are able to have honest relationships with others and ourselves. As a result, we develop a true sense of self. The soul is alive within us when we invoke principles in any given situation, instead of remaining attached to our opinions and points of view. By this, I mean principles such as honesty, integrity, courage, and service. When we are attentive to what is needed, rather than what we grasp for, the soul guides our thoughts, feelings, and actions.

As a result of the willingness to enter into this active process and to come into rapport with the deeper part of ourselves, rather than the personas with which we often identify, the principle of grace enters our lives. We are given the opportunity to come to terms with deeper aspects of our psyches without necessarily having to go through a crisis. Our lives need not be unraveled in order to learn. This process is not easy. Yet it is both vital and necessary if we are to develop institutions that will provide vehicles for healing in the future.

CHAPTER 7

THE EMINENT PLACE OF HEALTH CARE

Health care has become a commodity, increasing its resistance to change. People and their health are no longer perceived as the purpose for the health care system to exist. Rather, sick people have become the medium for health care commodities to continue their growth.

This very subtle change in the purpose of our health care system makes all the difference. Most physicians, nurses, and other health professionals genuinely care for their clients. However, a web of financial success is woven into the fabric or climate in which they work. This web will entrap and bankrupt us if it is allowed to continue its hold.

In order to perceive this web clearly, we need to understand the distinction between sincerity and truth. Most health professionals are sincere in wanting to help others. The spirit of service is strong in the health professions. Sincerity and good intentions must not blind us from perceiving the forces that are at work. Our collective attitudes about health care will keep us spending huge amounts of money, focusing on symptoms and specialization, without ever uncovering the root causes of our illness.

Many people today are becoming aware of what in psychological terms have been called shadow forces. Our shadow forces are the parts of each of us that shame or embarrass us, so we keep them hidden. We run, put on blinders, or overcompensate for our shadow forces. As a result of these denials, our lives are constantly undermined by what we refuse to look at and are not compassionately helped to see. The same principle applies to health care on a broader scale.

THREE AREAS OF HUMAN ENDEAVOR

There are three primary fields of human endeavor: the spiritual/cultural sphere, the political sphere, and the economic sphere. In other words, all of our work and activities fall into these three areas. Each has an equal right to exist.

1. Spiritual/Cultural Sphere

Educators, artists, and religious leaders fall within the spiritual/cultural sphere. Their purpose is to enhance our capacity for free thinking and creativity, and to contribute to the well-being of others. Income for these people is often agreed on in a collective manner, by boards of schools, religious institutions, or museums.

The spiritual/cultural sphere is the least valued in our country. Many people attempt to manipulate this area politically and economically for their particular fanatical or materialistic points of view. The result is often suppression of individual freedom and the capacity for free thinking.

A freely supported spiritual/cultural life is vital to the development of all of us. The kind of group process and community that can make changes in our culture will come from this sphere. A keynote of the spiritual/cultural sphere is education that is free of any particular product.

2. Political Sphere

This sphere of life embodies our rights, especially equality and democracy. The political sphere includes those who make, enforce, and interpret the laws. Politicians at all levels, police, armed forces, and the legal court system are part of the political sphere. This area receives much publicity in elections, and in lawsuits and other legal battles. This sphere, which is the natural meeting place of the spiritual/cultural and economic spheres, was the battlefield in the 1960s. Today it has been largely superceded by economic forces. When this sphere is alive and well in our society, each of us believe that the individual is a dignified member, equal to everyone else.

3. Economic Sphere

Most people in the United States, working at jobs that provide goods and services that meet consumer demand and that form the basis of trade, fit into this sphere. The country has come to depend on this third area for its sense of economic well-being. Just as we place an exaggerated value on physical symptoms in health care often to the exclusion of a person's inner health and well-being, so do we as a nation place supreme value on a consumer-driven economy of goods and services. The goal is to have more, be it objects of pleasure or years of life.

IN WHICH SPHERE DOES HEALTH CARE FALL?

The true home or calling of health care is in educating and supporting people to enhance their sense of well-being and insight into the relationship of lifestyle and illness. Health care stands alongside education, the creative arts, psychology, and spiritual disciplines in the first or spiritual/cultural sphere of human endeavor.

Yet this is not where health care falls today. With all the attention on cost control, insurance, technology, and pharmaceutical drugs, health care is now in the economic sphere. This has been true for at least the past hundred years, and especially so in the past 20 years. Health care is one of the top two or three fields in which investors have been able to reap large net incomes from goods and services provided.

The economics of medicine, rather than the health and well-being of people, drives health care. "A man cannot serve two masters." The master, the charioteer who directs, needs an attitude of service to enhance people's lives and health. Then the economics are arranged to serve this primary driving force. There is a general lack of education as to what illness and healing is about and the economic-based health care system is a monster out of control. The rampant fear of disease and the demand that all illnesses be fixed and made to go away regardless of the cost are clearly the fuel that feeds the monster, which threatens to devour those whom health care is intended to serve.

Here are some illustrations of our out-of-control health care system:

- One-third of the average American's lifetime health care costs are in the last year of life, and half of those costs are in the last two months.

- Neonatal ICUs save one-fourth of all premature infants who weigh as little as 18 ounces at a cost that runs to six figures, instead of costing microscopically smaller amounts that would be required to educate and support pregnant women in prenatal, perinatal, and postnatal care

- Physicians give more exotic and expensive drugs to patients to help them sleep, feel tranquil, and eliminate their pain, instead of integrating the much less expensive and often effective approaches of alternative medicine

- Two-thirds of the approximately 600,000 medical doctors in the United States are in specialties and subspecialties where procedures command large reimbursement, and human dialogue in consultation is much less valued economically

- Health care stocks have become a main source of profitability and retirement funds.

The retirement portfolios of many Americans depend on pharmaceutical companies and other health care stocks to make enormous profits. This is very significant because these same pharmaceutical companies make products that

61

not only do not contribute to our greater health and well-being, but are often actually detrimental to healing because they suppress symptoms and/or because the drugs themselves generate further toxins.

The more commonly profitable drugs treat symptoms. Because we are under the spell that relief of symptoms means cure of illness, we continue to take these drugs. Yet the underlying biochemical and physiological causes remain, which often derive from years of accumulated toxicities, deficiencies, psycho-emotional traumas, and spiritual emptiness. These biochemical and physiological causes create problems in other parts of our lives that are not fundamentally addressed by drugs. So at the same time that we require health stocks to make profits, we increase our propensity for chronic illness.

REMEDIES FOR OUR TIME

Returning health care to its rightful place in the spiritual/cultural sphere of our culture is a remedy for the current crisis. At the same time, we need to retain the positive qualities of our present system.

The purpose of all work is to promote human growth and self-actualization for the benefit of all. Each of the three main spheres of endeavor—spiritual/cultural, political, and economic—has its particular value in this process. In the same way, each of the parts of the human body has its particular role in the whole. However, when one part of the whole is permitted to run the show at the expense of the others, chaos and illness occur. This is true of the individual physical body and of the collective social body. Unfortunately, the situation today is that the more refined areas of the spiritual/cultural sphere, those types of work that support clients in developing a greater sense of well-being and sensitivity, are being trampled by the greed inherent in a commodity-driven health care system.

MONEY AND MEDICINE

There are three major ways that money is used in our culture: as purchase money, contractual money, and gift money.

1. Purchase Money

Most of us spend purchase money through daily transactions for such items as food, clothing, and entertainment. Each time we make a purchase we reach into the past, because purchase money is used to buy items that have already been made. The way we reach into the past is important to observe. This perspective of money in past, present, and future will be important as we proceed. The purchase of products is the driving force of the economy.

Purchase money is used to pay for commodities in the health care industry. These vary in cost and size from tongue blades to magnetic resonance imaging machines. Purchase money may also be used to buy vitamins, minerals, and homeopathic remedies. The demand for better technological and pharmaceutical commodities in health care is the major driving force in the upward spiral of health care costs. This includes the demand for more expensive goods such as total body scanners, transplants, implants, artificial enzymes, genetically engineered drugs, and more.

In health care, most people are shielded from and do not really have responsibility for the costs. Some other entity—government, insurance company, and employer—picks up the tab for us to be "fixed." We no longer have the monies to pay for a health care system that permits people to remain as children demanding to be fixed when their lifestyles of denial and rationalization lead to internal organ breakdown or accidents. We are all collectively responsible for these widespread attitudes.

It is important to grasp that we are a consumer-driven economy that depends on economic growth on people continuing to use their purchase money to buy whatever they want instead of what they really need. This is not freedom. Our unfulfilled desires from the past drive us into purchasing items that most often keep us addicted and in the past. State economies depend for revenue on cigarette taxes and gambling.

The health care system has thus far supported our illusions and fantasies and permitted us to hide from reality. There is a clear relationship between how individuals spend their purchase money and how the health care system spends money on goods and services. Much of people's daily purchase money goes toward items or activities that perpetuate imbalances: sweets, colas, gambling, tobacco, and toxic products and activities. As noted previously, these imbalances then manifest as illnesses or accidents. People then demand to be fixed.

A system of health care has evolved to meet this demand. The system greatly profits financially from the excessive focus on the physical by continuing to invent more complex and expensive mechanistic goods supposedly to rid us of our diseases. This is the modern version of the promise of Mephistopheles to Faust for eternal life. Meanwhile, people are becoming more ill. An increasingly expensive, technologically addicted and drug-oriented medical system would not be what it was today if we individually and collectively acknowledged that the true causes of illness are in our lifestyles, and took steps to change our lifestyles.

It is each and every person's responsibility to evaluate how he or she uses purchase money. Specifically, does the way one spends money daily on purchases of goods and services address real needs, or does it go to further habitual activities that are destructive to personal growth? Much money is spent in ways that keep us chained to the past. Our health care expenditures and demands reflect this, however adept we may be at blaming others.

2. Contractual Money

Fees that are agreed on between professional and client are contractual fees. Contractual money expresses the state of relationship between two people and the intention to create and maintain a certain type of relationship.

Fee-for-service medicine was based on this principle. The professional rendered care, and the client in exchange paid an agreed-upon fee or another form of mutually agreed upon exchange. Today this direct agreement has been fractured. Third parties such as government and private insurance companies have stepped in during the past 50 years to do the patient's negotiating with the professional.

This is in part due to:

- Rising technological costs that make much of the diagnostic and therapeutic procedures prohibitively expensive for most people

- Increasing specialization and the lack of value that is placed on human dialogue in consultations

- Our collective demand to be "fixed," and the resultant medical-legal framework that supports this demand.

It is widely estimated that 15 to 30 percent of all medical tests and procedures are of little to no medical benefit. This statistic was produced by technologically oriented conventional medical science. If we include the perspective of alternative medicine practitioners who do not use these tests and are often able to go to the core of the problem instead of merely giving symptomatic treatment, the percentage of unnecessary tests becomes much higher.

The key to the correct use of contractual money in health care and elsewhere is mutual responsibility, agreement, and mutual co-commitment. With purchase money we buy items already made in the past. With contractual money we bring ourselves into the present, in the form of agreements between people. As these agreements and commitments are constantly redefined, we build a process of living more in the present and less in the past. This is an integral part of the process of healing.

As stated earlier, widely used contractual agreements in health care today do not require individual people to change. A person can stay the same and continue to be insured against illness. Such agreements do not require people to make a commitment to themselves. Furthermore, many of the contractual agreements in medicine are not supported by the dynamic principles of group relationship, but rather by the mechanistic and materialistic concepts of business. This needs to be changed both locally and nationally.

Participants in the correct use of contractual money in health care need to understand the relationship between illness and healing. Patients and medical professionals need to change their lives and be responsible to themselves and to a larger whole or group beyond their families, church, or ethnic community. Healing comes from feeling connected to the creative process of life. Patients and medical professionals need to understand and appreciate that illness is a part of growth and purpose. Participants in contractual agreements in a health-promoting health care system would be required to define and be honest about their expectations, demands, denials, and lifestyle imbalances. The economics of contractual agreements in such a system would depend on these truths.

3. Gift Money

Michaela Glockler, M.D., in her excellent book *Medicine at the Threshold*, describes how a human being at core is intended to be philanthropic and open to the world, how the formation of a healthy body is the consequence of our interest in the world, and how the formation of a healthy soul is the consequence of our interest in other people. When we do not express these core qualities, the attendant suppression and contraction gradually become imprinted on our bodies and increase our susceptibility to chronic illness.

Each of us needs to develop interest in the world and in other people. If we have lost these interests, we must ask and find out why, and then be willing to receive the necessary assistance in restoring these healthy qualities to our lives.

Money that is freely given to support programs of social and cultural renewal, without demand for anything in return, is called gift money. Philanthropy is another word for gift money. Gift or philanthropic money is money given to build a better future. It emerges out of an interest in the world and in other people. Philanthropy has a reputation of something we can hope to fall back on if the social safety net weakens. It harkens back to the churches of earlier times that gave to the poor.

We need to become more observant of how we use our time and money. Just as in many other areas, it becomes too easy to give to organizations and expect the organization to take care of the needy while we stay in our addictive and illness-generating lifestyles. There is no individual development and responsibility, and no real sense of community.

At present, most of our money goes toward purchase money for goods and services. Money for contractual agreements between professional and client either come out of pocket or are partially paid for by government, insurance company, or employer in accordance with contractual law. Money for gifts, for contributing to the good of the whole culture, is scant because health care and other societal institutions are driven by the greed and mechanization of the economic sphere and the deception and inadequate social laws of the political sphere. The lack of gift money is an obvious reflection of how we are stuck in the past both economically and psychologically. Very few of our resources, daily thoughts, or imaginative faculties, are in service to the whole or to the future. Gift money helps build the future.

For there to be willingness to offer gift money, especially during difficult economic times, people need to focus on ways of transforming the first two uses of money in their individual and collective lives. Out of their focus arises the will to respond to future needs in transpersonal ways. To be effective, gift money needs to be given without a desire for personal recognition. It is gift money that helps support a solid spiritual and cultural foundation for the future.

As our use of purchase money changes to purchase more of what we truly need, and as contractual money agreements are based on mutual honesty and integrity, rather than collusions to continue hiding, then gift money will take care of itself. Building the future out of a living present will become a major focus for people's lives.

COMMUNITY BUILDING

Health care and education are presently at the mercy of the political sphere and the greed and management decisions of the economic sphere. This needs to change.

We need to make a commitment that the spiritual/cultural sphere of work is kept distinct and protected from the excesses of the other two spheres. People working together as communities, guided by the principles of group relationship, and developing agreements that are based on mutual responsibility can make this happen (see Chapter 8). The community needs to decide how funds from health care will be used within the community.

What occurs presently? Health insurance companies collect premiums, pay out a certain amount in health care expenditures for their subscribers, and mostly cover biotechnological expenses. These companies then invest the remainder of the money in stocks and bonds outside our communities, often in companies that produce products destructive to human health and the environment. They claim the right to do this because they are assuming financial risk for our health care. Our legal system supports this process.

The entire principle behind health insurance—sharing the burden of responsibility and risk—needs to be transferred to communities who are willing to work together. People in local communities and businesses need to develop common agreements on defining what is health care and how they are willing to support each other in a life-supporting health care program. Funds can then be collected. Perhaps a local HMO may be created, one based on entirely different principles from those in existence today. Community hospitals need to support communities, not major corporations.

Money that remains at the end of certain cycles can be re-circulated in the community. Instead of being invested in the stock market, money is invested in people's health and well-being. This is how gift money can support endeavors that will benefit all concerned. Then there is motivation for self-educative healing and preventive medicine within the community. There is openness to what works, instead of being told by a professional organization what is valid and what is not.

The pattern of third-party plans needs to be broken for any effective health care reform to succeed. Whether this third party is an insurance company or government, it allows professionals and clients to avoid defining their mutual responsibility and commitment in relationship. Third-party plans also permit health care to continue in an overly mechanized way. Furthermore, they encourage the climate of fear and hysteria that is deepening today as more people are uninsured, and as major insurance companies are shown to be on financially shaky ground. Third parties that were supposed to "protect us" from the costs of illness may not be available to us in the very near future.

HEALTH CARE TRIANGLE

It is not true that we either have to continue financing health care through private insurance or have a government-directed national health care system. The health insurance industry plays on many people's fears of big government inefficiencies and the fact that a government-run system would leave consumers at the mercy of political decisions that are made far away. These are correct perceptions with wrong motives. The real intention is to maintain economic control over people's health care decisions. Likewise, those who propose a national system ignore the weaknesses of central control.

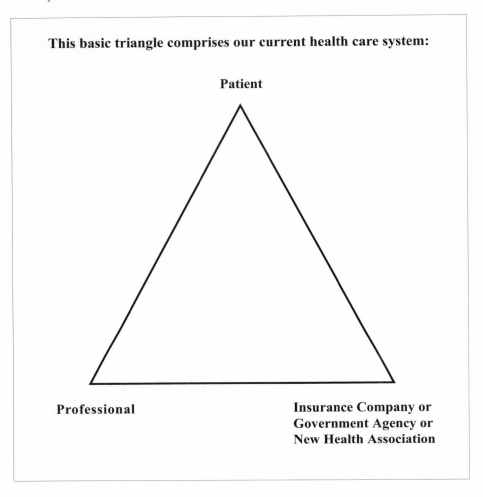

This basic triangle comprises our current health care system:

Patient

Professional

**Insurance Company or
Government Agency or
New Health Association**

There is a third force at work. That is the force of community. This is what needs to replace both insurance company and governmental agency in the health care triangle. This can take the form of health associations where providers and recipients of health care cooperate.

THE CHALLENGE

The challenge is to co-create an imaginative system that will permit health care to return to its rightful place in the spiritual/cultural sphere where it contributes to people's sense of well-being and sense of self. In uniting people who recognize the true purpose of illness in the process of self-healing, this will naturally happen.

It now seems clear that money is not the problem. Once we decide to wake up, stop denying and rationalizing, we will be willing to see clearly what the real problems are in health care. Separate and individual lives will evolve into mutual co-commitment that supports true individual genius. Over time, money will begin to reorient. There are no quick fixes. However, by developing an imaginative plan that is guided by basic principles, mutual agreements, and clarity of insight, we will develop a health care system that meets the needs of all human beings.

CHAPTER 8

SEVEN PRINCIPLES FOR HEALTH CARE REFORM

A new foundation for effective health care would support all of us in creating healthier lives. Such a new form of health care would provide guidance for each person to traverse the process of illness and its accompanying fears in ways that are deeply transformative and enable a person's soulfulness to be more present in everyday life.

In order to create anything worthwhile, we need directing principles around which we can gather material for the new form of expression. This chapter looks at seven main principles that need to be present and understood when we meet around these issues. Of course, with each of these principles there are obstacles to their manifestation, and it is important to look at these as well. In order to reach a resolution of potential conflicts here, we also need a supportive environment. When, with open hearts and a willingness to make needed and genuine changes, we bring together the principles, remove the obstacles, and provide a supportive environment, we will be creating a new foundation for health care.

The following sections describe the seven major principles necessary for health care reform, the potential obstacles to manifesting them, and the quality of a supportive environment for each. The seven principles are:

1. Change
2. Adaptability
3. Receptivity
4. Trust
5. Creativity
6. Quality
7. Sacrifice

#1
Guiding Principle: Change
Obstacle to Overcome: Inertia
Supportive Environment: Imagination
Like most established institutions, the institution of medicine has a tradition of being resistant to real change. It behaves like many individuals and

groups who recognize the personal and material benefits accrued from continuing with things as they are and have been. Resistance to change is a basic human weakness.

The image of the moon characterizes institutions like medicine. The moon reflects light but produces none of its own. Medicine as it is practiced today is obsessed with the security of repetitive routines, and as a result offers very little light to the process of real healing. There are certain established mechanical and dogmatic ways in which medicine is researched and practiced, ways that are supported in the economic and legal framework of current health care. Medicine is a system that is based on habitual and mechanistic thinking, constantly threatened by supposed outsiders, and has little room for fresh creativity.

Habit destroys artfulness. The art of practicing medicine dies to its routines. The unfortunate aspect of this is the great amounts of money invested in the continuation of repetitive habitual routines. By recapitulating the same old patterns even though they may be dressed in new terminology, the medical profession is like a rigid, stuck, dysfunctional family. Because many contemporary illnesses arise out of dysfunctional behavior patterns, can the medical profession really address contemporary illness when it refuses to transform these same aspects within its own nature?

Another aspect of habit is the quality of medical training with its emphasis on memorization and mechanical analytical thinking. Institutional resistance to change rewards inertia. The antidote is incorporating the principle that change is the law of life. The willingness to change from mechanistic thinking to objective observation guided by principles instead of personal points of view brings insight and flexibility instead of habitual thinking.

Children between the ages of birth and seven years old learn by repetition and imitation. Yet when this method of learning is carried into future life activities beyond this cycle of life, as in schools that teach primarily by emphasizing rote memorization of information, then the child's growth and development is affected and illness may result, as discussed in previous chapters. Arts-based education is the antidote. The same principle applies in medicine. What we see in many contemporary institutions including medicine is the unfortunate continuation of methods of learning that are appropriate to one cycle, but not to subsequent cycles of life. It is definitely time to change our limited mechanistic way of practicing medicine.

Up to one-third of our population may have obsessive-compulsive difficulties. These are repetitive and unconscious habitual routines that people incorporate in their work, eating, sex, or entertainment to give them a sense of control over their environment. How can a profession that is itself obsessed with control really serve millions with these types of problems? Pharmaceuticals, while modifying people's obsessive-compulsive behavior chemically, do little to bring about real healing.

When we create living and working environments that encourage imaginative thinking, we create pathways to healing by understanding in our cellular structure that change, not inertia and rigidity, is the prerequisite for healthy life.

#2
Guiding Principle: Adaptability
Obstacle to Overcome: Chaos
Supportive Environment: Real meetings

Another significant problem in health care today is chaos. An example of this chaos is the numerous systems for financing health care that confuse even the most knowledgeable. American hospitals employ many times more people in billing departments to recover outstanding debts than do Canadian and European hospitals and clinics. These business offices must deal with hundreds of different insurance companies and government agencies, each with certain bureaucratic rules, regulations, and forms to fill out. This is chaos.

Another example of this chaos is seen in the busy modern-day emergency department of many hospitals. More and more people use the emergency department as their source of primary care, reflecting the lack of real relationship between doctor and patient. The growing chaos and lack of rhythm in millions of people's lives generate much illness. The situation in the health care system reflects this chaos and further feeds it by only addressing illness in fragmentary and mechanistic ways.

Within this chaos of our times roams the Trickster, the Native American archetype mentioned previously that reflects the way we hide, manipulate, and fool ourselves and others. The Trickster thinks he can fool everyone by cleverly adapting to whatever situation he may be in without having to develop principles of his own. He moves in whatever direction is convenient at the time. This describes the way millions of people live their lives. Friends of the Trickster include families that do not seek truth nor encourage children to follow their dreams, schools that focus mainly on preparing intellects to fit into professional positions controlled by big corporations, and television advertising that trains people to be mindless consumers. Surviving through school as well as making it professionally involves becoming an adept Trickster in our culture. The Trickster brings us lessons to be learned. If we do not learn, the Trickster brings us the same lesson in another form.

The central illnesses of our time, especially cancer, immune system diseases, psychological, and nervous system imbalances, have arisen from the chaos in which we live. These illnesses cannot be addressed with new, sophisticated drugs, surgical techniques, or radiation therapies. If the institution of health care is to effectively meet the chaos in all those who seek help, then the profession needs to develop an antidote to the chaos in itself. How can this be done?

The underlying principle in transforming chaos is an adaptability that provides direction and purpose. The positive aspect of the Trickster is the character of the innovator. He ensures the free flow of clear information and ideas and provides an adaptability that brings change to the rigid habitual exclusiveness of medical care.

By embracing the principle of adaptability and making it part of our daily lives, we enter into meetings with each other in more responsible and capable ways. Most health professionals attend conferences that focus largely on technical information and require little individual expression. Meetings are focused more on entertainment and convenience rather than on healing, transformation, and growth. People usually leave these meetings the same as they were upon arriving. In more meaningful, real meetings, participants work together to develop imaginative thinking and living images of what is needed. Out of this process, the convergence of a free flow of ideas, a collective vision is developed. A new impulse enters people's lives, beyond the habitual thought patterns that many brought to the meetings. Something new has been created that will bring directed order to the chaos in health care.

#3
Guiding Principle: Receptivity
Obstacle to Overcome: Unwillingness to listen
Supportive Environment: Caring

A third obstacle to effective health care is the unwillingness to listen to each other, to receive the impressions of another person's life and illness process.

Many who seek help for illness are unwilling to receive the lessons their illness is attempting to teach them about the way they are living their lives. Indeed, the opposite is more often true. Instead of being willing to receive, we have become obsessed with the desire to take. This narcissistic gratification that is age-appropriate at an earlier time of life colors the lives of many adults, including professionals. There is a lust for more experiences and more information instead of a willingness to receive and integrate what these experiences bring to us. The passivity exhibited as we watch television or ingest an ample supply of food is an example of these attitudes.

Many people say, "My doctor never listens to me; he's always in a hurry." There is definitely more than a kernel of truth to this complaint in the modern office and hospital. Except for the initial description of symptoms, rarely is the patient given the opportunity to have any depth of dialogue with the physician about the progress of treatment. This is especially true if the physician believes that his treatment is successful as measured by objective tests, or if he thinks that the patient's comments do not match what he knows to be true about the illness. If the blood pressure is down or if the gallbladder is removed, then the physician feels his job is done. These attitudes are what have to change in order to make health care more humane.

How can we create a health care system to address these problems in a positive and constructive way? The emphasis needs to be on creating a caring environment, where time for caring is not constricted by cost-effectiveness. More than any food that hospital or clinic patients may eat, this principle of caring provides sustenance to those who strive to come to terms with illness.

The quality of caring by health professionals needs to be improved. This needs to happen not only in caring for patients, but also in the professionals caring for themselves and each other. It is easy to care for patients when one's job identity and personal income call for caring behavior. Yet there is a need to extend this quality of caring toward fellow workers with much more depth than the superficial ways in which it too often now occurs.

The principle that guides this caring environment is that of receptivity. This is often shown by our willingness to listen. The willingness to be sensitive and receptive to the experiences of another person shows caring. Receptivity and caring are acts of will. They require us to extend beyond the normal everyday narcissistic concern for our own lives and satisfactions to being willing to engage another person in the spirit of receptivity. To enhance this quality, we practice the qualities of observation and perception.

#4
Guiding Principle: Trust
Obstacle to Overcome: Pride
Supportive Environment: Social warmth

A fourth obstacle within the present system is pride. Pride has become something of a misnomer today because it is most often used in ways that suggest it is good to have pride. A person takes pride in their work or in their country or in their bowling trophies. A sense of accomplishment, self-confidence, and service is expressed.

Yet, like other characteristics, pride has its dark side. Pride can and often does become a sign of egotism, especially in the life of a professional. When pride turns to arrogance, many professionals become inwardly less flexible and more rigid. This personal pride grows out of inflated importance rather than soul-felt pride from a genuine feeling of service. In pride from position, others serve the position rather than the person as an individual. This is quite different from offering help because the professional is genuinely a compassionate and caring person who is trying to help people. Nurses across the country tell stories of physicians who walk into a busy emergency department and expect everything to stop for their convenience. A physician is often able to be demanding and intolerant and get away with it, as other doctors and I have experienced.

Healing is based on human warmth and trust. Many professionals do not realize that the common man and woman are able to distinguish between the professional concern of the doctor or nurse, and genuine human warmth. To engage consistently in the latter requires professionals to let go of position and participate in honest, warm dialogue with patients, colleagues, and the general public.

By people embracing and enhancing social warmth in therapeutic environments, the obstacle of professional pride will gradually give way to a genuine trust. Trust is sorely missing today. Patients often do not trust that the doctor is leveling with them. They suspect that he does not really know what is going on, or that he is ordering too many or too few tests, procedures, and drugs. Doctors are often worried that the patient will sue or go to another doctor if treatment does not bring about the desired results. Many professionals entered medicine because they lost trust in the wholeness of life. They entered a profession that enables them to escape into their heads as a means of becoming a worldly success. To restore trust will require much soul-searching and a letting go of over-identification with one's position.

As we create environments of social warmth, based on trust and honesty, we support healing of the pride and egotism that contributes to illness.

#5
Guiding Principle: Creative expression
Obstacle to Overcome: Intolerance
Supportive Environment: Self-initiative

A fifth obstacle or weakness that hinders the transformation of American medicine is that of intolerance. This intolerance takes various forms. There is intolerance by conventional medical authorities of therapies that have not been scientifically proven in their definition of acceptable studies. This intolerance actually springs from excessive mechanistic habitual thinking, along with the sometimes less obvious but still prominent desire to defend the economic and political position of the profession against intruders, who are then conveniently labeled quacks.

There is intolerance toward all those entities that make things difficult for the profession. Included are lawyers, government, insurance companies, many patients and their families, and nurses and other health professionals who are not available on demand. There is also intolerance on the part of many physicians toward patients who want to take initiative in their care and be active participants.

Finally, but not of the least importance, is the general public's growing intolerance for anything less than perfect or for the best and most expensive care.

The very qualities of initiative and enterprising character that are often descriptive of the successful professional are perceived as threatening to the physician's control and position when these qualities come from a patient. The true nature of the healing profession is to promote healing, not to become an entrepreneur, a businessman or woman. The health industry is one of the country's top investment and stock portfolio opportunities, and is thought to be recession-proof. Much of this depends on people continuing to become sick and needing drugs, surgery, and technical diagnostic procedures. While it is true that many physicians do not consciously think in this fashion and do indeed care for their patients, the system that they are a part of and benefit from sets these guidelines. The problem is not in doctors promoting their work in an entrepreneurial spirit. The problem is in putting this first, in promoting care that especially in chronic disease lacks credible results, and in being intolerant of other forms of healing.

Intolerance suppresses creative self-expression in those with whom we live and work. This plants the seeds of illness. We grow tumors because of internalized anger at not having created a life that is true to our souls.

Physicians and others in the health industry need to encourage in patients the very qualities that often have made them good businesspeople and entrepreneurs. Patients need to be encouraged to have the courage, initiative, assertiveness, and willingness to articulate in a clear fashion what has been hidden and may have subsequently contributed to their illnesses. This means encouraging patients to be creative, to think out of the box, to be open to ideas about healing they may not have considered. But to do this, to encourage this in patients, physicians and health professionals must be practicing this also. The physician and other high-echelon health professionals need to heal their own intolerances through a willingness to speak from good motives. They need to communicate in simple and honest language what the problems are and what they are able to offer.

#6
Guiding Principle: Respect for quality
Obstacle to Overcome: Gluttony
Supportive Environment: Artfulness

To the ancients a gluttonous person was one who ate too much, was always hungry, and was frequently overweight. Many people in this country are gluttonous to some degree. How does this image portray an obstacle to transformation of health care?

The gluttonous person is obsessed with quantity, always wanting to ingest more. Quantity rules over quality. Unfortunately, the institution of medicine and the health care industry has also become obsessed with quantity and appearance over quality. The number of milligrams in a drug dose makes all the difference. A particular drug is successful if it can induce the kidney to excrete more water or cause the heart to pump more efficiently. This is measured by expensive diagnostic technology. Therapies like homeopathy that do not fit into this paradigm of weight and measure are believed to be quackery.

The medical profession is also obsessed with information. The more quantity of information that physicians have at their disposal, the better they are able to help patients. Legions of specialists read volumes of journals weekly. However, information without wisdom is dangerous at worst, at best a waste of time, and often veils us from perceiving the whole.

There is gluttonous hunger for more patients. Physicians disproportionately migrate to population areas that have many well-to-do paying patients. The hunger for more patients translates directly into less time available per patient and is not the way to promote healing.

There is an underlying rigidity to this institutional gluttony. The gluttonous person is less flexible because of his accumulated quantity of either weight or possessions and therefore is less mobile.

There is wastefulness in society at large. The gluttonous expansiveness in medicine has taken on the negative connotation of enhancing more professional power, position, and prestige, rather than the positive expansiveness of benevolence, generosity, and wisdom.

How can principles be applied to create a supporting environment for the transformation of this institutional weakness into a positive and socially beneficent attribute?

The principle that health care needs to embody is that of respect for quality. The willingness to look at a patient's biographical picture of illness with its subtle attributes, rather than immediately trying to quantify the illness and make it into something objectively measurable and visible, is an example of this respect. Physicians need to strive to heal the inner rigidity and gluttony of the profession through the artful gesture of descending from the throne of position and connecting with their patients.

Respect in medicine is too often based on knowledge and money. This needs to be respect for the process of relationship that, through our illnesses, we are given an opportunity to rediscover. There needs to be a reverence and wonder for what each person who seeks help for a particular illness brings into the relationship with the physician. Reverence and wonder need to replace the current attitude of cost-effective convenience that immediately puts patients into disease categories. Furthermore, the obsession with volumes of information needs to be replaced with the open-minded quality of clear thinking and the willingness to develop an image and deep feeling of the patient's illness. In these ways, clinical facilities become supportive environments that encourage artful living, with respect for quality and a clear perspective and vision of life.

As we practice artfulness in our daily life and work, we naturally pay more attention to quality. This promotes healing in others and ourselves, and supports healing the gluttony that leads to illness.

#7
Guiding Principle: Sacrifice
Obstacle to Overcome: Avarice
Supportive Environment: Service

A seventh weakness of medicine that stands as an obstacle to renewal in health care is egoism and avarice, or covetousness. These strong words describe the profession as a whole. Avarice means theft of the future. When today's medicine is offering so-called cures to diseases that range from chronic heart problems to genetic diseases of the unborn, how can the word avarice be used to describe the health care industry?

The problem is that, according to conventional medicine, the future does not include encouraging the Self-Healing Personality. The cure for disease is expected to come from research laboratories that are steeped in secrecy and complexity. Dependence on people in professional positions will become even stronger as the addiction to medical and other information proliferates. Health care will become entrenched in even more mechanistic ways than it is today. And of course it will be even more profitable to investors who will not concern themselves about the increasing costs of health care for millions of people.

The reality is that the occurrence of life-incapacitating chronic diseases and psychological imbalances will increase in this future scenario. Illness will become a tomb of death for the living soul and spirit that have been ignored or relegated to religion instead of incorporated into a living model of illness and healing. The exclusively technical and mechanistic medical model of today, if carried into the future, will stand like a stalagmite in a cave: beautiful and aloof, the image of death. Human individuality will be chained to the death forces of rigidity and unable to find expression except through disease. Disease will be the reality, even though many people will continue to live their lives and appear happy. This is happening now.

It is time for these death forces in medicine to be confronted and transformed collectively by all involved. These forces rule our lives. The model needs to change into one that recognizes illness as an integral part of life rather than an invader that must be eradicated. It is the responsibility of those in professional positions to spearhead the transformation of illusions about medicine. Health professionals, trained in technical knowledge, need to penetrate these illusions and provide clarity as to how knowledge can be integrated with wisdom for the benefit of all.

Our cultural addiction to scientific and technical knowledge as the key to worldly success and bodily health is based on collective denial. As discussed in earlier chapters, the health care industry benefits greatly from this denial. It covets the future benefits from continuation of the denial and refuses to embrace the principles of service and sacrifice that are essential to a real healing process.

The controlling position of the professional must be sacrificed. The investigative character of scientific and technical laboratory-proven truth needs to retreat from its position of supremacy and become more of the observer of the wisdom that a person's biography reveals about illness. When this transformation occurs in health care, then professionals will have truly served by preventing the hardening death forces of conventional mechanistic science from possessing people's lives. Like Charon the boat master, who in Greek mythology carried Perseus across the River Styx into the land beyond Death, the medical professional may then be a guiding force beyond the land of death and into transformation through illness and healing.

When our deepest intent is to create an environment of service, and we are willing to sacrifice our old habits and hidden lifestyles, then our health institutions will no longer steal the future of healing.

METAMORPHOSIS

When each of these seven principles with their supporting environments are embraced and integrated into our health care system, then a true metamorphosis will occur. Through creating positive and supporting environments, these seven principles will effectively serve as antidotes to the major obstacles to change that come from both within the health profession and from the general public.

There will be much resistance. However, the process of maturation involves learning to live with resistance, and to understand and observe the ways in which this resistance manifests and affects us. By bringing about change with principles and honest reflection, new common law agreements can be developed among all participants in health care. In summary, there are two main tenets to these new agreements:

- Everyone is responsible for participating in their own healing and for changing their lifestyles when necessary. This means striving to understand the meaning of an illness and developing effective approaches that go beyond any specific therapy to transform it. This is not a dogmatic judgmental demand, and people are not punished if they choose not to participate. Rather, the tenet of this agreement is that neither the physician nor anyone else is responsible to fix the patient, regardless of compensation. This agreement recognizes that illness is a mixture of many causes, and that the major elements are our lifestyles, social and environmental imbalances, and heredity.

- Health professionals agree to surrender their position as the guardian of medical knowledge, a position that is most often used to control the therapeutic relationship and to maintain a position of success. They agree to approach the patient as a whole human being rather than as a heart or a stomach. They agree to be flexible and offer positive regard for the patient's situation, rather than striving to arrange the doctor-patient relationship so that it fits their own convenience.

When we have entered into these new common law agreements and successfully integrated the seven principles for health care reform, we will have transformed the chaotic and decaying present system into one that fulfills its destiny: to support all people in creating a living and dynamic balance between illness and healing, so that all have the opportunity to achieve their full human potential.

CHAPTER 9

HEALTH CARE REFORM
AND THE ELDERLY

I have taken care of many elderly people, both in the emergency department and in my practice. Many were quite frightened by illness and the limitations of aging. Others had confident lives and were facing the eventuality of aging and death with fortitude. One man with cancer in my practice was clearly not afraid of dying. I recall how impressed I was by his deep maturity about life, and how healing it was for me to be around him.

Today more than one-third of all spending in health care is focused on the 12 percent of the population that is older than 65. Many elderly people will end their current lives after long periods of debilitating illness. Over one-third of Medicare dollars and 10 percent of all health care dollars are spent on people who die within one year of treatment. Political and economic realities prevent most politicians from risking any attempts to change this trend because they fear losing an election. Most of the major players in the multibillion dollar health care industry—hospitals, pharmaceutical firms, medical technology companies, physicians, and insurance companies—depend on a continual supply of chronically ill elderly people who have given over their lives to a paternalistic medical profession. The chronically ill elderly and their families demand the best care at whatever the cost to the financial health of the nation. The new Medicare drug law will only worsen this situation.

Many people older than 65 believe that they have put in their time and that the nation now owes them and should take care of them. Indeed, Medicare and Social Security are called "entitlements" for people who believe they are entitled to government support by virtue of having gone through the Great Depression, World War II, and the Cold War.

The current elderly generation of people was born or lived their early lives in the Depression. These were times of tremendous unemployment and poverty. Because of this many have been very security conscious and devoted to work. The term "workaholic" arose when our current generation of elderly people was in their thirties, forties, and fifties, prime work years. Decades of work have not provided the happily-ever-after scenario that was the illusion behind the work ethic, however. Disillusionment with aging and with not living a fulfilling life has sadly left many elderly people prisoners in their

83

bodies. Older people often strongly identify their well-being with the condition of their physical body, unless they have experienced depth of love and fulfillment. As their life force declines with the years, many elderly people feel their lives are meaningless.

The identification that many older people place on their health and well-being, as defined by the condition of their physical body, has a major influence on the health care industry. If we begin to develop a system that delivers fewer technological advances and drugs to the elderly, this will be perceived as cold and as not providing what they need. And if we continue things as they are, we surely will bankrupt the health care system, especially as the current generation of "Baby Boomers" nears 65 years of age.

INNOVATION AND CREATIVITY

We need creativity in designing a new approach to health care for the elderly. In this approach, we become aware that it is more important to help aging people reawaken their often dormant soul forces than to keep their physical bodies going while the inner person recedes. By soul forces we mean inner development and connection to life. This basic principle needs to become the focus of all health care.

Physicians and others in the allopathic health care model have strong incentives to provide extensive mechanistic care for the elderly. Legal fears, financial rewards, mechanistic thinking, and social pressures are a few examples of these incentives.

Elderly people suffer in this arrangement. Chronic diseases are treated in mostly palliative or temporary ways. Suffering persists and often intensifies. People endure the side effects from drugs and drug combinations and the aftereffects of unnecessary operations. Many elderly people sit through hours in waiting rooms and undergoing expensive diagnostic tests, in search of magic diagnoses that can then be magically treated and resolved.

Elderly people are no different from any other age group in the United States in the numbers among them who deny and continue to live habitual lives of fear and resignation. Their situation in life is a consequence of what they have or have not done. This is not judgment or blame, but a reality we must acknowledge in order to make changes.

The current generation of elderly has, through a lifetime of experience, come to depend on institutions to deliver the good life. Many people today complain bitterly about the bureaucracy of institutions and how impersonal they are, yet continue to demand to be taken care of as if they are entitled to this care. Until this paradox is acknowledged and creatively transformed, our problems will persist. On one level, we all need and deserve to be cared for. On another level, to demand this as entitlement, regardless of social needs as a whole, is imbalancing.

Current approaches to health care of the elderly weaken all concerned: The economy suffers as more and more expensive procedures are demanded as a right; and there are fewer health care resources available to care for the young, the working poor, and the unemployed.

We do not serve a person, young or old, merely by eliminating pain and physical suffering while not addressing that person's whole life and needs. If we can reorient the great amount of funds that are currently channeled toward care for end-stage chronic diseases into other forms of alternative care for the elderly, then all will benefit greatly. We must honestly recognize that many elderly are in a process of dying that may go on for several years. We need an alternative to performing miracle operations and giving enough drugs to confuse or sedate most people, especially the elderly with their deteriorating livers and kidneys as a result of lifelong dietary indiscretions, overuse of pharmaceuticals, and other lifestyle imbalances and toxic accumulations. Instead of placing the elderly in custodial prisons to be ignored until they die, we would better serve them by creating facilities that help them to re-enliven and reawaken their often-dormant human qualities and creative capacities. We must enable them to step into the role of elders with much to offer to the younger generations. We must help them to age with integrity and honesty and be valuable contributors to society as they age, which is what all of us would want, given the opportunity. In this way, the aging and dying processes can become more conscious endeavors.

LIFE-REGENERATING PROCESSES

What is needed to bring about these changes?

- A social commitment to the elderly in such areas as re-education, home-care, proper nutritional counseling, applying the benefits of integrative medicine in Medicare, the creative arts, and honest straightforward dialogue about the aging process and the purpose of the latter years of life.

- A collective agreement to eliminate heroic and costly care for the elderly. Costly in this context means end-of-life efforts to prolong life for a few days or weeks, which most elderly people do not want, but which families, out of fear of loss, demand.

Presently, many elderly live alone, with families, or in extended care facilities. There is little to no exposure in any of these settings to life-regenerating processes such as: keeping the senses alive; creative arts; occu-

85

pations that put people in touch with the rhythms of the earth; proximity to children; opportunities for service; and proper nutrition and access to integrative medicine modalities.

1. Keeping the senses alive

Life is a journey into the world of the senses in the earlier parts of life, and then, depending on how we have lived, a gradual return into the world of inner development, which is the world of God. Understanding this is important in caring for the elderly, whose physical senses decay with age.

Many elderly people feel separate and alone. I have noticed in the course of my work that, more than other people, the elderly, when acutely ill or losing their sense of themselves, have a tendency to grab and touch others. Perhaps this is a response to feeling isolated and abandoned. Working with the sense of touch with the elderly—for example, providing opportunities for them to pet animals—may help heal their sense of separateness and aloneness.

Ease of mobility with its attendant sense of motion decreases with age. To replace this loss of outer mobility we need to develop an inner mobility that is based on sustained rhythm. Activities such as painting a picture or creating a garden can help with this.

As the sense of hearing diminishes, some elderly people have more problems with communication, and may become suspicious that others are trying to take advantage of them. We may help them to lessen this tendency not only with hearing aids, but also by encouraging them to recite poems, read from their written legacies, and create and perform drama. This enlivens the faculty of inner listening, which then becomes an antidote to the decrease in external hearing.

Many elderly today yearn for their younger years because they perceive life as more real when they could experience life through their physical senses, which decay with aging. With the awakening of the inner qualities of these senses, aging people can resurrect their lives in later years, and live without fear of physical decay. With aging there is a gradual decline of the life forces and a slow extinction of the senses. Developing ways to nurture the inner soul life through enlivening the inner qualities of the senses may be of greatest service to the elderly person, and to all people.

2. Creative arts

As an example, painting with watercolors that dissolve in water and into each other helps dissolve the inner and outer rigidity of elderly life that is often revealed in the hardening of the body and of attitudes. Creative movement can reawaken inner feelings of joy and self-expression.

3. Occupations that put people in touch with the rhythms of the earth

Occupations such as gardening help put people in touch with the rhythms of the earth with which many lose touch. Many elderly people go into service jobs, such as serving burgers, for example. This may be positive in the capacity to continue working with people. However, it may also be another way of avoiding being with oneself, of discovering who one really is. Many people go through their entire lives without doing this very necessary work. Working with the earth encourages inner reflection. The resignation that we often see on the faces of many elderly may be due in part to the sense of never having gone through the process of self-discovery. Many elderly people today have lived through time periods when these matters were not spoken about. Things that were kept hidden are now spoken of more freely.

4. Proximity to children

Building homes for the elderly that are near day-care centers where they can hear the joy of youth can help the elderly reawaken their childlike wonder and not be so isolated from people and from the inner feeling of earlier life cycles.

5. Opportunities for service

Many elderly believe they are entitled to be taken care of by society, to sit back and enjoy, with no social commitment. Egoism, excessive attachment to bodily comforts, and fear of bodily pain show us that many elderly are prisoners of their bodies and have given up. (This is, of course, also true of many people who are not elderly.) If there is to be any healing of the separative attitudes that elderly people may have cultivated in life and which have hardened their hearts, it is in situations of service. Recent studies have shown that elderly volunteers in hospitals generally have more vitality and are in better health than those who do not do volunteer work.. An increasing number of elderly people are either doing volunteer work or are employed at a paying job, and are benefiting from these occupations.

The service that can truly fulfill people in their aging years is mentoring. Earlier civilizations called this becoming an elder. Even in our youth-oriented culture, there are some people who look to the elderly for wisdom gained from experience. Of course, if the wisdom has not been developed over years, it does not suddenly appear. We need to encourage our generations of adults to look forward to old age, wisdom, and mentoring. This wisdom is developed by emerging from denial, living more authentic lives, and loving more deeply and unconditionally. These are qualities from which youths and adults could benefit greatly and sharing these qualities would bring joy to the elderly.

6. Proper nutrition and access to integrative medicine modalities

Many aging people are very deficient in essential nutrients and have significant levels of toxins in their bodies accumulated from multiple sources over the years. This makes healing much more difficult. There is great potential to help the elderly slowly improve in health and not be dependent on pharmaceutical drugs. Yet alternative medicine modalities are for the most part not paid for by Medicare or most insurance companies.

Our health care decisions need to be guided by principles and by lifestyle healing, not to make money for investors. There is nothing wrong with making money, as long as service to the health and well-being of others is placed first. Likewise, we cannot afford to continue to support those elderly or their families who continue to deny what is occurring in their lives. In Great Britain, a person who continues to smoke after a bypass surgery is not granted another surgery when the arteries close off again. This may sound harsh. Yet it keeps people honest and invested in their health care.

There are many pathological diseases of the elderly that are very real and need to be addressed. Sometimes these do require surgery, emergency care, or certain medications. However, there are many procedures, drugs, transplants, and ICU admissions that we need to decline. Monies that would have gone to these areas need to be refocused into extended care facilities that are not merely custodial, but promote education and self-healing, supported by alternative and complementary modalities.

In youth we put our energies into growth and development. In the middle years our efforts go into families, work, and relationships. After about age 63, it is in the time of life when spiritual development may arise, if we have prepared by not becoming too materialistic and mechanistic. The twin curses of our modern civilization are materialism and mechanism, and many elderly people have become deeply invested in them.

The goal in aging is not to keep the body functioning like it was decades earlier without any pain. The goal is to keep one's soul forces alive, or to re-enliven what has often been forgotten through years of habitual living and emotional suppression. Many elderly settle into egoistic lives of caring only about themselves and their families, and of placing too much importance on physical discomforts and imbalances. This, in some respects, is a return to adolescence.

Our commitment to health care for the elderly needs to be reoriented away from its present limited mechanical approach and toward an approach that recognizes the purposes and needs of this time of life. We need to be committed in spiritual, political, and economic ways toward providing elderly people with the opportunity to emerge from what often has become an inwardly dead existence, toward being more imbued with life. We have to be willing to accept that such a physical life may be shorter than it might otherwise be with conventional medicine.

The Native Americans were much more attuned to the seasons and the cycles of life than white people are. In Native communities, when it was sensed that life was over, it was over. The community was not held back because one person wanted to live beyond what all knew was that person's time to die. We have forgotten this, because we, in our so-called supreme modern intelligence, have lost touch with natural rhythms of the stages of life.

Today, family and relatives of elderly people often refuse to permit them to die. They may do this out of guilt or out of their own fear of death and of letting go. In this refusal the family does a great disservice to the elderly. Their attachments to holding on to an elderly father or mother make it more difficult for the elderly to emerge into a greater sense of individuality and feeling for life, and into a realization that there is no death, only life cycles.

By making an economic commitment to honor physical death and to honor above all else the life within the decaying form of an elderly person, we will nurture the soil of freedom. By perpetuating the present system that acts like a vortex and draws away our energy and funds in order to prolong physical decay without meaning, we hold the future in bondage to the past. When we permit our decisions and actions to be guided by clear thinking and real feelings rather than by emotional attachments, then we will be able to emerge collectively from the present crisis. And all will benefit.

CHAPTER 10

TOWARD AN ECONOMY OF HEALING

D uring medical school training at Children's Hospital in Columbus, Ohio, I became aware of an illness called lead poisoning. At that time, in the early 1970s, it was considered a relatively uncommon illness because a diagnosis of lead poisoning required blood lead levels far higher than the values recognized today. Lead poisoning is considered a serious illness that affects millions of people—children and adult—in the United States. It is a significant contributing factor in cardiovascular disease and neurological impairments. Lead-based paint in old houses is a major source of lead toxicity. And major cities such as Washington D.C. have been found to have pipes contaminated with lead.

Working in conjunction with a staff pediatrician, we organized a community-based effort to evaluate young children for blood lead toxicity. Teams of medical students and social workers went from house to house within a certain working class area of Columbus. We interviewed parents about the risk factors for their children becoming toxic with lead. It was my first real look at how people outside my middle-class bastion of doctors, lawyers, and successful businessmen lived.

We organized rides for the parents and children to a makeshift laboratory we set up at a community church, and drew blood on many children to determine lead levels. We then published our findings, which revealed that many more children were lead toxic than was previously believed. Some of the children were hospitalized for treatment. Without this treatment, many of them might have developed neurological and learning problems. Of course, from what we now know, many more children should have been admitted for treatment than were, because the research has shown that blood levels much lower than were considered normal at the time are actually toxic.

This work was followed by city council hearings on how best to deal with the lead-based paint so prevalent in old homes in the area. This was considered a greater contributing factor to many of these children becoming lead toxic than was exposure to lead-based gasoline or living near freeways. I recall sitting at the city council table, looking around at the participants, and realizing that there was no real intent to deal with this issue. I saw that the politicians professed to care for children, but in truth, were willing to sacrifice the health and well-being of children to special interests, in this case the building and construction interests that wielded considerable influence, and continue to do so in many areas to this day. I could see the built-in denial.

There was very little will at that time to do what it would take economically to make sure children were not being poisoned. It is worse today. If there really were a consciousness about children's health, there would be no vending machines in schools, candy bars and cola drinks would not be at the front of supermarkets, but behind the counter, along with cigarettes and Playboy magazines. Vaccination would have ceased a long time ago instead of increasing in frequency and the number of vaccines given to each child. What was missing then and is missing now is a commitment to an economy of healing.

What is an economy of healing? In the lead situation it would have meant marshaling resources to improve the interior of thousands of old homes that were toxic. We now know that the toxicity of these homes goes far beyond lead, to radon, mold, and electromagnetic interference fields. All of these are contributing factors to chronic neurological disease, learning disabilities, cancer, and other illnesses.

As previously discussed, affordable health care for everyone will require more than changing the mechanics of cost control. It will require us to change the economics of health care in our everyday lives, to define the value of health and healing, and to actively encourage alternatives to allopathic medicine so that we know where and how as a nation to place our health care dollars. Because health care has become a commodity that is driven by market forces of supply and demand, it is helpful to understand what economy is, as opposed to what it has become.

OIKONOMIA

The word "economy" derives from the Greek word oikonomia. This means "the management of the household so as to increase its value to all members of the household over the long run." The word "household," in a larger context, includes communities and institutions. The correct use of economy considers the costs and benefits of something such as health care to the whole community or the whole nation. The definition also embraces a long-term view. A long-term view and a consideration of the whole are as necessary for the healing of our health care economy as they are for the healing of each individual.

The lessons of our global economy and a global communications network are that everyone and everything is interrelated. In the same way, all illnesses in a person's life and all diseases within the body are interrelated, not separate disease entities to be treated by conventional medicine specialists. At the same time, effectively transforming our health care system will require changing the way we view the economy.

92

The definition of oikonomia, or economy, also includes the word "value." Effective health care change needs to include a redefinition of the value we place on health care, both individually and nationally. People cannot work without their health. It's that simple.

COMMUNITY VALUES

To change the economics of health care will require us to embrace what some have called "the moral force of shared community values." What exactly does this mean? To answer this effectively, we begin by examining the word "community."

Most of us view community as an extension of our heritage and family background, as occurs with a religious community or a local ethnic community. This type of community may be a positive source of strength for us. Community values are also seen nostalgically as small-town values that were part of our past. Like many things we hear, there is partial truth to this nostalgia, which makes for good political background. To the extent that we bring the positive and human enriching experiences of our heritages and families into community life, these communities can be healing.

However, many people left their small town behind at some point, either literally, or in their minds and emotions. They left because they felt constrained by the often-rigid conformity and restrictions to creative individuality. Or, they wanted experiences more stimulating than small towns could offer. They may have sought the anonymity of the city and university, but rather than moving toward creative individuality, their constrained feelings turned into intellectual and professional careers, or employment in large impersonal workplaces, or poverty.

We have now come full circle. Our country has evolved from a rural economy to an urban industrial economy to an information economy. Health care has paralleled this change. The health care profession has gone from the human orientation of the family doctor to a system of highly technical and impersonal physicians where specialists run tests and fix body parts. These specialists do not care to grasp with depth who their patients are as people, or the connection between symptoms and lifestyle.

There has been some movement toward holism. What was once ridiculed as the domain of holistic medicine—nutrition, exercise, and acupuncture, for example—is now accepted in mainstream medicine as if it had been discovered by conventional medicine. Sadly, the motives behind these attitudinal changes are more often financial than holistic.

Many who desire to return to that small town often express the need to slow down and have more quality time to be creative and to be with friends and family. We forget the conformity and intolerance of those times. Furthermore, the economy of this so-called idyllic past was very restrictive to many people, especially minorities and women. We cannot go back to that small town of heritage and "family values" unless we want to regress and see our health deteriorate further. Rather, we need to recreate the positive aspects of former values in a daily meaningful way that is health-sustaining and which takes into account the changes of the past 50 or so years.

We all desperately need true family values that nurture and encourage our growth and maturing. And we all would benefit greatly from the teachings of many ethnic and religious groups. But we also need to remember that most of us are still suffering from the "family secrets" that were kept hidden in families of the past and also in the present. Unfortunately, many of the ethnic, racial, and religious cultures in which we have grown up still preach separatism and superiority, not tolerance.

We need to heal our family secrets and our intolerances of heritage by creating new communities that embody the principles of oikonomia. In these new communities, where individual expression and creativity and healing the wounds of the past are valued and encouraged, we can evolve an effective health care system.

Healthy community consists of creative, honest, and self-regulating individuals who are drawn to work with and support each other, and who feel a common bond that may go beyond being related or connected in race or ethnic origin. The industrialization of America, the mechanization of health care, and the isolation of the family have all occurred at the expense of community. This is why the hidden multigenerational secrets of families are now being revealed. Many families are breaking apart. The moral values that gave strength to family structures in earlier times are by themselves insufficient for our present crises.

REBUILDING THE MIDDLE

We have to bring our public and private lives together in such a way that both are served by giving birth to a strengthened middle as a balancing force between the two poles.

What is the middle? In a human being the middle is feeling, the balance between thinking and action. Economically, the middle is new health care programs that incorporate the best of both public and private and that are at the mercy of neither.

The middle is also the principle of interdependence. Throughout our nation's history we have vacillated from one pole of behavior to the other, from dependence to independence. Out of misdirected idealism we have sometimes encouraged an indefinite dependence on government. Out of driven materialism we have encouraged a streak of independent individualism, which is often excessively selfish in motivation. Misdirected idealism and driven materialism actually support each other in a negative way, just as a clever intellect and a ruthless will work together to destroy many people's lives.

To prevent our culture from being torn apart and polarized, we have to work on strengthening this middle principle of interdependence and mutual responsibility. The seeds are already being sown in different areas. For example, new innovative programs are appearing in early childhood education. Teachers and administrators understand that children learn better in a cooperative and interdependent environment instead of the old system of dependency on the teacher and books that feed information to the children. In the field of psychology there is growing recognition that support groups allow people to heal in relationship with others, as opposed to focusing only on themselves. In group situations people risk being more vulnerable and learn to be more responsible for their thoughts, words, and deeds. Unfortunately, there is still great resistance to bringing the principle of interdependence into health care.

We need a new social contract for health care. Neither the government nor private insurance companies can pay for health care costs while people remain passive participants. Neither can the government, as the expression of collective will, continue to permit unbridled free-market forces, which have contributed significantly to rising health care costs, to continue controlling and fracturing health care for everyone. Especially since these are not really free-market forces, but are in actuality an oligarchy of physicians, pharmaceuticals, hospitals, and insurance companies that have greatly resisted permitting the free market to find a new level based on individual right to choose from a much larger availability of practitioners.

When health care entered the national stage in the second half of the twentieth century, both government (public) and industry (private) set up programs that promised to take away all risks of illness. This has not worked, because the motivation for human initiative and self-observation was removed. There is no balance and no reciprocity.

TRUE ECONOMY

The business picture in this country needs to change from corporate control and a primary concern with maximizing short-term gains for those with property and wealth to an economic environment that adopts the principles of oikonomia, true economy. The costs and benefits of business decisions to the whole community must be considered. When we combine oikonomia with new laws that permit and support any individual or family to seek health care from whatever trained practitioner they choose, then our health care will improve in quality and cost-effectiveness.

What must we do to renew our health care system so that it truly supports all people in their process of healing? This will require us to:

- Understand that our economic life is a living organism, not a dead collection of products and figures. For this economic life in health care to serve us, there must be more balanced involvement in the spiritual/cultural and political spheres of life.

- Establish spiritual corporations in health and medicine, guided primarily by spiritual principles. These will be legal entities that oversee the various levels of health care. They will take the place of both government-funded organizations such as Medicare and private corporations in health care with publicly tracked stock. They will be run by a Board of Elders and could resemble what we used to have as true not-for-profit corporations (not tax-exempt corporations). All corporations involved in delivering health care will only have shareholders who are directly contributing to the function of the corporation. Publicly traded stock companies in health care will not be effective in the future in their present forms.

ASSOCIATIVE ECONOMICS

This new approach establishes collaborative efforts among all who work in providing health care. It has the potential to spiritualize the economics of health care. Providers and consumers of health care would come together for decisions. Likewise, as discussed in previous chapters, we all need to redefine rules and decision-making in health care, and create institutions that reflect equality and dignity of participation.

By establishing such a new health care approach that combines principles of spiritual renewal, civility, and practicality, we will create a new economy of healing.

Changes are slowly beginning to occur in medical centers. "Soft" phenomena are being introduced into the debate on how we measure quality of health care. "Soft" phenomena include:

- Patient perceptions of their own well-being and quality of life

- Patient education in illness, as well as more active involvement in decision-making about treatment

- Rewarding practitioners who coach patients in self-help skills

- New provider teams that consist of psychotherapist, educator, physician, nutritionist, nurse, physical therapist, and energy therapist.

The principle guiding these changes is that the healing process works much better when patients are actively involved. Their sense of well-being becomes an important parameter, instead of the objective impersonal criteria so often used. Objective impersonal criteria are much easier to enter into computers for establishing billing criteria for insurance companies, hospitals, and government.

Our health care crisis has brought us to the point of decision. If the old hierarchical way is allowed to continue, we will experience greater illness without healing. Let's not allow our decision to be made by insurance executives, government bureaucrats, hospital administrators, or physicians. If we permit the mechanistic and materialistic trend in health care to continue and deepen, then we will have lost an opportunity to bring about this needed reformation.

There are three parallel and interconnected occurrences in the United States, and each is involved in health care:

- The United States is a microcosm of the entire world, with most of the world's racial, ethnic, national, and philosophical groups represented in our population. No other country is like the United States in this way.

- The major biotechnological and mechanistic models for world growth in the 20th century came from the United States. This has held us back from embracing the positive contributions of other modes of healing from older cultures.

- The American people are becoming more ill, in spite of what the media and conventional medical spokespeople say. Illnesses are being generated by imbalanced, toxic, and arrhythmic lifestyles, supported by what some have called the number one illness in the United States: denial.

Is something new to be born in the United States, which can then be returned to the rest of the world as an antidote for the separate and destructive over-identification with our different ethnic, racial, or religious backgrounds? As we develop uniquely creative ways of transforming our health care system and our approach to illness and healing, we will offer something of value to the world stage.

What will work?

A health care system that supports and encourages people to stop running from illness

1. Understand and become responsible for the sources of most illnesses in our unresolved psycho-emotional conflicts, toxicities, and deficiencies, which have grown out of imbalanced personal lifestyles and social priorities

2. Permit our unresolved psycho-emotional conflicts to transform, so that our families can become birthplaces of individual genius and strong sense of self, rather than the force fields where illnesses continue to be transmitted from one generation to another.

3. Create new health care provider teams that include physicians, psychotherapists, educators, nutritionists, nurses, physical therapists, energy medicine practitioners, and body workers (see Part II)

4. Back up these proposals with a commitment to restructure how money is spent in health care. This includes exploring innovative efforts to recirculate health care monies within communities that make the above commitments.

PART II:

COMPREHENSIVE MEDICINE

CHAPTER 11

21ST CENTURY MEDICINE

In the early years of the 21st century, we have three main approaches to health care in the United States. Conventional medicine, still predominately allopathic or pharmaceutically based, is the most widely known, and receives by far the most publicity and monies. Beyond this is a growing body of evidence and experience, which we are only beginning to tap, that comes from a wide variety of resources ranging from conventional medicine physicians to rainforest natives to color therapists. It is helpful to look at the three approaches.

1. Allopathic offices and hospital practices

These predominate in the United States today, still rule health care, keep it limited, unaffordable to many, and increasingly ineffective in healing chronic illness. Treatment is based largely on pharmaceutical drugs, surgery, and radiation. (This has been discussed extensively in Part I.) Allopathic medicine has been quite successful in surgery and emergency medicine, and the development of good diagnostic tools such as PET scans and MRIs.

2. Hospitals and physicians' offices that embrace some of the principles and practices of integrative medicine

There are now integrative medicine departments at hospitals such as Jefferson Hospital in Philadelphia and University of Arizona Hospital in Tucson. In addition, many more researchers and clinicians at major medical centers and teaching hospitals are beginning to apply the principles of integrative medicine. This is often still limited in scope by the rules and regulations of hospital practice, which is still largely pharmaceutical- and surgery-based. But we are now seeing more such faculty at integrative medical conferences presenting alongside practitioners with whom they would never have associated even five years ago. There is movement away from double-blind research toward the type of evidence-based research that is empirical and valuable. Medical Acupuncture is now taught at UCLA School of Medicine, and Medical Herbology is taught at Columbia University School of Medicine in New York City.

It must be added that there are employees of the Food and Drug Administration (FDA) and pharmaceutical companies who know this is the direction medicine needs to take, but whose jobs still depend keeping silent about this reality.

3. Private practitioners/clinics of integrative/comprehensive medicine

This is in a boom phase of development. Many physicians and other practitioners are opening offices at various levels of integration of different disciplines, including allopathic medicine, into a more comprehensive medicine. Public demand is driving this. The public is way ahead of the medical pharmaceutical establishment, insurance companies, and government agencies. This area of medical practice now includes, in addition to medical doctors, homeopaths, herbalists, osteopaths, chiropractors, energy medicine practitioners, and many other types of holistic practitioners.

A health care system that embraced and integrated the effective elements of all three of these approaches would greatly enhance the process of healing for millions of people. This is what we need and what comprehensive medicine is.

All three approaches have their place in healing. Physicians need to understand them all in order to work as part of a treatment team; for example, treatment could combine low-dose chemotherapy cancer with fever-inducing therapy, antioxidants, acupuncture, color therapy, and family systems therapy (see Chapter 13). A treatment approach that combines these and other therapies enables patients to recognize the fragments of their being that have become separated from the whole and which are, through the illness, demanding recognition and reintegration. This is what healing is all about.

This book is going to focus on the second and third approaches, mostly the third approach. Because of the present limitation (rigidity of thinking, finances, political control) of hospitals and medical centers, much of what needs to develop and flower as full comprehensive medicine offices will likely be delayed in these institutions. So while they gradually change, the focus of current needed change will be in the third area of approach -- private practitioners of integrative/ comprehensive medicine. It is these offices and their practitioners, and often their patients, who are most open to expanding from what now exists into a more far-reaching model of medicine that encompasses community and is not just limited to private practice or integrative clinics.

I imagine this model as an expanding model, like a flower unfolding from a bud, opening to the sun, expanding its field of expression. The first approach to medicine—the conventional, allopathic approach—involved the contraction of medicine into a small arena in the past one hundred years, as the West has forgotten other forms of medicine, or invalidated them for many reasons, as discussed in Part I.

Now, collectively, we are remembering the deeper sources of healing and creating bridges between these deeper sources and what we have developed in allopathic medicine. What is positive here is that we can now bring some of our observations and objective measurement tools from a century of allopathic medicine into the practice of traditional healing, or more recently developed holistic medicine methods.

THE TRANSITION TO COMPREHENSIVE MEDICINE

Holistic. Alternative. Complementary. Integrative. These words are often used interchangeably. The first word among these to gain acceptance by the American public was holistic, which is still a good description of comprehensive medicine. However, the word has gained a negative connotation in many circles, as has the term alternative. Many people prefer the word complementary. The term integrative has increasingly been adopted in the early 21st century. It means to integrate or bring together different forms of medicine and healing. Comprehensive medicine would take this to the next stage, integrating the best of all three approaches in a comprehensive, wise, and timely fashion.

With the rising popularity of integrative medicine in the United States, the word integrative is increasingly entering the lexicon of hospital, clinic, and insurance advertisements, designed to grab our interest. It does not necessarily follow that the product or medical approach advertised is truly integrative. Therefore, it is important to be increasingly observant and discriminative, and to seek a comprehensive medicine practitioner who can flexibly and ably move through all levels of medicine. Pay attention to your gut instinct, what you feel, regardless of the words you hear. Read. Do research. And pay attention to the energy behind the words.

When we are young, we are appropriately connected with and dependent on mother and father or other guardian for nourishment, shelter, and emotional support. As we grow into adolescence, we become independent as part of our growth, yet experience connectedness with others. Maturity brings with it an understanding that for continued growth, we need to develop skills in interdependence. The development of a world economy reflects this reality, even though it still operates according to a Darwinian survival-of-the-fittest model. David Deida, in his wonderful book *Intimate Communion*, speaks of these three stages of intimacy in our masculine and feminine natures, and how we often get stuck in our relationships at one of the first two levels—dependence and independence.

The same is true in medicine. Conventional medicine, along with any institution that is focused on control, is still at the dependent and independent levels. Physicians want people to be dependent on them as doctors of medicine, and physicians themselves want to be independent, specialized, and not have to answer to anyone else. They perceive insurance companies, hospitals, and government as threats to independence, as described in previous chapters, notably Chapter 5: The Three Phases of the Medical Institution.

For comprehensive medicine to become a success, not only economically, which it will, but also in improving the health and well-being of many more people, this principle of interconnectedness and interdependence needs to be consciously applied in practice with patients daily. For example, we now know that there are opiate receptors on immune cells. One way to treat cancer is to give low doses of an opiate called naltrexone, which will stimulate immune function. We know that lymph cells produce ACTH, which improves adrenal function. So when we can enhance lymph function with immune support, whether through homeopathy, supplements, deep breathing, or good sex, our adrenals grow stronger.

Intelligence
Is
Throughout the Body
in
Every Cell

Our bodies are permeated with intelligence. Please note that intelligence is not intellect. I remember the expression on Jodi Foster's face in the movie *Contact* when, in outer space, the character she played looked out the window in awe and wonder and said she had no idea. She was the skeptical intellectual who now could deeply feel the guiding intelligence of the universe, which many people call God. This intelligence is always communicating with all facets of itself at all time. To the extent that our behavior in health care and in life becomes cut off from this truth, we suffer the consequences.

For example, it is well-known that the microorganisms in us are part of this intelligence. Conventional medicine and even many integrative medicine practitioners labor under the illusion that these bugs are separate species, and that we can kill them off with antibiotics or garlic or other herbs or drugs. The reality is that these bugs are constantly exchanging genetic information, intercommunicating with each other in sub-molecular areas (this is what conventional medicine calls drug resistance). The reality goes even deeper. Not only are the microorganisms within us are constantly exchanging information with each other; they are exchanging information with our own cells. This changes our thinking and feeling because it shifts our biochemistry and physiology. As the "I" in us, our deeper sense of self, is weakened, it is no longer able to exert its influence to regulate these communications so that they serve the health of our bodies, souls, and spirits. This is why we become ill.

Until we feel a reverence, awe, and wonder for the deeper Intelligence that guides all of our life processes, and we open our fields to being receptive to receiving understanding and wisdom from this deeper Intelligence, and then implement this receptivity in the way we practice medicine, our health will worsen.

COMPREHENSIVE INTEGRATIVE THINKING

The practitioner of comprehensive medicine needs to ask the following basic questions and be honest about the answers:

- What is really at work in my patients?
- What is the mystery of life that this illness is revealing?
- What are the patterns of illness in this patient's life?
- Do I really care to see this?
- What is my commitment to healing?
- What is the task of illness?
- What is illness teaching us?
- What does recovery mean?
- Can we remain the same person and get well?

Dr. Thomas Rau of the Paracelsus Klinik in Lustmühle, Switzerland, depicts disease and the relationship of conventional medicine and what we call alternative or complementary medicine in his picture of the Disease Iceberg.

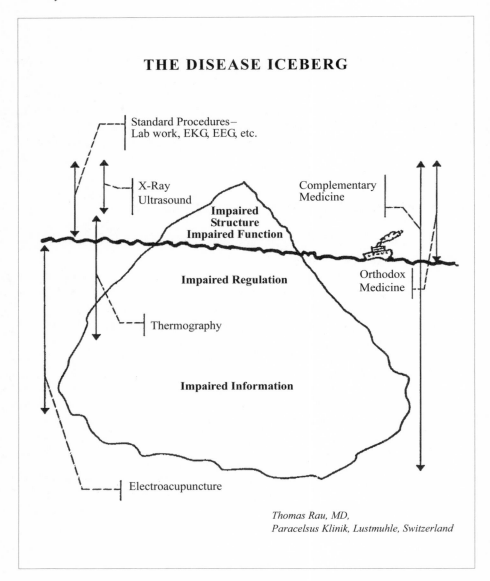

THE DISEASE ICEBERG

Standard Procedures—
Lab work, EKG, EEG, etc.

X-Ray
Ultrasound

Complementary
Medicine

**Impaired
Structure
Impaired Function**

Impaired Regulation

Orthodox
Medicine

Thermography

Impaired Information

Electroacupuncture

Thomas Rau, MD,
Paracelsus Klinik, Lustmuhle, Switzerland

The current situation of health and medicine is like the iceberg in water with only its tip visible above the waterline. Most of the iceberg is underwater because we do not notice our patterns of illness for many years, until unpleasant symptoms of chronic illness manifest. During this time, we often develop what can be called functional symptoms: fatigue, aching, digestive problems, hormonal imbalances. After more years, enough tissue changes occur for our symptoms to be labeled a disease, the diagnosis achieved through increasingly expensive laboratory tests, X rays, and MRIs. Though a little more of the iceberg may be exposed above the waterline, the disease is still the top of the iceberg. This top portion of the iceberg, unfortunately, is the focus of patients' and medical professionals' attention. Volumes of information are published about our diseases. Most of the practice of medicine is shortsighted and centers on this quantifiably visible, yet small part of the whole process of illness.

The part of the iceberg that is underwater symbolizes all that contributed to the slow development of illness. What lives beneath the surface is our biographical records, the story of how we have lived our lives, the development of our personalities, how we have made our choices, how we have dealt with our stresses, our pain, our sorrow, joy, and shame, our relationship choices, and what we have kept hidden. Both the medical profession and most people choose to ignore these important parts of ourselves. Most of us spend considerable energy trying to keep these parts suppressed. Yet these parts increasingly well up to the surface and cause major lifestyle disruptions. They may appear as addictions, obsessions, compulsions, depression, accidents, or chronic diseases of internal organs.

The medical profession's denial is in the decision to ignore, or only give a passing glance toward the workings of these underwater forces, both in their own lives and work as well as in those of their patients. Doctors talk about ways that a disease can disrupt physical organ functions and how a particular new miracle drug can reverse certain effects and supposedly restore the person to health. This focus of thinking does not require physicians to think about the life of the patient.

After all, it is not cost-effective to listen to a patient for long. What a statement this is about our current attitudes toward health and illness. Most people go along with this collusion because of fear of and dependence on outside authorities to whom they have given control over their lives.

This iceberg picture is a very good illustration of the problems with conventional medicine and how comprehensive medicine goes deeper. The part of the iceberg that is above the water is the area dealt with in conventional medicine. Allopathic medicine focuses too much on impaired structure in its diagnostics and treatments. There is some effort made to look at function, for example, stress EKGs, glucose tolerance tests, and pulmonary function tests. But the results are interpreted only in terms of what surgery or drug to give the patient.

Integrative medicine looks more closely at impaired function. This is a function of time, as opposed to the space of structure. Integrative medicine practitioners measure the function of an organ over a period of time, instead of only seeing what the organ looks like on an X ray or CT scan. Whereas conventional medicine has only a few tests that evaluate based on function, integrative medicine draws on a wide array of testing to determine liver and gastrointestinal tract function, heavy metal toxicity, and other important functional parameters.

Today, what is called integrative medicine is still largely focused on impaired function and how to fix it. Most of the instructors at such major organizations as ACAM (American College for Advancement in Medicine) work effectively at this level. This takes us below the water in Dr. Rau's iceberg diagram, which is good. However, we must go even deeper.

Where medicine really needs to go in order to become an effective and affordable healing force is below the water on the iceberg. It must address the idea of impaired regulation. What does this mean? When we move from lying down to standing, the cardiovascular system regulates to keep our blood pressure and pulse steady so we do not lose consciousness. Between meals, a healthy liver and adrenal glands regulate to keep blood sugar steady enough so that we do not lose consciousness. If because of heavy metal toxicity the cell membranes of our bodily cells are unable to regulate inflow of nutrients and oxygen and outflow of toxins, then nutritional supplements become much less effective and fatigue continues. This is impaired regulation, and it involves the autonomic nervous system. There are diagnostic and therapeutic modalities in integrative medicine that address this level of regulation.

Below the area of impaired regulation is impaired information. Our bodies function well if they receive the right information and in correct sequencing on a cellular, sub-cellular, and DNA level. Cellular and sub-cellular function develops a state of impaired information when cells become toxic with the wrong information (heavy metals, chemicals, radiation, electromagnetic fields, for example) or deficient in the necessary information (too little chromium, for example). All of these physical level changes are regulated by the impaired subtle and not so subtle information we receive from our upbringing. And so our psycho-emotional patterns work their way into our biochemical system over years. In comprehensive medicine, there are many therapies that help to heal the state of impaired information.

In summary, the four levels that need to be addressed in comprehensive medicine include:

Impaired Structure
Impaired Function
Impaired Regulation
Impaired Information

When the field of comprehensive medicine deeply embraces all four of these levels, then deep healing will be available to more people. There are many practitioners in the United States who are already doing this work. Bringing such practitioners into the full expression of comprehensive medicine, which includes inviting their participation in therapeutic teams and financing therapies is our challenge.

THINKING COMPREHENSIVELY: AN EXAMPLE

How can practitioners or those investigating their own issues or symptoms think in these comprehensive and inclusive ways, in order to discover the real causes of illness? Let's say, for example, a person with anxiety and depression seeks help.

In this person's medical history, there may be the overuse of antibiotics, the effects of immunizations for measles, the effects of food allergies to wheat protein and cow's milk protein, and the overgrowth of yeast-like fungus (Candida) in the intestines. All produce a weakness in the protective layer of cells, the mucosa, that lines the intestinal tract. This is the impaired structure.

This often leads to symptoms of irritable bowel: flatulence, distension, constipation, and diarrhea. These are functional disturbances. In addition, the regional nerve ganglia, which are places in the body where nerves come together, become toxic and unable to function well. One of these is the celiac ganglion, deep in the upper abdomen. The ganglia are like small brains that regulate function of organs and tissues in their areas of influence. There are ganglia in the pelvis, head, neck, and lower back as well. Over time, their dysfunction leads to chronic pain and disease.

The ganglion imbalances are relayed to the brain, and more specifically to the limbic brain. This is the part of our brain that is connected to and processes our emotions. Our neurotransmitters change when the ganglia do not function well. This is an example of how depression and anxiety can and do have their origin in gut dysfunctions resulting from our lifestyles.

Levels of Dysfunction (Stress Burden)

- Impaired Structure: Intestinal mucosa
- Impaired Function: Celiac ganglion
- Impaired Regulation: Limbic brain
- Impaired Information: Neurotransmitter disruption

So the damage to the lining of the intestines leads to damage that ascends from ganglion to limbic brain to neurotransmitter.

CHECKLIST FOR COMPREHENSIVE MEDICAL THINKING

- Diagnose and treat problems on structural, functional, regulation, and deep information levels
- Apply body-mind-spirit dynamics
- Treat toxicities and deficiencies
- Individualize care

109

- Apply therapies that support healing
- Do no harm
- Perceive patterns of imbalances
- Think in terms of fields (See Energy Medicine in Chapter 13)
- Be flexible, dynamic, creative, and inclusive

IMPROVISATION VERSUS INNOVATION

Improvisational thinking is a type of thinking that goes beyond what we today call innovative. Dennis Klocek, anthroposophical author and teacher, describes the difference between innovative and improvisational thinkers. As he explains, when we say someone is innovative, this means he or she is at the frontier of new developments that will make all of our lives better, or at least more fun and interesting. Yet innovation today has become quantitative and technical. It has come to mean the manipulation of things that already exist, packaging things in new ways, adding a few new twists, most often for the sake of consumerism. This characterizes most new pharmaceuticals and new techniques in surgery. While such developments may be interesting to the intellectual mind and beneficial to the pocketbook of investors, they do not really contribute to the health and well-being of people, and may even cause further problems.

In the integrative health field, one can palpably feel more enthusiasm, more creativity, and improvisational thinking. The willingness exists to observe a phenomenon and perceive it as part of a greater pattern, a greater truth beyond the intellect. Instead of coming up with an idea that becomes "my" idea that can be patented, there is the attitude that "this idea came to me and needs to be shared with many." Whereas innovations are often deemed valuable when they are cost-effective, sleek, and upbeat, creative improvisations often require risk-taking and collaboration and are labor-intensive. Labor costs are perceived as a necessary evil in many businesses, but health care is not like other businesses. It has descended into the business realm and must be lifted up to the realm to which it rightfully belongs: the sphere of enhancing human health, well-being, and creativity. The burgeoning field of integrative medicine is leading the way in health care creativity.

Imagine what it would be like to be part of an improvisational theater. Spontaneity and collaboration become the norm. Children practice improvisation all the time. In adults this behavior is called goofy or weird, and we default to our safe and economically rewarded behavior of innovation.

Another way to look at this is as the relationship between gravity and levity. The past hundred years or so have seen the development of pharmaceuticals and surgery as the primary approaches in allopathic medicine. Medicine is weighed down by its own gravity, its very limited perception of health care as only being on the physical level, manipulating biochemistry with drugs and changing structure with surgery. Because of our adoration of allopathic medicine, we are all weighed down. Epidemics of chronic, incapacitating illness are our evidence.

Our culture materially rewards innovative cleverness in professionals. If this continues, our health care and its financing will collapse. Improvisational thinking and the emerging field of comprehensive medicine bring a much more promising future to conventional medicine.

Comprehensive medicine brings a feeling of levity back into medicine. This is an uplifting enthusiasm that seeks to bridge the tremendous and often valuable intellectual research of allopathic medicine with creative improvisational thinking that is based on being open to inspiration from higher intelligences.

For example, herbal medicine is ancient, long practiced, and proven in indigenous cultures. Yet until recently it was slandered by conventional medicine. Pharmaceutical companies cannot patent the herbs that grow wild, so they influenced conventional medicine and society into believing that herbs are harmful. This is so even though in 1998, as noted previously, the Journal of the American Medical Association reported that adverse reactions from prescribed pharmaceuticals was the fourth leading cause of death in the United States. Today, major hospital research is confirming the effectiveness of herbal therapy. Collectively, we are listening more to our intuitive knowingness that nature is an important part of healing.

Other examples abound of creative, improvisational, risk-taking thinking. Dietrich Klinghardt, M.D., Ph.D., of Bellevue, Washington, is very creatively improvisational, continually refining and remolding his approach to energy medicine, integrating and acknowledging the teaching and experience of other researchers. His work involves a warm and intimate perception of phenomena in nature and in the human being, and his thinking perceives the unfolding deep intelligences or archetypes that are behind the veil of the visible. Larry Dossey, M.D., has contributed much in the area of non-locality, demonstrating the healing effects of intercessory prayer independent of distance. This principle of non-locality, which Rupert Sheldrake has also described so well in his books, will also eventually be shown to apply to radionics.

As both a board-certified emergency physician and an integrative alternative medical doctor for more than 20 years, I have attended conferences on both allopathic and integrative medicine. Often there is an enormous difference, and not only in content. Both types of conference contain intellectual information. However, the integrative conferences have more success in converting the chilling wasteland of quantities into the warm, intimate connectedness of qualities. The warmth of enthusiasm is based on a deep knowingness that this is the right path of practice. It is unusual to experience this at allopathic conferences.

The field of comprehensive integrative medicine is the frontier. There are still those in this field who think innovatively, and who try to apply the same formulas to everyone in order to sell their particular product. But many of the new technologies in integrative medicine, from thermography, to heart rate variability, to improved laboratory diagnostic approaches, are very creative and contribute to our understanding of the human healing process. Many of these are still not recognized or financially supported by the medical establishment. But this is changing. More physicians in conventional medical institutions are recognizing the need for these changes and coming forward with creative new research.

We need to think in these terms: gravity and levity, innovation and creative improvisation. Then we can begin to turn the wheel of health care in this country more toward supporting healing and regeneration.

I once saw a picture of the prophet Ezekiel, kneeling, looking up, his head pierced through the veil of the ordinary world. Now he was able to perceive the beauty of cosmic laws, the awesomeness that stands behind our physical world and supports our existence. It is to this world that we look for healing, to step out of formulaic and mechanistic medicine and take the risk to be creative and improvisational. This is where comprehensive medicine is moving us if we let it, and why so many patients and practitioners are heading in this direction.

CHANGES FOR THE DOCTOR

How does a physician become a comprehensive integrative medical doctor? It is not just starting to prescribe vitamins and minerals in the office or clinic. Rather, becoming this type of doctor requires the physician to begin to think and act differently with patients. Otherwise, and this is already in danger of happening, the word "integrative" (and "comprehensive" as well) will become a hollow shell of what it really needs to be.

There are three basic areas to address:

1. Doctors' thinking must gradually become more fluid, open, tolerant, inclusive, and unbiased. This means not being intellectually rigid. They still employ technology in practice, but now this technology enables them to see beyond disease and into the functional changes that begin long before physical disease develops.

2. Doctors' feeling natures become less egoistic and more open and compassionate toward people who come to them for help with illness. These are the practitioners who hear the whole of life, who listen with intention to their patients' stories, who develop a sense of what their patients' lives are about and the deeper meaning of their patients' illnesses.

112

3. Doctors' actions reflect a willingness to treat based on individual needs rather than based only on convenient formulas and protocols. They become more of the healer who awakens the deeper process of healing in others because they are already doing this work in their own lives.

In addition, the comprehensive integrative physician needs to be mindful of what the word "integrative" means. Principles of community, equality of responsibility, and working in effective group relationships need to be embraced (see Chapter 5).

AN EVOLVING PRACTICE

In my comprehensive medicine practices, I have worked with other individuals. One is a psychotherapist who embraces many nontraditional and effective approaches such as Reichian mind-body dynamics, color therapy, EMDR (Eye Movement Desensitization and Reprocessing), and the family constellation therapy of psychologist Bert Hellinger. Massage therapists, colon hydrotherapists, movement therapists, and acupuncturists have also brought their energies to our collective efforts.

All of us share a deep commitment to this work, this calling. We love to exercise our faculties and gifts with our patients. We are always having "aha's" as one of us has a deeper insight into what is going on with one of our patients. Our hearts and minds have become more open in doing this work.

Economically, our office still uses some traditional procedures, such as standard employment arrangements, medical insurance, and insurance billing. These will be necessary for some time. There is the inspiration of therapeutic communities such as the anthroposophical center in Spring Valley, New York; Paracelsus Foxhollow Clinic in Louisville, Kentucky; and health associations that various practitioners have set up in other places in the United States as examples of the changes to come.

INTEGRATIVE CLINICS AND INTEGRATIVE PHYSICIANS

There is another perspective on the word "integrative" provided by Silena Heron, N.D., a well-known and respected teacher and practitioner of herbal medicine who lives in Sedona, Arizona. There is a difference, she says, between an integrative medical office and an integrative practitioner. In the former, we may find a number of different practitioners of various fields in complementary and alternative medicine. The physical structure of an integrative medical office may consist of a physician who does nutritional medicine and homeopathy, a massage therapist, and an acupuncturist. This approach is what is growing in medicine today.

Then there are integrative physicians. These physicians practice in an integrative fashion. This means that while they are with a patient, they are doing the internal work of integrating their observations of the patient with their knowledge and experience in many fields of integrative medicine. They are seeing the patient from a homeopathic perspective, an anthroposophical perspective, from the point of view of an herbalist, a nutritionist, an energy medicine practitioner, and whatever other areas in which they have trained. Many of these perspectives are described in Chapter 13.

Such physicians feel joy and gratitude that life has given them the opportunity to exercise these faculties in the service of people on their healing paths. They may only see six or seven patients a day, because they are aware of the tremendous inner work it requires to do this deep integrative work with patients. For these reasons, Jacob Teitelbaum, M.D., director of the Annapolis Research Center for Effective CFS/Fibromyalgia Therapies, advises such physicians to see patients for only up to 28 hours per week. Dr. Teitelbaum devotes considerable time to his own internal process of healing and regeneration.

Integrative practitioners are daily striving to be flexible enough, open enough, fluid enough to move freely from one level of healing to another. This is the comprehensive integrative physician of the future. Many physicians, deep in their psyches, know that they are not really practicing medicine the way they want to. They have become aware that their training is limited. They have families to support and positions in society. It takes courage to listen to these inner thoughts and to begin to open up to the possibility of being a much more fulfilled and effective practitioner. This is the courage called for in these times.

CHANGING THINKING

Physicians need to change their thinking in three main areas: from organs that are separate to organs that interrelate; from humans versus nature to human symbiosis with nature; and from quantity to quality.

1. From organs that are separate to organs that interrelate

Most of us physicians learned about organ function in detail in medical school. However, we learned about the structure, physiology, and biochemistry of organs as separate entities. This information is accurate, but it is not the whole picture. The organs are deeply interrelated.

Endocrinology, the study of glandular function, most embodies this interrelatedness. In Chinese medicine, it becomes much more obvious how organs are interrelated. The organ is not just in a physical area of the body but has a sphere of influence throughout the body through its particular meridian points that impact the autonomic nervous system (see Acupuncture in Chapter 13).

There are various levels that comprehensive physicians can work on. For example, much in integrative medicine today begins to approach the level of seeing the effects of more subtle liver imbalances on biochemistry. This can deepen practitioners' understanding of the patient's situation if they can incorporate the principles of Chinese medicine, anthroposophical medicine (based on Rudolf Steiner's work of almost a century ago), or the deeper constitutional pictures of homeopathy and how each applies to organ functions (see Chapter 13).

2. From humans versus nature to human symbiosis with nature

This is the evolution of thinking from the perception of microorganisms as something to be killed with antibiotics to a perception that respects the delicate interaction of our own human cells with the millions of microflora in the body. This is no more obvious than in the intestines. When this deep understanding becomes part of daily thinking, doctors will not be so quick to prescribe antibiotics.

A practical example is in the diagnosis and treatment of children's ear infections. Most often, ear infections are treated with antibiotics. Not only is this frequently ineffective, but it may also cause many problems in the biological terrain of the intestines and immune function.

Comprehensive physicians look deeper. They may work on the food allergy level and apply an understanding that if these children have cow's dairy products removed from their diet, many of these ear infections will not occur. In a deeper way, they may perceive that the bacteria typically treated with antibiotics are merely doing the work for us that we refuse to do. This means that these ear infections are misplaced digestion: that which was unable to be digested and assimilated in the intestines is displaced into the mucous membranes of the ears. Fluid builds up in the wrong place, instead of its correct place in the gut. The bacteria then feed on this misplaced fluid, and symptoms of ear infection occur. Rather than giving an antibiotic that kills microorganisms and strips away protective linings in the gut, the physician gives a homeopathic remedy that supports immune functioning or one that helps the body to reabsorb this misplaced fluid. This is comprehensive integrative thinking. Allopathic medicine is finally also coming to the conclusion that antibiotic treatment for ear infections is not the answer in many cases. This is good.

Unfortunately, in its arrogance, it gives no credit to alternative and integrative practitioners who have known this for decades.

3. From quantity to quality

Comprehensive physicians open their perceptions from focus on limited and strictly quantifiable measurements to subtleties of energies, words, and gestures in a patient's visit. They become more open to the effectiveness of energy medicine. In a deeper way, as part of working with patients, comprehensive physicians train themselves to perceive the subtle and invisible forces that are at work in the patient's life and illness, how these forces work their way deeply into the constitution and biological terrain of the patient, and what these forces mean to a person's life and fulfillment.

EDUCATION FOR PHYSICIANS IN COMPREHENSIVE MEDICINE

In the summer of 2003 I attended a week-long conference given by Dr. Klinghardt. It was held in a retreat center on an island north of Vancouver, British Columbia. The sessions were several hours long each morning, afternoon, and evening. Much information was provided on examining the interrelationships of illness and the neurological system, the toxicities and stored emotional traumas. At the beginning of each session, Dr. Klinghardt took out his guitar and led the group in singing. Singing enlivens our parasympathetic nervous systems and helps us relax, so we can learn better.

As a matter of fact, Dr. Klinghardt starts the day at all his conferences with singing or qi gong movement. Initially, the singing made me feel somewhat uncomfortable. "Why can't we dispense with the New Age singing and just get down to business?" I would wonder. Yet gradually I began to see the reasons for the singing. I experienced a feeling of joy, of openness, and I was brought into my body and out of my head where professionals love to reside. This is in stark contrast to most other conferences I have attended, even in integrative medicine, and especially so in the uptight and overly serious allopathic medical community.

An anthroposophical physicians' conference in 2002 that I attended was held in the upstairs of an unfinished barn in Wisconsin. By then, this did not seem abnormal to me. Yet I still could not help but feel amazed that this group of highly intelligent doctors, some of whom were cardiologists and other specialists, were sitting on chairs in a barn, hearing the animals downstairs, and talking about illness, healing, and remedies to use in different situations. What a wonderful change of scenery.

The recent ACAM (American College for Advancement in Medicine) conferences in Washington, D.C., and Las Vegas, Nevada, were held in much more traditional settings and people were more formally dressed. This level of workshop is much safer for physicians who are beginning to make the transition to integrative medicine. They come to hear speakers who are well-respected in their fields and who are doing honest research. Talks are often presented with a sense of humor that springs from the enthusiasm and knowingness that this is where medicine needs to go. The enthusiasm of those attending the conference was also apparent.

116

THE CHALLENGE OF COMPREHENSIVE MEDICINE

The field of integrative medicine now includes many disciplines, including homeopathy, anthroposophical medicine, nutrition, Chinese medicine, and so on. The challenge in developing a new, more comprehensive medicine is developing the capacities and intent to bring the different approaches we learn into relationship and communication with each other, perceiving the picture of illness they portray in a patient, and crafting therapeutic programs accordingly.

Depending on how we do this, with the correct rhythm and timing for each patient and with clarity of thought, we can help a patient to heal. But let's not deceive ourselves. None of our therapeutic approaches heal. What heals is awakening the often-dormant will to heal within each patient.

Each patient's mirror of life has cracked into pieces. The work and fun of comprehensive medicine is to create a picture with each patient of how the mirror of life cracked and how it can be put back together, so that a sick person can regain a clear image of his or her life and begin to feel better. To do this effectively requires more than just gathering information. It requires us to be able to create a bridge within ourselves between intellectual information and imaginative thinking.

What is imaginative thinking? In Chinese medicine the physiological and psychological themes that are related to each meridian system are imaginations. They have living images that have lived through time.

What else is imaginative thinking, and how can we bring about a synthesis in ourselves between information and imagination so that both our lives and those of our patients can be enriched? Imagination is the attractive cohesive force that we place at the center of the process. Then we gather information around it. Imagination gives us focus. Imagination is the life that we breathe into our accumulated information, like the way we blew bubbles as children, expanding each bubble into a unique sphere that had a life of its own. As we imagine, we breathe pneumena (spirit) into phenomena (information). This helps us to be able to relate in different ways to the same information each time we use it, so that we do not look at a patient as just another rheumatoid arthritis patient or another irritable bowel patient.

Imagine reading late one afternoon, looking up, and seeing the sunlight streaming in the window. The table and the vase look different because of this light. Intellectually, the vase is familiar—so familiar that it normally slips beneath conscious awareness. Because of today's light, however, you see the vase and table in a way you have not seen them before. This is objective imagination.

Through cultivating objective imagination, we become adept at being able to live and move between two worlds: the obvious, physical world of information, objects, and people; and the subtle world in ourselves and in nature, which is infused with soulfulness and spiritual forces.

We can be with a patient on a particular day and at the same time be able to hold a breadth of vision of the person's entire life before us and perceive the person as a soul/spiritual being who is experiencing physical problems. We can be open to inquire inwardly about the relationship between this patient's life and the illness he or she has. To do this requires inner effort by the practitioner.

PAST, PRESENT, AND FUTURE

In order to heal, people must be able to integrate their pasts with their present. To do this, the past needs to be objectified. This is accomplished in office visits by taking a history, conducting a physical examination, and running objective tests. Then we support the patient between visits with treatment programs and exercises. The goal is to help patients develop new life rhythms. Treatment programs can take many forms. They can range from supporting improved sleep and giving amino acids that inwardly strengthen a patient's emotional state to giving certain exercises to tap acupuncture points four times daily.

We cannot fight disease. This is a basic fact that allopathic medicine has not yet understood. We help patients begin to remove obstructions to healing with detoxification and nutrients and the development of authentic focus for their life energies. Over time, the old areas of trapped energies and forces die of attrition because the patients are no longer feeding them with their habits and imbalances.

For practitioners, imagination keeps our thinking inwardly mobile, adaptable, and flexible. This is necessary so that we are constantly dissolving the rigidifying or hardening tendencies that develop in people who rely too much on the intellect. When we allow our imaginations to flow in our lives and in our practices, then we are able to support others to do the same.

The problem today is information without imagination. We harden with intellectual information without imagination. Premature hardening or sclerotic tendencies are the basis of all chronic disease. If we as comprehensive practitioners do not address these tendencies in ourselves, we will be less able to help our patients.

There is a saying: Intellect is the shadow of light. As discussed in an earlier chapter, the shadow in Jungian psychology is that which is hidden from conscious awareness, that part of us that we keep hidden from ourselves and from others. Professionals in our culture are rewarded for what they know, rather than for who they are. As a result, professionals become too comfortable with intellectual information. This shields us from perceiving the greater light of consciousness that embraces core images, improvisational thinking, and depth of feeling and compassion.

To give an image of where we are today, every five hundred or so years there is a renaissance. We are just entering one in our current times. Just as the darkest time of the day is before the dawn, so the past 50 years have seen a hardening of the intellect and more entrenched mechanistic and materialistic thinking in medicine, which has affected everyone. Early in the twentieth century, great visions for healing were offered by people such as Enderlein, Reich, Steiner, Dinshah, Tesla, and Rife, among others. They planted seeds but were mostly unsuccessful in their times because of the illness of mechanistic materialism in medicine that was developing. This illness is what keeps our health care system in financial crisis and ineffective in healing.

Now we are in a battle to bring health care and technological medicine back into the stream of life. Part of this involves bringing thinking from abstract, intellectual, mechanistic, and formula-based to imaginative, intuitive, creative, and fluid. The latter type of thinking is inwardly mobile, constantly producing one form out of another. This is what is termed pleomorphic. A good image for this type of thinking is a lava lamp where the forms are always changing shape in the medium of fluidity, producing one form out of another.

The way we think about fats in our food provides an illustration of the different thinking modes. We are increasingly becoming aware of the importance of avoiding trans-fatty acids in our foods, in spite of the efforts of the margarine industry over the past 50 years. But let's go beyond this. When we think imaginatively, we can perceive a relationship between the amount of trans-fats in foods and the premature development of intellect. As Patricia Kane, Ph.D., of the Haverford Clinic in Haverford, Pennsylvania, and others teach, with high consumption of this type of fat, we increasingly find in the nervous system very long-chain fatty acids, which are more rigid and lead not only to chronic degenerative neurological conditions but also to many other problems. When we eat healthy oils and fats, Dr. Kane reminds us, we help the cell membranes in the nervous system to remain fluid and flexible so that our nervous systems and thinking can remain clear.

"All things brought to us as information, data, and facts need to be interpreted and considered anew by our deepest forces."
—Rudolf Steiner

INCURABLE ATTITUDES WIELD INFLUENCE

"There are few incurable Illnesses.
There are many incurable attitudes"

This is a very important quote, and I cannot recall where I first heard it. It reminds us that while there is a growing interest in integrative medicine, there is still much resistance to its development. Dr. Joseph Mercola, in his free Internet newsletter (www.mercola.com), which I highly recommend, documents and updates the realities of integrative medicine virtually every week.

There are still many incurable attitudes that wield much influence. The Medicare Law of 2003 blocked the government from bargaining with pharmaceutical companies for cheaper drug prices. Dr. Mercola on his website, www.mercola.com, describes these developments in much more detail. The lead article in the New York Times business section on October 26, 2003, entitled "Generous Medicare Payments Spur Specialty Hospital Boom," describes the tremendous increase in heart hospitals across the United States, eager for patients who have had and will continue to want open-heart surgeries, angioplasties, cardiac catheterizations, implanted pacemakers, and defibrillators. These are obviously areas where the money is in medicine. These hospitals are increasing in the face of mounting evidence that these procedures miss the point in heart disease. Working with the chronic infections in the coronary arteries (for example, infections from oral periodontal infections made worse with heavy metal toxicity from dental fillings and magnesium deficiencies) could bring the number of people needing surgical procedures, and the costs, way down (for more on this, see Dr. Garry Gordon's website, www.gordonresearch.com).

As comprehensive medicine becomes the future of medicine, these types of hospitals will become extinct, or we may be extinct if they continue to prosper for too many more years.

WHAT TO DO IF YOUR DOCTOR HAS RESISTANCE TO INTEGRATIVE MEDICINE

This is a problem that many patients who use integrative medicine have when they go to an allopathic doctor for a specific health issue. At some point in the interview, a patient feels conflict and wonders how she is going to discuss what she has learned and observed with her doctor. She fears that the doctor will discontinue working with her as a patient because she is working with a holistic doctor as well. Or the doctor may become irritated and the patient worries that her care will suffer. Or she may feel disloyal to her doctor who has provided care to her for many years.

Here are some suggestions for dealing with these issues:

1. It is your right to choose who your doctors are. Your doctors are your partners in your healing process. They do not control your life. Part of this conflict is your need to get over dependence on authority and get over acting out of fear.

More allopathic physicians are aware of integrative medicine, and some are becoming more knowledgeable in this area. After all, most of the integrative medical doctors were at one point more conventional allopaths. Try not to be intolerant, because this could draw out your doctor's intolerance of anything outside the way he or she practices medicine. Remember that the reactions to what you are doing and the questions you ask are often also based on fear. You may want to give your doctor some literature to read on the area of your illness care that is a concern, and ask his or her opinion. If you project anger that your doctor is this or that, then he or she will have a much more difficult time working with you in this new arrangement. You can also invite your allopathic doctor to call your integrative medical doctor.

2. Keep in mind these points:

    - Do what you feel is right for you.

    - Make every attempt to be inclusive with your allopathic physician.

    - Do not act out of fear.

    - Act out of trust in your intuition and your sense of what you need.

CHAPTER 12

COMPREHENSIVE MEDICINE ASSESSMENT AND TESTING METHODS

This chapter details the objective evaluation methods that are useful in a comprehensive medical practice. Objective evaluations help us to recognize the areas in our body that are in distress. Our current health care system is filled with a myriad of testing procedures that provide information about the internal workings of the body. Comprehensive Medicine expands the range of testing in order to evaluate objectively the deeper areas of impaired function, impaired regulation, and impaired information.

The four areas of testing in comprehensive medicine are:

A. Physical examination

B. Office testing procedures (examples)

- o Thermography (computerized regulation and infrared)
- o Autonomic nervous system assessment (heart rate variability)
- o Iris evaluation
- o Biological Terrain Management (BTM)
- o Bio-Energy Testing (BET)
- o Dental Panorex
- o Autonomic Response Testing (ART)

C. Self-testing

- o Urine and stool evaluation
- o Coca pulse test
- o Basal body temperature

D. Laboratory tests

- o Hair mineral analysis
- o Blood profiles

123

     o   Heavy metal evaluation
     o   Comprehensive Digestive Stool Analysis
     o   Amino Acid Profiles

Several pages in this chapter describe self-testing. Information is included on observing urine and stool, and measuring body temperature. These tests offer valuable information about the functioning of our internal terrain.

Some tests needed for prescribing effective therapies are sent out to laboratories. Examples are hair analysis, stool tests for parasites, and 24-hour urine hormone assays, as well as routine tests done at local laboratories. Many of us have had X rays and lab tests at conventional hospitals and laboratory facilities. Sometimes these conventional tests are necessary, and a comprehensive medical practitioner will suggest them.

Tests are part of a comprehensive evaluation. It is important to remember that no single test or evaluation gives the whole perspective. By looking at our lives from different perspectives, the comprehensive medical physician is able to develop a picture of the patient's imbalances. This is true holistic medicine.

A. PHYSICAL EXAMINATION

The initial part of the objective evaluation is a physical examination. The examination combines approaches from conventional medicine with very helpful techniques gleaned from Chinese medicine, modern neural therapy, and iris diagnosis. The meridian approach to diagnosis is a very helpful guide in evaluating a condition and recommending therapy.

The physical exam also consists of a thorough evaluation and mapping of the mouth. As stated in Part I, the teeth are connected to the rest of the body, and problems in a particular tooth can contribute to an illness or an imbalance in one's overall health.

Particular attention is given to a neurological evaluation. Information is sought about the condition of the autonomic or unconscious nervous system, as well as indications of heavy metal toxicity of the nervous system.

It is also important to evaluate any scars present from prior accidents or surgery. These scars can create imbalances in the autonomic nervous system, leading to organ dysfunction and disease.

B. OFFICE TESTING PROCEDURES

THERMOGRAPHY (CRT)

Computerized regulation thermography, or CRT, is an objective, noninvasive, and safe way of evaluating the body's functions. CRT, also simply called thermography, represents one of several objective diagnostic evaluations in integrative medicine. It is a medical imaging method that supplies information as meaningful as that obtained through an MRI or X ray. More than 1,500 physicians in Europe use CRT. Current medical journals contain more than 12,000 citations and studies on thermography.

CRT evaluates body functions by a direct temperature measurement probe instead of by measuring thermal radiation. This scanning method is far more precise than any other thermographic system. The complete autonomic nervous system is mapped out as the probe projects to and from each organ or tissue. With this form of thermography, we can finally see what the body is doing long before it becomes dysfunctional enough to create an irreversible problem. CRT does not diagnose disease; rather it identifies patterns that lead to disease so that these patterns can be successfully treated.

How Does Thermography Work?

Each internal organ and gland has a corresponding point on the skin. A technician, holding a direct temperature measurement probe, measures the temperature of 68 points on the body. Measurements occur simply by touching a probe against these 68 points. There is no discomfort. Next, the patient partially disrobes, which gives the body a chance to cool. These same points are measured again ten minutes later.

CRT measures the difference between these two measurements at each of these 68 points over a ten-minute period. When each of the internal organs that are correlated to these 68 points is functioning optimally, there is normally a change in temperature between the two measurements. Dysfunction in these internal organs or glands is revealed by an abnormal response in the second measurement, which is taken after the body has been mildly stressed by the cooling that partial disrobing produces.

By the patterns of the temperature changes at each of these 68 points between the first and second measurements, we are able to evaluate accurately the internal functioning of the organism (the person being tested). We can see how adaptable the patient is to change. In addition to revealing disease patterns, thermography enables us to perceive imbalances in the system before these imbalances become pathological diseases. This is true preventive medicine.

Why Is Thermography Helpful?

In chronic disease, there are often factors that block successful treatment. These include:

- Infections in the teeth
- Low-grade chronic viral or fungal infection
- Heavy metal toxicity

- Chronic psychological imbalances
- Intestinal toxins and dysfunction
- Immune system weaknesses
- Lymphatic obstructions
- Food allergies

With thermography, we can see if and where these imbalances are found in the body.

Remember that no illness occurs in isolation. There are always patterns of dysfunction. These eventually lead to symptoms of illness, often only after years of dysfunction. It is these patterns of dysfunction that the holistic practitioner attempts to identify in order to provide guidance toward a successful treatment program. The results of the thermography evaluation, together with other diagnostic testing, are needed to design an effective treatment program.

Remember that healing requires a change in lifestyle. Many of the imbalances in function we may see on a thermogram are due to lifestyle imbalances that have been in place for many years. With thermography, we can identify the patterns of illness that these lifestyle imbalances have impressed upon the system. Then, treatment can be more ably guided in a successful direction.

Mammography Versus Thermography

A major asset of thermography is in the area of early detection and confirmation of breast cancers. In a German study, 54 percent of breast cancer patients were correctly diagnosed by history and physical examination. The number rose to 76 percent when mammography was added. However, when computerized regulation thermography was used, the accuracy of diagnosis rose to 92%. Many women today are concerned about the effects of accumulated radiation from routine mammograms. That concern is addressed by instead using thermography, which involves no radiation, and ultrasound when necessary.

With thermography, we do not have to rely on mammographies. And with the growing controversy on the radiation exposure from repeated mammographies, as well as the not insignificant percentage of false-negative results, thermographic screening becomes increasingly attractive. However, it is always important for women to do thorough manual evaluation of their own breast tissue, and to have the practitioner do likewise.

INFRARED THERMOGRAPHY

Another form of thermography is called infrared thermography. This is a noninvasive diagnostic system using digital infrared thermal imaging to detect subtle changes in structure and function before pathology develops.

It also provides information about a patient's response to treatment. Localized or full body imaging occurs in seconds, and it is safe, with no radiation involved.

AUTONOMIC NERVOUS SYSTEM ASSESSMENT (Heart Rate Variability)

The heart rate variability (HRV) test is well researched and provides a quick and easy assessment of autonomic nervous system function. The autonomic nervous system (ANS) regulates the heart, breathing, circulation, body temperature, digestion, metabolism, and hormones, among other vital functions.

As illness materializes, or as the body gradually stops functioning normally by physiological and biochemical standards, the autonomic nervous system stops functioning optimally. Since this system regulates our internal organ function, without a healthy autonomic nervous system it is difficult to heal or maintain a healing condition.

The two parts of the ANS are the sympathetic and parasympathetic nervous systems. The sympathetic is our arousal system. It activates a fight-or-flight response when the body detects danger. The parasympathetic controls calming responses, such as sleep, relaxation, and nurturing. Many people's parasympathetic systems have been weakened, and this may be seen on the heart rate variability test. Strengthening programs are then designed as part of a therapeutic program.

The HRV test lasts about ten minutes. A strap is placed around the chest that monitors 442 heartbeats, both when lying and standing. The machine measures the intervals between each heartbeat. In good health there is normally a very small but detectable variability of time between each heartbeat. When we stop functioning optimally, this variability narrows and gradually becomes rigid.

With this autonomic nervous system assessment, we can see how much functional reserve the patient has. This guides us in how much therapy can be tolerated at this time. We can also see the level of functioning of the patient's general physiology.

IRIS EVALUATION

The iris is the colored part of the eye that surrounds the pupil. By observing this part of the eye, a trained practitioner is able to perceive markers and patterns as to a patient's:

- Constitution—its strengths and weaknesses

- Tendencies toward imbalances and diseases, or to concentrate toxins

127

- Personality and cognitive processes, i.e., mind/body interre-lationships

- Quality of connective tissue

The markers and patterns observed in the iris offer an opportunity to understand certain inherited strengths and weaknesses, according to Scott Moyer of BioEclectic Research Foundation in Santa Rosa, California. By making choices within the boundaries of our strengths and weaknesses, we have the opportunity to live a creative and balanced life. Iris diagnosis helps us to identify the therapies/activities/expressions that will balance our constitutional weaknesses.

BIOLOGICAL TERRAIN MANAGEMENT (BTM)

Biological Terrain Management, or BTM, is a quick, *easy, and effective* lab test to evaluate one's biological terrain. Using freshly voided samples of a patient's urine and saliva, the office will run tests that show how a person's body is functioning. The results of this test has proven invaluable to practitio-ners in correctly prescribing for one's particular biochemistry and physiology. BTM's are often repeated weekly or biweekly, or even more often in more seriously ill patients, in order to objectively evaluate the effectiveness of treatment and see what is the next step in treatment.

The test also helps the practitioner to see which acupuncture meridian is most stressed and which is most deficient at the present time. He can then ap-ply meridian treatments to help correct these imbalances, so that the patient may move more in a direction of healing.

This technology was developed by Timothy Ray, O.M.D., of BioRay, Inc. in Los Angeles, California. The great value of this test is in its ability to evaluate what therapy to use at each level of a patient's therapeutic process. The image of peeling off the layers of the onion is very helpful here. When we heal, we are peeling off these layers. At each level there are new issues with which we must work.

The test pays little attention to the name of a disease. This is still being done all the time in allopathic medicine, and still very often even in alterna-tive medicine, where we are taught to take CoQ10 for heart failure or Glucosamine for arthritis. These can be very helpful in such situations. But by addressing the underlying biological terrain, the self-healing forces in the body become more active, regardless of the name of the disease.

Tests like the BTM will soon revolutionize the practice of medicine in the world.

BIO-ENERGY TESTING (BET)

Frank Shallenberger, MD in Carson City, Nevada is using a very promising approach to energy medicine. He calls it Bio-Energy Testing, or BET. This test uses an FDA-approved analyzer of pulmonary (lung) gas, an analyzer often used in conventional medicine. The patient's expired air is tested at rest, and then again after a few minutes on a stationary bicycle. Dr. Shallenberger has expanded upon the way that conventional medicine uses this machine and transformed it into a wonderful tool for energy medicine diagnosis. With this test, the practitioner is able to accurately determine why a patient has decreased energy, and then prescribe an individualized therapeutic program that will enhance energy production in the patient's biochemistry and physiology. All diseases are pathological conditions which develop because our cells, organs and self-regulating internal systems become dysfunctional. This leads to a decrease in energy, and then to disease.

The BET is also an excellent wellness and preventive medicine evaluation. Dr. Shallenberger feels that the new paradigm for medicine of the future is that there is one disease: decreased energy production, and one treatment: increasing energy production. In Dr. Klinghardt's model at the end of Chapter 13, Dr. Shallenberger's diagnostic approach with the BET as well as his main treatment approaches which increase energy production, are mainstays in Levels One and Two. This is a Healthy Medicine system.

DENTAL PANOREX

A significant part of biological medicine is the connection between the teeth and the body. More specifically, the condition of the teeth and the bones of the jaw are intimately related to bodily health and well-being. Such dental procedures as metal amalgam fillings, root canals, and jawbone cavitations can be contributing factors to illnesses elsewhere in the body. For this reason, part of an initial evaluation includes a dental panorex. This is an X ray of your total mouth. The significance of any findings is reviewed at an initial appointment.

AUTONOMIC RESPONSE TESTING (ART)

The body and every cell within it is an antenna of electromagnetic energy. If this energy is working optimally at all levels, then we are in good health. We are absorbing and utilizing foods and supplements well, sleeping well, feeling energetic, and so forth. When this energy becomes deficient, we experience symptoms of illness. Proper regulation of this electromagnetic energy is what contributes to our state of health and well-being. Regulation is the capacity of the nervous system to recognize a stress stimulus and adapt to it. Most people have what is called restricted regulation. This means that the capacity to respond to stress is blocked. The cause of blocked regulation may be heavy metals, food allergies, environmental toxins, structural problems, or psycho-emotional stresses, among other factors.

Autonomic Response Testing (ART) is a form of muscle testing that determines how our autonomic or subconscious nervous system is functioning. Through ART, a dialogue is created with the subconscious in the body. ART was developed by Dr. Dietrich Klinghardt (see www. neuraltherapy.com).

Dr. Klinghardt has developed increasingly ingenious ways of using our understanding of light and physics in muscle testing to make it more accurate in testing our state of regulation, or whether it is open or restricted. Tapping (see "Tapping" in Chapter 13), incorporating color-tinted glasses, or moving the eyes in certain directions (Shapiro's eye movement desensitization and reprocessing, or EMDR) can help keep autonomic nervous system regulation open and functioning better. This enables more nutrients and oxygen to reach the sub-cellular levels they need to reach in order for you to be able to heal.

In another part of the test, when the patient is holding certain fingers together, we can test muscle response to tell how well the nervous system is processing data, or processing the information it is receiving.

We pay particular attention to scars or teeth extraction sites. These are focal areas of infection or nervous system irritation. These focal areas have non-absorbable material in the connective tissue that is detrimental to our health. A devitalized tooth, with impaired lymphatic drainage, is an example of a focal area of infection. Muscle testing can identify the problem, determine if it is related to organ malfunction elsewhere in the body, and help us develop a treatment plan.

As we go on in the testing, the tester may also put his hand on various areas of the patient's body. These areas correspond with internal organs and acupuncture meridians. This helps us to find current blockages and then discover what the body needs to heal. In addition, the organs that test weak often have deeper emotional issues that are contributing to ill health. For example, the kidneys may be weak because of electromagnetic stress, a root canal on a tooth that corresponds to the kidney meridian, heavy metals, or a deep level of fear and insecurity that is being held in the body regardless of how much cognitive therapy a patient may have received.

Patients leave with prescriptions for tapping certain acupuncture points to keep these areas functioning better, with a pair or more of color-tinted glasses to wear daily for a short period of time, as well as with their particular herbs, homeopathic remedies, and supplements.

There are also other ways of doing autonomic response testing. We refer here to acupuncture point testing devices such as those made by Vega and Best. Many practitioners are able to use these machines with accuracy in diagnosing and treating conditions. They can also be combined with muscle testing. While these forms of testing and treating are largely outside of conventional medicine, we are witnessing the beginnings of an integration process. For example, at Jefferson Hospital's Department of Integrative Medicine in Philadelphia, there are physicians who utilize muscle testing and presenters from Germany who introduce particular testing machines that could be employed in the department.

Other forms of energy besides electromagnetic can be used in testing, as in devices that use photon or light as a medium of testing. These will come into increasing use in the next decade, and may enable us to do deeper testing to determine where hidden infections lie in the sub-cellular, intra-nuclear, and DNA structures. Even good kinesiology is often unable to reach these levels.

The future is very promising. These testing and treating methods will enable practitioners to go even deeper on the iceberg diagram (see Chapter 11), deeper than structural/chemical and functional/physiological levels of testing, and into the areas where the physics of light and sound will enable us to see how the various parts of our bodies communicate with each other.

In my experience, as I do this deeper work, I gain a much deeper appreciation of how little we really know, and how much our arrogance can get in the way of helping people to heal. Our cells, as well as the microorganisms in them, are communicating at levels and speeds that are far beyond what we can do with each other daily in our interactions. And their intelligence in adapting to changing circumstances makes us appear rather foolish in our presumptions that we can so easily manipulate body chemistry and physiology with drugs or even supplements. Our habitual and increasingly rigid lifestyles appear in clear opposition to this deep adaptability in our cells that is the hallmark of healing.

As energy medicine is integrated into our medical model, and we come to deeply appreciate how mysteriously our bodies operate, and feel reverence and awe and wonder, the dividing line between spirit and matter dissolves. We develop a science of the spirit. And we learn to apply this science to all levels of human life, from medicine to agriculture to business. These are all areas of human endeavor and opportunities for healing.

C. SELF-TESTING

URINE AND STOOL EVALUATION

Urine Evaluation

Determining the pH of urine is one of the best and least expensive ways of evaluating one's acid/base condition. This may be done either by testing the first morning urine. Use pH paper purchased at a local store and observe the color change after you dip the paper in your urine.

The optimal value for urine is 5.8 to 7.2. For non-vegetarians or lacto-vegetarians, the normal range is 6.4 to 6.8. For vegetarians mostly on raw food, the normal value is about 7.0.

Ideally, observe how it feels when the urine is at certain pH values, as revealed by a home test. An optimal value should appear when feeling relaxed, able to focus, and think clearly, with no tightness in the muscles.

When you discover the 24-hour urine pH at which you feel the best, take note of the foods eaten, especially the acid/alkaline ratio of these foods.

Saliva Evaluation of pH

It is also possible to do saliva testing to determine your pH level. Collect some saliva and measure its pH before eating in the morning. Collect saliva before meals. The normal pH of saliva is 6.8 to 7.4. The pH should become more alkaline (higher numbers) after eating, all the way up to a pH of 7.2. If the morning saliva is less than 6.2, that is too acidic. If it is between 5.5 and 5.8 and does not rise after eating, that indicates that you are in a very acidic condition, lacking alkaline reserve, and likely to be quite depleted in minerals.

Stool Evaluation

Observing your stools is an important way to determine the health of digestion. The best way to perform this test is to evaluate stools over several days to a week. The following are what to look for in evaluating your stools and what their condition may indicate.

Question: Do the stools float?
Underlying condition: If yes, indicates fat digestion problem

Question: Is the stool whole or in pieces?
Underlying condition: Whole stools indicate good digestion

Question: Does the stool break up in the toilet bowl?
Underlying condition: If yes, indicates digestive imbalance

Question: Are there fibers visible in the stool?
Underlying condition: If yes, indicates protein digestion problem

Question: Does it stick to the bowl?
Underlying condition: If yes, indicates fat digestion problem

Question: Does the stool have a bad odor?
Underlying condition: If yes, indicates intestinal putrefaction or fermentation

COCA PULSE TEST

The Coca pulse test determines sensitivity and reactivity to foods. Count the pulse for one full minute, eat a very small amount of a food, wait a couple of minutes, and then count the pulse again. If the pulse rises by more than four beats per minute, there is probably an "allergy" to that food. This test is different from what is measured by standard blood tests for food allergies. The Coca pulse test measures the reaction of the autonomic nervous system to the stress of a food. This test is more significant than an allergy test. It detects subtle functional changes.

Be aware that there is much more to allergies than reactions such as hives, swelling, or difficulty breathing. Those reactions are created by an overflow of antibodies. However, we may react to foods and chemicals in other ways that do not show up on conventionally designed tests. Be aware that it is difficult to heal an allergy without first cleaning up the intestines and changing the diet.

BASAL BODY TEMPERATURE

Basal body temperature evaluates thyroid function, though abnormalities in this test may also be due to a low functioning pituitary gland. Purchase a basal thermometer. Then do the following:

- Shake down the thermometer to below 95° F and place it by the bedside at night.

- Upon waking, place the thermometer in the armpit for a full ten minutes and remain still.

- After ten minutes, read and record the temperature and date.

133

- Do this for at least three days, preferably at the same time of day.

- Keep a record of the results.

Low body temperature may indicate low thyroid function, and may also reveal low pituitary function.

D. LABORATORY TESTS

HAIR MINERAL ANALYSIS

Assessing the mineral and heavy metal content in the hair is often a good way to evaluate body chemistry and how we handle stress. We can also see toxic blockages of enzyme function, as well as nutritional deficiencies. Minerals and heavy metals in the body are only partially present inside cells. Therefore, measurement of urine or blood is often not accurate.

The amount of a mineral in the hair does not necessarily reflect the amount in the body. The values of the hair analysis do not necessarily tell us whether there is too much or too little of the mineral in the body, but rather how the body is utilizing the mineral in its metabolism. In other words, a high calcium level does not mean we have too much calcium. Rather, it may indicate a low thyroid function, and a need for calcium supplementation until the metabolism improves.

Hair mineral analysis helps us to prescribe supplements correctly. By helping to balance body minerals, correct deficiencies, and improve glandular function and digestion, our body is much better able to heal. Hair analysis also gives a picture of our metabolic function over the past two to three months.

Since the body compensates and adapts in layers, as we move toward health, we may actually at times go backward in layers. The first hair analysis may not reveal the deeper problems. Often it requires reevaluation with several hair analyses over a year to monitor progress. For example, as nutritional supplementation improves health, heavy metals may begin to be excreted by the body and show up in the hair, though these metals were not initially present in hair. (We recommend having a hair analysis only with a laboratory that does not wash the hair sample before testing.)

Hair mineral analysis also provides measurements for heavy metals. A healthy metabolism prefers minerals to metals. For every body function there is a preferred mineral. But if that mineral is not there, the body will take the next best option. For example, if we are deficient in zinc, which many people are, the body will hold on to cadmium, which is a very toxic metal, in order to metabolize. A hair analysis comes in the form of a graph of the metals and minerals found in the hair sample. What is most important is the pattern on the graph. For example, high calcium and magnesium, coupled with low sodium and potassium, suggests that a different dietary and supplement program will be needed compared to low calcium and magnesium and high sodium and potassium.

BLOOD PROFILES

A basic blood test panel is a good idea. Tests such as a CBC (complete blood count), chemistry panel, cardiovascular risk profile, thyroid panel, and hormone panel may be familiar. While standard blood tests at conventional medical laboratories may report test results as within normal limits, other good medical laboratories such as the Body Bio Corporation in Millville, New Jersey, provide much more depth of understanding in their test analyses. The patterns of relationships within test results often reveal functional imbalances before they become diseases.

HEAVY METAL EVALUATION

Many people today have some degree of heavy metal poisoning. These metals cause problems because they block enzyme systems in our metabolism, and prevent other vital trace minerals from being effective. When heavy metals are present, we are more predisposed to develop chronic diseases.

The heavy metals that are commonly seen in excess in people's bodies are:

1. **Mercury:** Mercury poisoning is more common than most people realize. The main source of toxicity is the presence of mercury amalgams in teeth.

2. **Lead:** Lead poisoning has been implicated in many diseases, including chronic nervous system and digestive problems. The main sources of lead poisoning are lead pipes, lead in paints, and of course, lead in gasoline, although this is a less common source in the United States since gasoline was made unleaded.

3. **Aluminum:** Aluminum has been implicated in attention deficit disorder in children and in Alzheimer's disease in the elderly. Sources are aluminum cookware, many canned foods, and aluminum-containing deodorants and antiperspirants. There is even aluminum in some common table salts.

4. **Cadmium:** People who smoke or have smoked extensively and those who work with paints or metals may have cad-

mium poisoning. Cadmium toxicity is less common than lead, mercury, aluminum and copper toxicity, however.

5. **Copper:** Copper toxicity is common and may contribute to anxiety. There are many sources of copper in our environment like copper water pipes. Copper toxicity is higher in vegetarians. Dr. Larry Wilson (www.drlwilson.com) has published a good book on hair mineral analysis called *Nutritional Balancing and Hair Mineral Analysis.*

These metals do not act in isolation from other body imbalances. For example, because tissues are more acidic in today's environment, we pick up more aluminum from external sources than if our tissues were more alkaline.

There are several methods of testing for heavy metals. These tests vary in price and effectiveness. Tests include:

- **Hair analysis**. This is a good test for aluminum, lead, cadmium, and copper. Hair also tests well for some common necessary minerals, such as zinc, calcium, and magnesium. The only major metal that hair will not accurately test for is mercury.

- **Urine analysis** (after administration of an oral or intravenous chelating agent for heavy metals, such as EDTA or Metal-Free). A chelating agent is a substance that will bind to the heavy metal and carry it out of the body. This test is both diagnostic of how toxic our body is with these metals, and also therapeutic in that it detoxifies our body of metals.

How do we treat heavy metal toxicities after they have been identified?

1. Strengthening the adrenal glands aids in the detoxification of metals.

2. Homeopathic remedies and herbs such as cilantro, taken orally, can pull certain heavy metals out of the body.

3. Supplements that detoxify include antioxidants, zinc, selenium, and other minerals; chlorella can replenish the mineral base and chelate mercury.

4. Adequate amounts of sulfur-based amino acids and proteins are important. If these are deficient, the body will hold on to mercury in order to have adequate metabolic enzyme function.

5. Dental work by a biologically oriented dentist to have mercury amalgams replaced with composite fillings reduces the ongoing exposure to mercury.

COMPREHENSIVE DIGESTIVE STOOL ANALYSIS

This is a commonly used test in functional medicine, a subsection of integrative medicine. The stool is collected and sent to one of a number of good laboratories in the United States. Valuable information is obtained about digestion, bowel function, and microorganism overgrowth.

These tests, when performed in a timely fashion, offer the practitioner the capacity to see deeper below the surface to the mass of the iceberg, and often discover imbalances that standard medical tests miss.

CHAPTER 13

COMPREHENSIVE MEDICINE THERAPIES

A s you will see, the therapies offered in comprehensive medicine are many. They go far beyond the limitations of conventional pharmaceutical and surgical medicine. The goal of all therapies is to help us heal. What does this mean? In comprehensive medicine it means waking up our capacity to react. The process of becoming ill takes years. In these years we gradually become deficient in our capacity to react, to throw off toxins of all kinds, to self-regulate our bodies and our lives. The goal of comprehensive medicine therapies is to restore these capacities.

While there are many technical therapies, there are also numerous subtle approaches that utilize energy therapeutics. And though there is a growing body of published articles and books with volumes of facts, the reality is that the effectiveness of the latter therapies requires of the practitioner an artfulness of application, a devotion to and reverence for this work, and a sharp and inclusive mind.

Comprehensive medicine therapies discussed in this chapter are grouped according to the following categories. Each category lists and describes representative examples, but by no means is exclusive.

A: Nutritional and Physical Alternative Medicine

- Nutritional Supplements and Intravenous Therapy
- Herbal Medicine
- Digestive Enzymes
- Oxygen Therapies
- Chelation
- Colon Therapy (Colonics)
- Functional Medicine
- Cranial Osteopathy
- Bowen Therapy

B: Energy Medicine

- Homeopathy
- Anthroposophical Medicine

139

- Biological Medicine
- Acupuncture
- Ayurvedic Medicine
- Neural Therapy
- Magnetic Field Therapy
- Microcurrent Therapy
- ElectroBloc for Pain Control
- Color Therapy
- Color Auriculotherapy
- Sound and Healing
- Infrared and Far-Infrared Light Therapy
- Matrix Regeneration Therapy
- Chi Machine

C: Energy Psychology

- Tapping
- Applied Psychoneurobiology

D: Soul Healing

- Systemic Family Constellation Therapy
- Soul Healing: Other Examples

A. *NUTRITIONAL AND PHYSICAL ALTERNATIVE MEDICINE*

NUTRITIONAL SUPPLEMENTS

This is a very large and important area of care. Without addressing nutrition, other areas will be less successful. Chapters 15 and 16 are full of helpful information regarding food intake and illness.

There are many ways of taking and prescribing supplements. These vary from practitioner to practitioner. And there are many supplement manufacturers. Good rules to follow are:

1. Work with someone who individualizes a supplement program

2. Take only what is needed for the healing layer being worked on. We all have layers of imbalance and illness built into our biochemistry and physiology. A supplement may be very

140

good, but it may not be what is called for at the present level being addressed

3. Keep digestion working while on supplements

Key nutritional issues that often need to be addressed are:

- Mineral imbalances, which can be measured in hair analysis

- Fatty acid (omega-3 and omega-6 oils) intake, which should vary according to time of year and illnesses being treated. The work of Patricia Kane, Ph.D., of the Haverford Clinic in Haverford, Pennsylvania, and Body Bio Corporation in Millville, New Jersey, (www.bodybio.com) is invaluable here. Amino acid supplements, especially for psychological problems and food cravings, which virtually no one has (some humor is required here). The contributions of Julia Ross, M.A., author of *The Diet Cure* and *The Mood Cure*, have been invaluable.

There is much research in nutritional therapy of chronic diseases, even at many major medical centers. Examples include:

- Coenzyme Q10 and Parkinson's disease
- Gluten sensitivity in chronic illness
- Amino acids and addictions, food cravings
- Modified citrus pectin and cancer

Many resources and publications reveal the extent to which nutrition plays a central role in the treatment of chronic illness. Yet most allopathic medical doctors either know virtually nothing about nutrition, or become condescending toward patients who bring such research to their office visits. This must change.

INTRAVENOUS NUTRITIONAL THERAPY

Thanks to the work of Jonathan Wright, M.D., and Alan Gaby, M.D., intravenous (IV) nutritional therapy is now widely used in integrative medical practices. It is not yet available to a wider number of patients in hospitals and allopathic medical offices. With an IV, we can introduce high-quality vitamins, minerals, and homeopathic remedies directly into your circulation. This means they do not have to be absorbed through the intestines and liver.

Intravenous therapy is helpful for people who are debilitated or chronically fatigued, who do not have good digestion and absorption, or who require more intensive therapies over a shorter period of time than oral therapy provides. Intravenous therapy, such as high doses of vitamin C in cases of cancer, is becoming an effective mainstay in many successful treatment programs.

HERBAL MEDICINE

Herbal medicine is an ancient approach to healing that is becoming more widely applied and integrated into health care today. There have been many research studies at major centers verifying the effectiveness of herbs in the treatment of acute and chronic conditions. This has been, of course, a fact known to natural medicine practitioners for centuries.

There are many brands of herbal products. How effective the herb or herbal combination is depends not just on the herb, but also on the source and preparation of the herb.

The combinations of herbs in herbal formulas are safe and almost always without the side effects of prescription drugs and over-the-counter drugs. In these combinations, some herbs strengthen, some give tone, some normalize function, and some relax and support elimination. The herbs in each combination function as a whole, producing a balanced effect on these different functions. Please use these herbs in their recommended doses. Initially, take only a small amount to make sure there is no reaction.

DIGESTIVE ENZYMES

Many people are deficient in digestive enzymes. Enzymes are metabolic catalysts. That is, their presence is required for many necessary metabolic reactions to occur in the body, and to do so with correct timing. If there is a deficiency of these enzymes, it then becomes more difficult to absorb and utilize nutrients from food. Health food stores are filled with literature on this common problem.

Most people with chronic disease and/or digestive problems have deficiencies in digestive enzymes and stomach hydrochloric acid. Our modern way of life leads to these deficiencies. Foods that are processed, pasteurized, microwaved, and cooked have had their enzymes destroyed in these processes. Also, even if digestive enzymes are present in the food or in the body, they are often unable to work effectively because the internal biochemical terrain is too acidic.

Most modern American diets lead to this acidity from eating the wrong foods. When they feel uncomfortable, people take antacids and other similar products that give temporary relief but only make matters worse by further imbalance of the internal biochemistry. In addition, the often fast-paced way people eat prevents digestive enzymes from working effectively. For example, lack of sufficient chewing will not release enough amylase from the mouth to enter into the upper stomach.

There are many brands of digestive enzymes that can be effective. Most contain combinations of amylase, protease, lipase, and cellulase. In the body, these are necessary pancreatic enzymes for maximum absorption of food nutrients. In supplements, you can buy these enzymes in a non-vegetarian form or a vegetarian form (the same enzymes are derived from plants). There are many store brands, as well as brands sold only through practitioners. In a comprehensive therapeutic program, doctors discuss with patients the advisability of using digestive enzymes.

OXYGEN THERAPIES

Oxygen has a wide range of uses in the expanding field of effective therapies. Except for oxygen through canulas and masks, and hyperbaric oxygen treatments for burns and carbon monoxide poisoning, allopathic medicine has not taken advantage of these therapies. Intravenous ozone and hydrogen peroxide therapies, when administered correctly, are an effective treatment for chronic and acute illnesses. They are legal on a state-by-state basis. Hyperbaric oxygen chambers are a key part of integrative medicine. They are used successfully with stroke patients, cerebral palsy, and other chronic neurodegenerative disorders, and are indicated in other conditions as well.

CHELATION

Chelation is a well-established therapy in integrative medicine, and courses are regularly taught by ACAM (American College for Advancement in Medicine). Over the years, many physicians have been threatened or had their medical licenses taken away for using chelation with patients. This is changing for the better. Thanks especially to the research of Dr. Garry Gordon, M.D., chelation therapy has evolved beyond what most doctors have used it for, as a roto-rooter therapy for blood vessels, and into its key role as an important therapy in heavy metal detoxification. Virtually all people in the United States have heavy metal toxicity. Dr. Gordon teaches physicians an effective five-minute EDTA IV treatment for evaluation and clearing of heavy metal toxicity.

COLON THERAPY (COLONICS)

It may be that the majority of chronic and degenerative diseases have their origin in long-standing dysfunction of the digestive organs. Breast-fed infants have a population of 99 percent Bifidobacterium bifidum in the colon. After weaning, their intestinal flora changes to become primarily of Lactobacillus acidophilus. However, the colon flora of bottle-fed babies contains many unnecessary bacterial species. This leads to lessened immunity, and thus to the following common illnesses of childhood: colic, allergies, asthma, and otitis media. Receiving foods that are too complex early in life, especially cow's milk products and wheat, are significant contributing factors to childhood illnesses and many chronic adult illnesses.

The colon is much more than an organ of elimination. Many vitamins and minerals are absorbed through the walls of the colon. Some, such as vitamin K and several B vitamins, are synthesized in healthy colons that have a majority of beneficial Lactobacilli. The type of bacterial population in the colon is an important determining factor in the health of the entire body and mind.

As noted previously, our predominant medical system approaches all bacteria as invaders, enemies that must be eliminated. Antibiotics are specifically designed to kill these bacteria that are believed to be the cause of infectious disease. As a result of the overuse and overdependence on drugs such as antibiotics, anti-fungicides, and anti-parasitics, the microorganisms within our bodies have grown much smarter. They have developed capacities of mutating into strains that are much more disease producing than earlier forms.

Our colons have been forced to bear much of the brunt of our culture's obsession with this quick-fix pharmaceutical treatment approach. Unfortunately, that has now made us more vulnerable to disease than ever before.

Establishing healthy colonic microflora is essential to attaining good health. Many people today use laxatives, which drain the body of valuable minerals and harm the colon in other ways. Others believe that bulk agents such as psyllium seed or oral Lactobacillus supplements help cleanse the colon and improve function. However, these efforts are often not effective enough when used as the primary or initial step in improving colon function.

What is often required is colon therapy. Colon therapy has become a mainstay in the treatment of many chronic diseases. A trained colon therapist administers the therapy. Up to six initial treatments are typically required to clean a colon that has become toxic. Some colon therapists take two additional steps. They reacidify the colon, because Lactobacilli require a slightly acid environment in which to grow. Then they implant live Lactobacilli in the rectum. It is important to ask a colon therapist if he or she is trained in these latter two effective approaches.

144

FUNCTIONAL MEDICINE

Functional medicine, spearheaded by Jeffrey Bland, M.D., of Gig Harbor, Washington, is a growing area of integrative medicine. Functional medicine involves evaluating and treating based on the status of organ and tissue function, instead of looking only at structure, as with an X ray. Certain laboratories have developed tests that permit the practitioner to evaluate liver function, for example, by seeing how well the liver detoxification pathways clear a pre-measured amount of a substance that the patient takes orally. Other examples are cardiovascular risk profile tests and heavy metal challenge tests with EDTA that involve measuring the amount of metals in a six-hour collection of urine (see Chapter 12).

The patient is evaluated in this way over time. Then treatments are administered in the form of homeopathic remedies or nutritional supplementation that improves organ function and detoxification pathways. By doing this, the biological terrain is improved and the patient's capacity to heal is enhanced. Functional medicine that evaluates and treats based on physiological response is an improvement over the predominance of structural and chemical medicine, which is the foundation of surgical and drug-oriented allopathic medicine.

The objection that some raise about functional medicine is that it is still primarily treating with supplements. While this is often better than drugs, the level it is addressing is still primarily the physical level. We must evolve our approach to healing and include much more of what is called energy medicine, which is covered later in later sections.

CRANIAL OSTEOPATHY

A three-year-old little girl was scheduled to have eye surgery, a shortening of the eye muscles, then eye-patches for three weeks, while strapped into a crib at the children's hospital. The parents were told that she would probably need similar surgery at least twice before completing high school. She was taken to a cranial osteopathic medical doctor for help. He found that the left occipital base of her skull had been pushed forward and up high, probably at birth, and that due to pressure on the visual cortex, the eye muscles could never work properly. He added that all serious visual disturbances in children were usually the result of cranial compression that occurred during birth, or from a fall. Following the visit, the cranial osteopath requested that the little girl's thick glasses be removed since he believed her vision would improve greatly overnight. The next morning her 20/400 vision was 20/20, and the strabysmus had completely resolved.

A wondrous, steady, rhythmic flow of cerebrospinal fluid pulses eight to ten times per minute throughout life, matching our respiratory rate while we are in deepest sleep. Named the primary cranio-respiratory mechanism, it is the only known constant rhythm in the body, not changing with physical or emotional activity like the heart rate, respiratory rate, and lymphatic flow, which vary from moment to moment. The origin of this pulse is not yet known, but has been directly viewed by anesthesiologists during brain surgery. Cerebrospinal fluid is held next to the brain and spinal cord by a thick fascial membrane known as the dura mater, strong mother that flexes and extends with the slow pulsations. CSF completely remakes itself every four hours, delivering one hundred ten nutrients to the brain and the spinal cord.

Cranial pulsation is palpable with very light touch anywhere on the body since all fascia in the body is interconnected. Fascia continues from the dura, wrapping around the bones, muscles, and organs, suspending and separating. Very elastic, it shortens and binds when impact or injury occurs, as a protection, a kind of splinting. Until it is released it can pull on the connecting fascia, and circulation of all fluids can often be impeded. During birth, dura mater can become pulled up on one side. Results can include chronic ear infections, visual problems, digestive disturbances, reading difficulties, headaches, developmental delays, behavior differences, auditory discrimination, and scoliosis, to name a few.

Chronic ear infections are often resolved with cranial therapy once the compression on the Eustachian tubes is relieved and they drain properly. Occipital stress is visible in many ADHD children: on profile the line of the neck moves straight up the back of the head with no rounding out of the base of the skull. Pressure on the brain stem can cause the nervous system to chronically stay in "fight or flight," causing impulsive behavior and poor sleep. Once the occiput floats back and self-corrects, a positive shift happens. Many stressed children and troubled teens transform, relax, follow the rules, and sleep after good cranial osteopathic treatment. Increased self-esteem follows.

Most autistic children have a compressed fourth ventricle, the small chamber in the center of the brain where new cerebrospinal fluid is made every four hours. One non-verbal six-year old initiated his first conversation after two cranial sessions, with appropriate questions and full sentence answers.

Adults also benefit greatly. One fifty-four year old client who experienced a lifetime of headaches was free of them after two sessions. Then her hair, which had been gray for twenty years, came in dark brown at the roots. Hyperactive adults verbally describe the deep relaxation that occurs for them after cranial therapy.

All osteopathic medical students now learn craniosacral technique. Those who teach them claim that about 4% are really enthusiastic as they learn, and just a few of those actually include it or make it the core of their practices. Learning to palpate the subtle mechanics of the CSF hydraulic system requires concentration and attention to the flexion and extension patterns, the patient's respirations, temperature changes of the skin, sensation of fascia unwinding outward in a spiral, and ever-changing symptoms. Techniques are taught to other health practitioners one-on-one by individuals, in weekend, or week-long seminars and workshops. Many practitioners continue learning in study groups where they share case studies and work on one another to refine techniques.

Research has shown that 95% of all human beings need cranial therapy for optimum health. The amplitude of the cranio-respiratory mechanism is now considered one of the best measures of overall health. Many homeopathic practitioners have learned the techniques themselves or have brought a cranial practitioner into their office, finding a great synergy between combining the homeopathic and cranial therapies. Many pediatricians in Europe do cranial assessment on each visit to keep the fascia freed up: after birth, then through the falls a toddler takes while learning to walk, bike accidents, and on. They educate parents that even a minor fall or blow to the head, back, or tailbone can cause fascia to splint and disturb the symmetrical flow.

The touch is extremely light; most are taught to spread the weight of a nickel over the palmar surface of the hand, and that any touch heavier than that interferes with the flow of CSF. Anxious parents of newborns are told that the touch of the cranial therapist's hands will be less pressure than a hat on the baby's head. Midwives, grandmothers, and other wise women all around the world work immediately and through the first days of life to resolve the overlapping plates that have telescoped during birth to allow the head to be born. They have done so for ages. It is a lost art that is returning, slowly, and we look forward to the time when all newborns are assessed and assisted with correcting the cranial geometry immediately for best brain development, coordination, and happiness in their lives.

This is adapted from an article written by Ann Szaur, N.D. She may be e-mailed at ann@annszaur.com.

BOWEN THERAPY

Bowen Therapy is the name for a bodywork technique that was developed by Tom Bowen of Australia from the 1950's into the 1990's. In the words of one teacher, Gene Dobkin, who teaches the Neural Touch branch of the Bowen Legacy, and from whom much of this written material derives, Bowen has been called bodywork without the work.

Unlike other therapies like massage and chiropractic, Bowen works much more subtly and energetically with what is called the body's "fascia." This is the tissue that surrounds all organs and tissues of the body. The whole body is wrapped in layers of this fascia. It is said that the fascia remembers, so problems can stay stored in the fascia for years.

The fascia is continuous throughout the body, so problems and solutions can travel from one part of the body to another. Over time and with the multiple stresses of today's life, this fascia changes from its healthy, fluid like state

147

to more rigidity and stiffness. In relation to principles of wellness, if the fascia becomes dehydrated it can shrink up to 10-15%. This puts stress on many organs and tissues.

The fascia is like a liquid crystal. There is constant ongoing communication all over the body via this liquid crystalline matrix that supports us. Similar research has demonstrated that the substance inside our cells and DNA is in constant intercommunication via vibratory frequencies through this liquid matrix. Bowen is an energy therapy in that it applies very subtle applications of touch to effect changes in the physics of this liquid matrix so that it can move towards its original health state. With subtle movements of the thumb or fingers at specific areas, the therapist can help to liquify this fascia and let this liquifying movement ripple out to blockages and help dissolve them.

There are certain moves with Bowen therapy in which the therapist very gently helps to define the patient's body to them by outlining the osseous or bony tissue with the fingers. It is taught that this gives the body a reflection of itself, whereby it can heal itself. This is similar to some cognitive therapy approaches, in which the therapist encourages the patient to speak spontaneously of thoughts and feelings, thereby helping the patient to be able to reflect upon himself. It is also similar to compresses used in anthroposophical medicine, in which the patient is able to feel his boundaries with the application of a compress.

Bowen may be seen as a transition therapy from more physical therapies to energetic therapies. Because it is so subtle, and works with the physics of the liquid fascia crystalline matrix of the body, Bowen therapy resembles homeopathy. In homeopathy, less is more. This means, as we will see in the subsequent chapters on homeopathy, that a more diluted preparation of the original substance can have stronger therapeutic effects, even when there is none of the original substance present. This is what confounds modern medical mechanistic quantity-fixed thinking. The same applies to Bowen. It is a physical therapy that uses the principle of less is more.

Practitioners of this therapy apply a slight movement of the fingers at particular points on the body to effect changes in the muscles and joints, as well as in endocrine and autonomic nervous system function. It is completely safe. Various schools of Bowen teach how to apply this gentle and non invasive work to help the body to reset itself. The particular movement that is taught involves gentle rolling moves done across superficial muscles, tendons, and nerves. It is an elegant therapy, meaning that it is simple, involves less work, and has deep and lasting effects.

The reader may do a web search at www.bowendirectory.com and find more information about the several schools for learning Bowen therapy.

B. ENERGY MEDICINE: THE NEXT STEP

The next big area that will transform our method of health care is energy medicine, which employs a wide range of therapies and diagnostic and therapeutic equipment. Many practitioners in Europe and some in the United States have been using energy medicine techniques for years. Examples are electro-acupuncture, acupuncture, and homeopathy. But the field is much more than this. The focus of energy medicine is in the areas of impaired regulation and impaired information.

Energy medicine is addressed in Klinghardt's *Holistic Integrated Map (Model) to Health & Healing* at the end of this chapter. Another individual who is addressing the subject is Dr. James Oschman in his book *Energy Medicine: The Scientific Basis*. I strongly encourage the reader to read this book.

Dr. Oschman reminds us that "while pathology may manifest as chemical imbalances, the underlying problem is electromagnetic." Unfortunately, the money in pharmaceuticals is in biochemistry, and biochemistry is still where a big percentage of money is in much of today's integrative medicine, as well as in the form of nutritional supplements.

There has been a great deal of improvisation in energy medicine since the late 19th and early 20th centuries. If the techniques developed had been integrated into mainstream medicine during the last one hundred years, they would have saved many lives and helped millions of people heal diseases. The work of Babbit, Tesla, Reich, Rife, and many others was largely suppressed and persecuted in the second half of the 20th century. Thus far the therapies they developed have been considered fringe, and have been either ignored or ridiculed by conventional medicine and the media. This will change rapidly in the coming years.

These techniques and more fall in the category of what author Richard Gerber, M.D., calls "vibrational medicine." The idea is that diseases and disorders alter the electromagnetic properties of molecules, cells, tissues, and organs. Many hands-on therapists and therapies such as polarity therapy and therapeutic touch work directly with these altered electromagnetic properties. In *Energy Medicine*, Dr. Oschman covers a wide range of energy-based therapies and techniques that need to be incorporated into mainstream integrative medicine. These include:

- Brain wave biofeedback

- Patients are taught to change their brain wave patterns. This in turn can help them improve their attitudes, sleep, biochemistry, and physiology

- Magnetic field therapy (discussed in the next section)

- Hands-on healing

- Therapeutic entrainment

- Practitioners train themselves to enter into a healing state with a patient

- Color Therapy

Energy medicine and energy psychology are fields that reflect what we now know is an interface between medicine and physics. For the past one hundred years, medicine has been under the spell of an exclusive biochemical, mechanical model. With the interface of physics and medicine, we now understand that there are many reactions in the body that take place at speeds far faster than biochemical reactions or synapse transmissions of nerve impulses.

As Karl Maret, M.D., of Heart Mind Communications (www. heartmind-communications.com) has stated, our DNA communicates by light photons, and our bodies are really energy resonators. He describes our cell membranes not just in biochemical or physiological terms, but also as a symphony of sounds that inform nerves and connective tissue of our bodies. Because we are 60 to 70 percent water, this works like a giant liquid crystal.

This water forms a liquid crystal net within us that holds the body together. Depending upon how the water molecules in our body are clustered determines how healthy we can be. Water in clean springs in nature has a low number of molecules clustered together. So this type of water, when ingested, can much more easily pass through the cell membranes and enter our cells, thereby helping the intracellular energy factories function at a higher level. Tap water, on the other hand, is highly clustered water. So anything we can do, whether it be: taking good water; to working with sound, color, or magnetics; that helps our bodies to restructure water; will enhance our healing process.

We need to think more in terms of the effects of energy and less in the narrow, restrictive biochemical model that is predominant primarily on a pharmaceutical drug level, but also on a nutritional supplement level. The more we, practitioners and patients, can work on the level of energy medicine and energy psychology, the more we can influence our metabolism, our absorption and utilization of nutrients, and help in our process of detoxification and rebuilding.

At this time, early in the 21st century, many more energy medicine therapies are being practiced across the country. Some are covered here.

HOMEOPATHY

Homeopathy is a safe, effective, and inexpensive approach to healing. It is widely used in the treatment of most modern acute and chronic illnesses and psychological imbalances. Homeopathic medicine is also especially helpful in treating childhood illnesses. Homeopathy is true preventive medicine because it helps the practitioner to recognize and treat functional problems before pathological disease changes occur.

Homeopathy operates on the principle that there is a therapeutic correspondence between processes in nature and illnesses in people. Homeopathy discovers this correspondence through what is called "The Law of Similars." The clinician takes an extensive history, much more than is seen in mainstream medicine. After having put together a composite of the patient's symptoms and signs, in a process that sometimes requires two hours, the practitioner then strives to discover what substances in nature will produce this similar composite picture when given to a healthy person. These substances are then administered in a potentized form to the ill person to promote healing. The idea is that every illness has a counterpart in nature that will awaken a therapeutic process.

The focus of homeopathy is not just the relief of symptoms, rather the healing of illness. This is accomplished by awakening a patient's latent inherent capacities to heal. The homeopathic practitioner seeks to understand and develop a picture of the intricate relationship between symptoms and the client's totality of being: physical, emotional, mental, and spiritual. The extensive initial interview helps the practitioner to acquire this necessary insight into a client's illness and its biographical circumstances.

After this in-depth evaluation, how does the homeopathic practitioner arrive at the remedy program that will awaken a healing process? As the biography unfolds, the homeopathic practitioner strives to perceive the similarity or correspondence between the patient's illness, and the homeopathic remedy that best fits that patient. Homeopathic remedies are most often prepared from the specific remedial capacities of particular plants or minerals.

These capacities are released from natural substances by qualified homeopathic pharmacies through a process of what is called potentization—the dilution and succussion, or repeated rhythmic motion, of a substance from nature. This preparation process releases latent forces that have been held inactive in the chemical bonds of that substance. These dormant or sleeping forces, which we are now able to measure scientifically, are brought to life in this process of potentization. They are then turned into a pellet or liquid that may be taken safely.

When correctly prescribed, homeopathic remedies bring into activity the forces of healing that lie dormant in every person. This often results in an enhanced sense of well-being, vitality, and capacity for clear thinking.

Many of the homeopathic remedies used in the United States are imported from Europe. In certain countries in Europe, homeopathic remedies must meet strict government criteria in order to be sold. These European remedies are made from preparations of fresh, whole plants, rather than dried plants or parts of plants. This makes them more effective. They are picked at different times of the day and different seasons of the year, according to when their alkaloid or active component is strongest. Special equipment, including thin-layer chromatography, is used with each batch of many of these remedies to ensure that alkaloids are still present and that the specimens are not contaminated with heavy metals.

Homeopathic remedies are not prescribed for the purpose of symptom relief. Unfortunately, many people take supplements, herbs, and homeopathic remedies with this goal in mind. Many people believe that if they take a certain remedy and their uncomfortable symptoms disappear, then the remedy was a success. This may sometimes be true, if the underlying disease was healed at the same time. However, it is possible for symptoms to disappear with natural medicines, while the underlying imbalance in the body's chemistry remains and worsens. Keep in mind that homeopathic remedies and other therapeutic modalities are prescribed to help the body heal, not just to alleviate symptoms.

Classical Homeopathy

In the Unisys or classical approach to homeopathy, a classical homeopath will, over several hours of a patient interview, find the single best one remedy for the patient. Experienced classical homeopaths have had very good results. The reader may refer to my book Rhythms in Time: The Homeopathic Future for more in-depth descriptions of both classical and drainage/combination homeopathy.

Homeopathic Combination Remedies

These are most often combinations of remedies from plants and minerals, and they may also be derived from animal and even occasionally human tissue. They are generally of low potency, which means they will be gentle, yet still effective.

Many people are ill because of years of suppressive therapy and a buildup of toxins in the body. Repeated courses of antibiotics, other pharmaceutical drugs, surgeries, inadequate coping with stress, chemical exposures, heavy metal accumulation, inadequate eliminations, and poor nutrition are all contributors to illness.

Combination remedies encourage a process of detoxification by opening biological eliminatory pathways that may have been closed for many years. These remedies reactivate dormant enzyme systems in the body and encourage the organs of elimination—especially the liver, kidneys, skin, and gastrointestinal system—to function better in their role of eliminating toxins from the body. The term for improving this function is called drainage. Many combination homeopathic remedies are either low-potency drainage remedies from herbs or minerals or combinations of both that increase the circulation to specific organs. By increasing the circulation, these remedies improve the metabolic function of the organs of elimination.

A remedy program is highly individualized, depending on many factors and taking into account the individual's history, physical examination, and laboratory tests. Combinations of remedies are suggested to provide slow and gentle improvement over several months. The combinations often change monthly or every six weeks.

The purpose behind prescribing these combination remedies is to promote detoxification and drainage of toxins from key body organs. The subtle energetic effects of the remedies induce biochemical changes in ways that are gentler and more effective than is often the case with conventional medicine.

Elimination of parasites is typically part of an initial program. Most people have parasites in their systems. Viruses and other microorganisms may hide within the parasites and be very difficult to eliminate without first treating the parasites. This is especially true in many chronic diseases. At the same time, parasites will always be with us. They digest decaying tissue in the body. So it is important to work toward eliminating the toxic material in the body that, when it decays, becomes food for parasites and other microorganisms. Unfortunately, many stool tests for parasites do not find parasites even when they are present. And, many of the natural herbal approaches are not always effective, especially in eliminating parasites that are hiding in places in the body other than the intestines.

The signs that combination remedies are working are increased bowel movements, increased urination, and a general sense of feeling better.

Acute Remedies

Acute remedies are prescribed for acute conditions such as sore throats and bronchitis. Though single remedies may be taken for these conditions if there is a clear picture of the remedy, often combination remedies are also very effective. Acute remedies are safe to use and do not suppress illness. Symptoms improve because the remedies strengthen the immune system. Take as directed.

ANTHROPOSOPHICAL MEDICINE

After a summer homeopathic course in the 1970s, I was invited to the house of one of my instructors, the late Dr. Henry Williams, in Lancaster, Pennsylvania. While the others sat around the dinner table, I wandered into a library-like front room of the house. There were many old books and I felt as though I were in some archive of ancient books; it felt like home. I began to look through some of the books. Most of them were written by Rudolf Steiner, of whom I had not heard before. I quickly became fascinated with his writings, and have continued to be so to this day. There are books I have read, or speakers I have heard, that I feel a connection with, as if when I read the books, I am drinking from a deep fountain. Steiner's anthroposophical medicine, about which I read a little that day, seemed more like a deep cosmology. I have studied it extensively since then and still feel that I have much to learn about this remarkable medicine.

Rudolf Steiner, who was also known as the genius behind Waldorf education and biodynamic gardening, developed anthroposophical medicine in the early twentieth century. Anthroposophical medicine is practiced much more widely in Europe, where entire clinics and hospitals employ this approach. With the growth of alternative medicine in the United States, anthroposophical medicine is gaining in interest and practitioners.

Anthroposophical medicine is most similar to homeopathy. Both of these disciplines use potentized remedies that are generally from mineral or plant sources. Both are highly individualized approaches to patient care. Likewise, both operate on the principle that there is a therapeutic correspondence between processes in nature and illnesses in people. However, there are some differences in how this principle is practically applied.

As in homeopathy, the anthroposophical practitioner focuses upon the totality of the client—physical, emotional, mental, and spiritual. The practitioner learns how to perceive the dynamic interactions between these parts of every person, and how these interactions alter our organ function, physiology, biochemistry, and ways of thinking and perceiving.

Through trained observation and asking pertinent questions, the physician is able to recognize subtle organic disorders involving the four major internal organs: heart, kidneys, liver, and lungs. These subtle organ imbalances may be detected long before they manifest as physical symptoms that are measurable by laboratory methods or seen on radiological procedures. The signs of these imbalances may be perceived in the person's temperament, persistent thoughts, fears, food cravings, body movements, or facial expression, to give some examples.

Each of these four organs is much more than just a mass of physical substance with biochemical and physiological activities. Each organ represents a corresponding temperament and character quality that may be observed. In other words, each organ presents a psychological-physical picture that lies somewhere along a spectrum of illness and healing. The composite picture of each person—which organs are over-stimulated and which organs are suppressed—is then put together in a diagnostic picture of illness.

Through this composite picture, the physician is able to perceive how a person's soul and spirit are blocked from being integrated with the physical body. It is in this respect that anthroposophical medicine is truly holistic. The subtler parts of oneself—soul and spirit—are not just abstract ideas that are relegated to religious institutions or psychology while medicine fixes the problems of the physical body. Soul and spirit are an integral part of anthroposophical medicine.

The separation of mind and body is the great illusion of our time. In reality, our state of health and illness is determined through experiencing ourselves through our physical body as soul-spiritual beings in daily life. When we are working to integrate our physical, soul, and spiritual selves, then we are engaged in a process of healing.

Anthroposophical physicians are able to educate their patients about the inner significance of a particular illness. Healing comes from understanding the relationship of an illness to the whole of one's life, and then, based on this understanding, taking steps to change one's lifestyle.

Based on these principles, the anthroposophical physician designs a therapeutic program. Unlike homeopathy, which is limited to potentized remedies, anthroposophical medicine is an entire comprehensive system of healing. In this sense it is more similar to traditional Chinese medicine, which is much more than acupuncture.

In addition to potentized remedies such as those used in homeopathy, the anthroposophical physician may also prescribe other modalities of healing. These include artistic therapies (sculpture, painting, music, and movement), therapeutic massage, baths with certain oils and preparations, and/or counseling. Each of these is prescribed according to a similar understanding of a patient as a being of body, soul, and spirit. For example, in addition to a combination of potentized remedies, a patient may be given a certain therapeutic eurythmy (see the section that follows) exercise. Experience and Dr. Steiner's indications have taught the physician that this particular movement is often helpful in improving the function of the liver, for example.

The counseling used in anthroposophical medicine is comprehensive. It includes exploring the biographical origins of an illness. As a process of growth in consciousness, without which there is no healing of illness, patients learn how to observe objectively what they often subjectively experienced. Conversely, without a comprehensive therapeutic program that supports inner organ development, counseling will fail.

The patient is an active part of the therapy, rather than just a passive recipient of medicines. The healing of illness is inseparable from the development of insight and the awakening of a conscious, purposeful will to redirect one's life. Anthroposophical therapeutic programs engage all aspects of a person in the process of healing.

There are many facets to anthroposophy and anthroposophical medicine, including a community of professionals in Spring Valley, New York, committed to working according to these principles. What I noticed and what attracted me when I visited this community were its economics and how the practitioners worked together. The physicians are not necessarily paid more than others working in the clinic. Income is based on need, balancing the individual's needs and the needs of the clinic and the community. Further, there is value placed on physicians not always working in the clinic as a physician. Sometimes, they are in the biodynamic garden working with the herbs they use in the clinic with patients.

I am reminded of the mother I overheard in a grocery store telling her son that carrots do not grow in stores. We in medicine are too often removed from the source points of our healing techniques and methods.

Therapeutic Eurythmy

Eurythmy, developed by Rudolf Steiner, is a type of movement therapy that is not well known in the United States. As a movement therapy, eurythmy is often placed in a category with yoga and tai chi.

Therapeutic eurythmy, however, is different. The word "eurythmy" means visible speech. The movements of this therapy correspond to images of the vowels and consonants of language visible in movement. We learn speech and language today in abstract ways, with very little living feeling for what lies in the words. So with eurythmy, we bring the pictorial back into language. Specific movements that correspond to vowels and consonants have been found, when practiced for a short time on a regular basis, to effect changes in physical structure and functioning.

Therapeutic eurythmists train for six to seven years. They often work with a physician in patient care. Initially, they observe how patients walk, talk, and hold themselves. They listen to the patient's concerns. Then, over a seven-week period, they gradually lead the patient through certain movements that correspond to an A, or an R, or an L. During the seven-week cycle, they gradually work the patient into a prescription of usually three to four letters. The patient practices the movements corresponding to these letters several days a week for 15 to 30 minutes.

Therapeutic eurythmy has proven valuable in a wide variety of clinical conditions, including eye problems, lower back pain, hyperactivity in children, and cancer.

Therapeutic eurythmy is a form of energy medicine. It brings alive the energy field and enlivens what I referred to earlier in the book as forces of levity, to help counter chronic disease conditions. Unlike many of the other therapies in energy medicine, therapeutic eurythmy is not about passively receiving a therapy. Rather, patients actively give themselves their own energy medicine daily, by prescription.

Therapeutic eurythmy is practiced more extensively in Europe than in the United States, including in hospitals and major clinics.

Developing Rhythms of Healing Through Biography

Another anthroposophical approach to therapy is biography. Developing a life biography guides us toward gaining a greater understanding of balance and how to incorporate healing. Biography is defined in the dictionary as the detailed story of a person's life and achievement. Biography as it is used in anthroposophical medicine is this and more. It is a detached recollection of the various threads that are woven together to collectively become one's life's influences. This process of recollection is a necessary ingredient of true self-healing. The physician attempts to reawaken the forces of self-healing with homeopathic, anthroposophic remedies and proper rhythms of nutrition, and the presentation of a basic picture of the delicate balance between health and illness. However, the patient must actively partake in this process so the experience of illness that initially brought him to his present life circumstances can become a vessel through which his life is transformed. Developing the biography is an imaginative way of creating this vessel.

Biography is the perceptive picture of the attempts of each person's spiritual self to shape a personality into a receptacle necessary for the manifestation of that individual's life purpose. In biography, we bear witness to the inner self's striving to become fulfilled in daily life. When the inner life is unable to express itself through our personality, the way that we meet the world, then disease may occur. As stated earlier, illness is often intended to dissolve or shatter our resistance to a greater outward manifestation of our inner lives. For example, those who exercise vigorously understand that often they must break down and destroy muscle tissue that has formed under different and perhaps more limited life circumstances, and then rebuild the muscles according to the more expanded image of life that they are now attempting to manifest: a new self-image.

What are these resistances? Resistances can take form as habits, traits, fears, and inabilities that seem to appear as shadowy figures following us and influencing our activities and relationships. It is out of these shadows that illness often grows in our lives. In biography, we take account of the chemistry of our shadows, asking:

- What role has hereditary lineage played in the development of the illness?

- To what extent have environmental, social, economic, occupational, and educational conditions influenced the development of imbalances?

In the responses to these questions are often found the threads that have become entangled and created blockages to the full expression of our life purpose. Composing a biography can reveal these blockages. Biography is an ongoing, dynamic process. To be successfully developed, biography requires an enhanced receptivity, a quality of listening to life, and an openness to confront ourselves.

Conventional biographies are limited. Often one observes in those who compose a biographical sketch of themselves an enhanced self-centeredness, only serves to further harden the personality and intensify the illness. This is evident in the attitude that "all these things have happened to me."

Obviously, this approach will not serve those who seek to solve the riddle of illness in their lives. As a biography is composed, it is important to make an attempt to survey the past with an objective and detached view. Remember that this biography will provide the tools with which to do self-research into the aspects and timing of significant events and relationships that have helped shaped your life.

Seven-Year Cycles

As the biography is developed, events may be perceived as occurring in seven-year cycles. Life's unfolding involves a series of births and deaths. Each seven-year period marks a new birth and death. What is ordinarily called birth is only the birth of the physical body as it separates from the protective maternal organism. It is also the death of a prior existence in the womb. The laws of heredity play an important role in this cycle, as do the nurturing forces that work at first through the mother and then through the home environment. It is in this period of infancy that the organs are given form. The last of these are the teeth, the hardest substance in the body. The change of teeth marks the time of the second birth, usually beginning at about seven years old. At this time, the teacher at school enters as the mediating force between the child and the world. Puberty signals the third birth, around the age of 14, beginning the period of adolescence.

After this point, the succession of births continues to unfold but are less physically conspicuous than with the change of teeth or pubertal sexual changes. These changes may be seen to manifest on more psychological levels. They are far subtler and outwardly less obvious, but nevertheless potent inwardly throughout all the adult life cycles. If what needs to be completed within a certain cycle is not finished, a residue may remain that can inhibit further development in future cycles of life and eventually precipitate illness as a way of making these residues more obvious to a person.

As the various aspects of an individual's biography are recalled, it is important to be mindful that every person and illness will be different according to when in the cycle of life the illness arose. For example, it is a very different experience if a person has the measles at seven years of age compared to at 27. Not only is the actual age important but also the life cycle the person is currently in as well as the lifecycles that have already been experienced. We are born to a particular family, into a specific country/race, were educated in such a way, belong to a certain religion, have had such and such experiences, past illnesses, certain important encounters, and so on. Begin to take note of these factors in such a way as to see what has occurred in what life cycle and under what circumstances.

Illnesses are often of a group nature. These illnesses include epidemics, environmental illnesses, cancer (an illness of humanity), and various cultural psychological illnesses such as anorexia nervosa. It is vital, then, to review one's life in the context of what groups one has been involved with throughout life. The first group for most of us is the family—father, mother, and child, or single parent and child, or adopted parent, or foster home guardian. This is followed by school, work, social groups, and so on. Take note of illness and its relationship to the group dynamics going on at the time the illness began.

If illness grew out of the stresses of the workplace, become aware of the quality of work. What aspects of character are strengthened in this work? What elements are weakened or kept back? Has the repressing of certain strivings or aspirations provided soil in which illness can grow? This is undoubtedly so for many people.

Just as history records different stages in the development of civilizations and biology perceives the growth of a plant through successive cyclic levels of growth, so a human life unfolds and manifests according to specific rhythms. Indeed, the origins of illness can often be traced to a chaos that has entered human life, both individual and collective. This chaos often grows out of a resistance to develop constructive rhythms of living that reflect laws that guide all growth on the planet. We need only listen attentively to various music compositions to appreciate the imagination and inspiration that evolves out of working in accordance with certain laws of cycle and rhythm.

The illnesses that have brought us to seek help have often grown out of past rhythms that have become imbalanced and chaotic, and no longer serve us in a constructive way. We need to develop a new rhythm of life at this time. To do this correctly, we must begin by recollecting the past in proper perspective. Therefore, when writing accounts of life and its significant turning points, inscribe these within the framework of seven-year cycles. In this way, the inherent plan of life can become more apparent.

We can approach a health crisis by asking biographical questions to reveal the light of conscious awareness that might otherwise remain hidden in our shadowy aspects. Illness then becomes a gate to walk through to discover a deeper richness in our lives. While good homeopathic care provides an initial basis for healing, conscious application of biographical principles lays a foundation for bringing forth our innermost dreams and sense of purpose into man-ifestation.

The reader can learn more of the anthroposophical approach to biography in *Phases*, by Bernard Lievegood, M.D., available at the Steiner Books website (www.steinerbooks.com)

BIOLOGICAL MEDICINE

We are faced today with a growing epidemic of acute and chronic diseases and infections. While modern hospital-based medicine has been very successful in surgical techniques and emergency medicine, in large part it has been unsuccessful in bringing forth therapies that help us heal from chronic disease. As a result, there has been a tremendous growth of alternative medicine therapies, many of which are very helpful.

A number of these alternative approaches have been integrated into biological medicine, which has developed in Europe over the last 45 years. Biological medicine is an effective and successful approach to the healing of disease, and combines homeopathy, acupuncture meridian principles, nutritional understanding, and a host of other diagnostic and therapeutic modalities under one comprehensive and truly integrative pattern of healing practice. Biological medicine supports each person's inherent processes of self-healing and internal regeneration

Biological medicine is effective in treating almost any illness and is also an excellent preventative approach. Illnesses that are commonly treated by biological medicine practitioners include:

- Allergies
- Asthma
- Chronic fatigue syndrome
- Fibromyalgia
- Thyroid problems
- Rheumatism and arthritis
- Autoimmune disorders
- Cancer
- Tooth and jaw infections
- Heavy metal toxicity
- Chronic stomach and intestinal problems
- Children's illnesses such as autism, ear infections, and hyperactivity
- Chronic infections such as Lyme disease
- Cardiovascular diseases such as hypertension
- Common hormonal disorders of both women and men

Rather than merely treating and suppressing symptoms, the practitioner of biological medicine works in an active partnership with a patient to discover and address the deeper causes and underlying patterns of illness within the matrix of life. In biological medicine, there is a deep trust in the natural intelligence of the body/mind/spirit unity of each person. The focus of the practitioner of biological medicine is to help patients remove the accumulation of blockages to the full expression of their innate natures.

The guiding principle of biological medicine is that illness develops out of the imbalances in the biological terrain that comprises our internal milieu or environment. These imbalances are usually precipitated by a combination of causes, including environmental toxicities, heavy metals, nutritional deficiencies, electromagnetic disturbances, dental and other hidden body infections, as well as unresolved psycho-emotional and spiritual conflicts. A combination of these imbalances, occurring in differing patterns in each of us, will generate dysfunctional patterns in our biochemistry and physiology. We become aware of these dysfunctional patterns through symptoms. By the time symptoms occur, our inherent capacities at self-regulation have become weakened. Due to the accumulation of toxins that eventually impregnate and weaken the function of many cells in our body, our energy decreases, our immunity becomes deficient, and our thinking becomes impaired.

The biological medicine practitioner, often working in tandem with a good biologically oriented dentist, conducts a comprehensive patient evaluation. In addition to in-depth personal interviews and a physical examination, the practitioner may suggest certain objective diagnostic tests. These include computerized regulation thermography, autonomic nervous system assessment, a panoramic X ray of the mouth, and specific blood and urine evaluations that can reveal weaknesses in the function of your internal organs and tissues. It is only by addressing these imbalances in the biological terrain that we have the possibility of healing, and not merely suppressing symptoms. In recent years, these evaluations of body function have been able to define metabolic abnormalities of illness long before pathological disease occurs. This is true preventive medicine.

The wonderful multifaceted nature of biological medicine is that it integrates traditional ways of healing from ancient cultures with modern technologies. The practitioner is able to craft a unique, effective program of healing for each patient that is based on sound principles of scientific observation.

The therapies employed embrace a wide spectrum. These include more physical approaches such as nutrition and supplements, herbs, physical/structural therapies, and dynamic and energy-oriented methods such as homeopathy and acupuncture. Therapies also often include remedies to improve the biological terrain by helping to reestablish a "right relationship" between the body's tissues and the host of microorganisms that live within us.

The biological practitioner also works to uncover hidden, yet frequently present, dental focal disorders that are impacting health. In addition, the practitioner helps patients determine the inner psycho-emotional dysfunctions that are affecting their autonomic or unconscious nervous system, glands, and organs. Because illness has often taken decades to develop, the process of healing often requires time, patience, and a fundamental change of lifestyle.

As Dr. Dietrich Klinghardt explains, the attitude toward healing in biological medicine is not "How can I kill such and such microorganism?" The attitude is rather "How can I assist patients to improve their biological terrain?" so that they may tolerate the presence of certain microorganisms without being weakened.

Biological Medicines

Remedies used in biological medicine can help to balance the acid/base and internal biochemistry, and strengthen the immune system. This rebalancing of the internal terrain is an essential part of the healing process. Rebalancing the internal terrain increases the effectiveness of homeopathic and other approaches of natural medicine. These remedies are sold under the product line name of Sanum or San Pharma.

The internal environment of the body—the biochemistry and physiology—is altered by many changes, including:

- A diet rich in refined carbohydrates, animal foods, and trans-fatty acids

- Drugs, chemicals, and other carcinogens

- Lifestyle and thinking patterns which are out of balance.

When this altering of internal ecology occurs, otherwise harmless and primitive microorganisms that normally live in symbiosis or harmony with the body cells and tissues are permitted to evolve into higher toxic phases within their growth cycles. In these states they may cause tissue destruction. When destructive tissue changes occur, chronic diseases develop: arteriosclerotic vascular disease, hypertension, arthritis, diabetes, multiple sclerosis, and others.

Biological medicines have the capacity to help our bodies revert these harmful and destructive microorganisms to their more primitive and harmless forms, which can then be excreted by the body. Biological medicines strengthen eliminatory organs, including the intestines, kidneys, and skin, and also stimulate and strengthen immune defenses.

Biological medicines are bio-regulators. This means that they

- Change our internal environment beneficially

- Interrupt the ability of other disease-producing microorganisms to harm the body, both in acute and chronic diseases

- Control the amount of toxins being produced by harmful microbes in the body

- Help the body heal and stay healthy

The medicines are helpful in both acute and chronic conditions. There are different medicines for each type of condition. They can be taken concurrently with homeopathic and herbal remedies. In chronic diseases, where they are most often prescribed, they need to be taken in conjunction with other medicines that help to balance the body chemistry.

Biological medicines are named to represent the harmless primitive forms of the microorganisms they are designed to heal. For example, if the package reads Penicillium Notatum, this is not penicillin. In thousands of patients who have taken these remedies, mostly in Europe, there have been no allergic reactions, even in those who are allergic to penicillin.

How Biological Remedies Work

After years of lifestyle imbalances—poor diet, unmanageable stress, heavy metal, and other toxicities, chronic infections, lacks of exercise—people accumulate decaying material in their bodies. Eventually, because of excess acidity in the interstitial spaces, which creates conditions of low oxygenation of tissues and impairment of cell membrane function, the internal terrain and eliminatory organs become weakened. When this occurs, the microorganisms we normally live with in symbiosis are attracted to the decaying material that the body can no longer eliminate.

In a healthy body, we have a symbiotic relationship with our microorganisms. This means that when the tissues are healthy, and the interstitial space is not too acidic, the microorganisms help us. They remain in their benign, primitive phases of growth. In chronic acidic conditions, they develop into pathogenic forms. This leads to symptoms of acute illness.

To heal chronic illness, the internal terrain of the body fluids must be restored to a less acidic, less toxic, better-oxygenated condition. The biological remedies that are prescribed are the primitive phases of the pathogenic microorganisms present in most diseased tissue. These primitive phases, when taken as remedies, have been shown to induce the pathogenic, or disease-causing forms of the same microorganisms, to change back into harmless forms and be eliminated from the body. By doing this, we change the internal environments of the cell and cell membrane so they can function better.

Biological remedies can improve the body's capacity to regulate. This means the body is able to recognize changing conditions both internally and externally and adapt to them. We are then able to maintain a balance in both body chemistry and in daily life. The goal is to help reestablish an internal equilibrium on all levels—cell, tissue, organ, and organism. Biological remedies establish this internal equilibrium either by altering the structures within the cell to improve cellular chemical activity, or by changing the nature of the fluid matrix between the cells in a beneficial way.

Note that biological medicines are much more effective if the biological terrain is becoming more alkaline. Eating more alkaline-producing vegetables, taking green drinks that alkalinize, or both, will help accomplish this.

To reap their full effectiveness in chronic illness, biological medicines do need to be taken over a long period of time, sometimes six months to a year. They most often work slowly and gently, like homeopathic remedies. It is possible to have some minor discomforts, such as intestinal gas or a slight decrease in energy, for a few days to a week after first beginning them. This is a minor nuisance compared to how much they can help.

ACUPUNCTURE

Acupuncture is a therapy that dates back thousands of years. It is part of a more comprehensive approach to healing from China, a traditional Chinese medicine which includes herbs, pressure point therapy, movement therapies such as tai chi and qi gong, and therapy with food according to patterns of what are called yin and yang foods.

Until recently, acupuncture was not accepted in the West. This has changed dramatically over the last 20 years. The University of California at Los Angeles School of Medicine now teaches acupuncture to interested medical doctors, and it is taught in most naturopathic schools, also.

It has been found by Dr. Klinghardt that acupuncture points have correspondences to the autonomic or subconscious nervous system. In addition, the meridians (energy channels) that these points access can be influenced by colored light. Some researchers have discovered that light enters the body through the acupuncture points and meridians.

There are two main schools of acupuncture: Traditional Chinese Medicine (TCM), and Five-Element Chinese medicine.

This is a very brief description of this growing and effective field of integrative and comprehensive medicine.

AYURVEDIC MEDICINE

Ayurvedic medicine is an ancient form of healing that originated in what is now the Indian subcontinent. Like both Chinese medicine in the East and anthroposophical medicine in the West, Ayurvedic medicine is a whole systems approach to healing. It includes foods, herbs, movement, and medicines. These are prescribed for patients according to the patient's constitutional type, of which there are three: vata, pitta, and kapha, along with overlaps of these pure types. The reader may find more on this ancient and effective system of healing both on the Internet and in bookstores.

NEURAL THERAPY

Neural Therapy is the name given to a form of therapy that promotes healing through the nervous system. More specifically, nerve anesthetics, such as lidocaine or procaine, are injected into areas around specific nerves or in areas of the skin that correspond to specific organs or acupuncture meridians. These nerves are part of what is called the autonomic nervous system (ANS). Neural Therapy was developed by Dr. Dietrich Klinghardt (see www.neural-therapy.com).

The ANS is the part of the nervous system that is unconscious, that is, not under the control of our conscious will. Whether we are awake or asleep, the ANS regulates breathing, circulation, body temperature, digestion, metabolism, and hormone function, just to name a few of its functions. In illness, the autonomic nervous system loses its capacity to function optimally. Neural therapy can help eliminate regulatory imbalances in this system, leading to improvement of general health and well-being.

An organ never becomes diseased in isolation. Illness always involves the whole individual—body, soul, and spirit. The task of the physician is to improve the capacities of the patient to self-regulate on all levels.

Because the autonomic nervous system extends into every area of the body, by injecting scars over organs, or sometimes deeper tissues, we can improve the capacity of the body to self-regulate.

In illness there are disturbances present in the autonomic nervous system. Disturbances at the cellular level can be measured as imbalances in self-regulation: a too acidic (very often) or too alkaline (rare) environment, inadequate oxygenation, or mineral deficiencies, to name a few. The fine endings of the autonomic nerves and of the blood vessels terminate in the fluid that bathes every cell. Therefore, disturbances at the cellular level are ultimately carried by the entire nervous system.

Inflammations, injuries, bacterial infections, foreign bodies, and scars from surgery can block the function of the nervous system in specific areas of the body, affecting cellular and organ function and leading to symptoms of illness. Skillful injections of anesthetics can reverse these adverse effects, restore cellular function, and remove any blockages to healing.

Neural Therapy Helps Pain

Sometimes people get enmeshed in a cycle of pain from which they have difficulty extricating themselves. An initial injury or painful area develops, with subsequent spasms, leading to decreased circulation to the area. As a result, there is a decrease in oxygenation and toxic elimination. This creates the conditions for more pain and spasm.

A larger cycle of pain is also created. After the injury or painful area develops, with subsequent spasms, people may have difficulty sleeping or relaxing. They may take pain medications or pharmaceutical sleeping pills. Over time, these medicines can compromise the liver's capacity to detoxify and function correctly. Long-term acetaminophen can especially be a problem for the liver. This leads back again to more pain, and the cycle continues.

Neural therapy, in combination with other therapies, can help break this cycle of pain and help the body to reset the signals to recovery. Once this cycle of pain is broken, blood supply to cells is improved, waste products are moved to organs of elimination, and spasms and pain are relieved.

The nervous system is a power grid that links all cells and all organs together. Every cell in the body is a tiny battery that has an electrical charge. As long as this electrical charge is maintained, the body functions normally. When exposed to an accumulation of stresses from various sources, the electrical charge in the cell collapses. When this occurs in enough cells, symptoms of illness appear, especially pain and fatigue. With neural therapy injections we can repolarize and recharge the cells in an area of illness, and thus support the process of healing.

With neural therapy injections, we attempt to treat the source of a problem, rather than just the immediate symptoms. For example, scars from a childhood tonsillectomy may in adulthood be a source of illness in another area of the body, and this illness may not appear for years. A scar from other types of surgery or from a miscarriage can do the same. Not only do scars cross and interfere with the function of acupuncture meridians, there are also stored emotions connected with these scars. The potential exists for these scars to cause problems in distant areas of the body, sometimes years later.

The main goal of treatment is to improve the capacity to self-regulate. Self-regulation means that the body is able to recognize changing conditions both internally and externally, and then adapt to them. When self-regulating, a balance is maintained both in body chemistry as well as in thinking, feeling, and action in daily life. The goal is to help reestablish an internal equilibrium on all levels: cell, tissue, organ, and organism.

Scar Therapy

Cells that are cut, as in surgical scars, give off abnormal electrical signals for the rest of a person's life. These electrical signals then travel via nerves to other areas of the body. Excessive electrical energy generated somewhere in the body will find a way to express itself elsewhere in the body as a dysfunction. For example, an electrical signal constantly generated from an old appendix or gallbladder scar may be a contributing factor in problems such as asthma, headaches, or other symptoms of illness that are distant from the original scar.

We can often reverse these dysfunctional effects. We find the scars that are causing problems and inject them with procaine, or treat them in other noninvasive ways, such as with red lasers or wheat germ oil. The stress on the body decreases, which helps the body in its efforts to self-heal.

Before going to the office of a practitioner of neural therapy, a patient should make a list of his or her scars and where they are located. Also record the age when these scars were incurred, and any emotional events that were occurring at the time of the scarring, or whether the surgeries were emotionally difficult.

The scars that hold the most potential for improving health and removing blockages to healing after being treated are those from surgeries with anesthesia, and especially from surgeries that were emotionally difficult.

Sources of scars that can be problematic include:

- Umbilicus (from cutting of umbilical cord)

- Circumcision

- Tonsillectomy, appendectomy, hysterectomy, gallbladder and other surgeries

- Wisdom teeth and other tooth extractions

- Tattoos

- Immunization areas, especially if there were reactions

- Bone fractures, especially if they require surgery or metal plate insertion to hold bones together

MAGNETIC FIELD THERAPY

Most of us have deficient magnetic fields. This directly impacts on cellular function. Our electromagnetic (EM) fields are weakened by electromagnetic pollution in the form of electrical wiring in homes, especially near our beds, and by televisions, microwaves, overhead lights, electrical poles, cell phones, cordless phones, mixed dental metal fillings, and more. There is a significant increase in childhood cancer among children who are regularly exposed to the EM fields of power lines in many cities. Magnets placed under bed mattresses, along with removing overexposure and getting enough sleep, can help correct our deficient magnetic fields.

Magnetic field therapy is a form of energy medicine that includes the use of magnets and electrical devices to generate controlled magnetic fields. Orthopedic surgeon Robert Becker, M.D. uses weak electrical currents to promote the healing of broken bones.

CORRECTING GEOPATHIC DISTURBANCES

Geopathic. What does this mean? To most people, it does not mean much.

Yet the influences of what are generically called geo-pathic disturbances upon our state of health and disease are profound. The ways that this area of discussion is becoming most known is in the debate over the role that cell phones may play in the development of brain cancer. Of course this is much too simplistic an approach, one that only serves to diminish to role that geopathic stress plays in our lives. Studies have shown that children who live within a hundred yards of cell phone towers, which means most children in big cities, have abnormal EEG brain wave patterns. Other studies have shown that food is altered in its nuclear structures when it is microwaved. Dr. James O'Dell of Louisville, KY, has described how frequent exposure to microwaves is an important risk factor in the development of muscle weakness and in digestive problems in babies. This has become widespread without much research into how this affects our health. We can recall how watching an atom bomb being exploded was downplayed in the deserts of New Mexico during World War II, with the subsequent increases in blood cancers of those who were too close. How much have we really changed, or how much are we still permitting ourselves to be lied to, not wanting to think about the potential dangers of cell phones and microwaving foods because it would interfere with our convenience-oriented lifestyles?

There are case histories of patients with brain tumors, leukemia and chronic fatigue syndrome who responded favorably to treatment once issues of geopathic stress were addressed. In addition to cell phones and micro-waves, geopathic stress may include one or more of the following:

- **Underground water:** This means literally underground streams that can come up near the surface of the earth close to the place where one is sleeping in the bedroom, for example. This can have deleterious effects on health. Sometimes underground caverns with their metal charge, may also affect the biochemistry and physiology of those who live above them.

- **Electrical fields in a house or office**. This can range from having the head of one's bed next to an electrical outlet, to an excess of electric fields in a house, to sitting too long in front of a computer screen, to being indoors all day exposed to conventional fluorescent lights.

- **Disturbed magnetic fields**. This can occur if one is sleeping on beds with metal springs. There may also be magnetic fields generated by the earth under one's home or place of work.

Each and all of these can lead to changes in cellular oxidation, hormone function, chemical reactions, and other changes in the human body.

They are a big and largely ignored factor in the development of chronic illness. Sometimes the causes can be discovered with relatively inexpensive equipment that may be purchased locally. To determine other problems, such as underground water and caverns, may require a person who is trained in the art of feng shui. It is in these instances that we can see the importance of working consciously on both Stage 2, that of energy medicine, and also Stage 4, soul healing. For working with these subtle yet very real and sometimes harmful effects that derive from the earth places us in a different attitude and relationship with the earth and its forces. This is the realm of shamans, as we will discuss in Part D of this chapter.

In the future, no one will purchase a home without this thorough research being done first. These realities will be well accepted. And to do this correctly will require us to use our deeper knowledge of the human being that we acquire in Biological Medicine. For example, Dr. Rau of Paracelsus Klinik in Lustmuhle, Switzerland, describes that certain types of people, what in Ayurveda are called Vata types, are more vulnerable to geopathic stresses. So are people who are heavy metal toxic (many of us), kidney type of people in Chinese medicine, and women ages 35-60 years old.

Good food, supplements, correct homeopathic and biological remedies, may help lessen the effects of these adverse geopathic stresses. But they ought not to be discounted, especially in our large cities.

Finally, to put this into perspective, be mindful that the most important energy field we have in our lives, beyond these geopathic fields, is the field we create with our own minds and beliefs.

MICROCURRENT THERAPY

As described by Dr. Klinghardt, the energy medicine known as microcurrent therapy generates high-frequency wave patterns in low frequencies. Biological wavelengths are oscillated in ways that are nutritive to the nervous system. Microcurrent is used in lymphatic detoxification, organ improvement, the treatment of specific infections with frequencies, and improving psychological function. Microcurrent speaks the language of cells, sending information that the cells can understand and use in frequencies. This improves an individual's energy and detoxification regardless of the illness.

Microcurrents are extremely small pulsating currents of electricity finely tuned to the level of the electrical exchanges that take place at the cellular level. We can look at every cell in the body as a mini-electrical generator that generates electrical currents. By working with these currents, microcurrents allow the body to heal itself. Microcurrents support and help many different functions of the body.

These currents have the ability to penetrate the cell as opposed to going around the cell, as other stronger devices do. The "Arndt-Schultz Law" states that weak stimuli increase physiological activity and very strong stimuli inhibit or abolish activity. Think of watering a delicate flower with a water hose that is on full blast as opposed to watering it from a little glass of water and letting the water seep slowly into the soil.

Microcurrent increases the production of ATP, which is the stored cellular energy that the cell uses to function. It also increases blood circulation. Microcurrent allows the body's own natural healing process to take place. Protein synthesis is increased, which will assist in tissue repair. The polarity of the cell can be balanced. Absorption of nutrients is increased as well as elimination of waste products. In other words, homeostasis is restored, and increased fivefold. The biological processes of the neurological, endocrine, and musculoskeletal systems are affected. Microcurrent is the same type of current that flows through the human body. It has extremely low amperage that operates below the threshold of pain. People normally do not feel anything during a treatment.

170

Microcurrent can help:

- Decongest lymphatic fluid
- Mobilize metal
- Control pain
- Reduce pain from TMJ (temporomandibular joint) syndrome
- Normalize cellular function
- Balance the meridians
- Treat eye problems

ELECTROBLOC PAIN CONTROL THERAPY

Another form of energy medicine, ElectroBloc is an electric pain control therapy developed in Europe, and now approved by the U.S. Food and Drug Administration (FDA) for use in pain control. Certain types of electrical stimulation are applied to nerve ganglia in the sympathetic nervous system. Unlike TENS units, the beneficial effects of the ElectroBloc treatments last long after the treatment has ended.

Each treatment takes 20 minutes. The patient is connected to two electrodes, one near the site of the pain or the nerve ganglion that needs to be stimulated, and the other typically on the opposite side of the body. The amount of current that goes through the wires and into the body is gradually increased. The patient controls the amount of current based on what is tolerable. For the most beneficial effects, it is best to tolerate as high an amount as possible without discomfort. Treatments are either daily or several times per week depending on the condition. In severe situations, daily treatments for two weeks are advisable. As improvement is noticed, the frequency of treatments is decreased.

COLOR THERAPY

Light and color have been used throughout history to effect beneficial changes in the human body. Light/color therapy was reintroduced in modern times by Dr. Dinshah P. Ghadiali in the early twentieth century. Like many other geniuses of that time (Rife, Reich, Enderlein, Koch, to name a few), he was persecuted for his work, despite the fact that there was extensive research documenting the beneficial effects of colored light.

Color therapy is a growing and dynamic field of energy medicine. Tony Cocilova of LifeForms, a company in Prescott, Arizona, has developed a photon machine that enables the practitioner to transmit colors at different frequencies through a small penlike tip instrument and into acupuncture points on the ear or the body. The book *Light Years Ahead*, edited by Brian Breiling, documents the volumes of research being done with color and healing. On a deeper level, Dennis Klocek of the Rudolf Steiner College in Fair Oaks, California, teaches practitioners to discover the colors that a patient avoids or dislikes, and slowly begin the introduce these colors into a patient's daily life. He states that the substance of the soul is color. What color does a person not allow into his soul? Colors help the practitioner and patient to see the hidden emotional patterns that we can remain stuck in, and which may impair healing.

Color therapy also is playing an increasing role in energy psychology. In these applications, the practitioner determines particular colors and frequencies that a patient will either view through a machine, or wear in the form of colored glasses in order to bring balance to emotional issues often stored in the limbic brain. This is an important part of healing. For example, the hypothalamus is part of the limbic brain. The hypothalamus in turn regulates pituitary function, which in turn regulates our hormones. So by working with color in appropriate and effective ways, a practitioner can have significant effects on body physiology and biochemistry.

COLOR AURICULOTHERAPY

Colored light placed at acupuncture points helps restore balance to the flow of chi, or vital energy, through the body's meridians. Pulsed light, as opposed to a constant light source, has been found to increase the response of the body to this therapy. Organisms become more receptive to colored light when it is pulsed. This therapy is noninvasive, painless, and simple to administer. Color auriculotherapy is a form of acupuncture that recognizes that there is a map of all the body's acupuncture meridians on the ear, and that light enters the body through acupuncture points. Practitioners may effect changes in meridian function by applying light and color on the ear points, or on standard body points.

SOUND AND HEALING

Just as color is a form of energy medicine with well-demonstrated research and beneficial effects in healing, so sound is another form of energy medicine that has shown many promising positive effects.

Vibratory frequencies have been used in both conventional medicine and alternative medicine to treat physiological problems. For example, dissolving kidney stones with high frequency sound waves is a well-established medical therapy. Ultrasound therapy is used in treating many conditions.

There are many practitioners of sound healing in the United States. Some work with voice and musical instruments. Others work primarily with voice imprints to find the notes that are missing in a person's voice. They correlate these missing notes with imbalances in organs, and then create audio-tapes for patients that are specifically designed to correct frequency imbalances.

One of the most well known sound healing methods is the Tomatis method. Tomatis was a French physician who developed the "Tomatis Method and the Electronic Ear." Through observation of factory workers and opera singers, he developed three laws:

1. A person can only reproduce vocally what he is capable of hearing. So changes in the ear will immediately affect the voice, and vice versa.

2. By retuning or re-educating the defective ear to hear missing or faulty frequencies, these are instantly restored to vocal expression

3. Controlled auditory stimulation can alter one's self-listening and phonation.

Tomatis emphasized that his method addresses the problems of listening, not hearing. He stated that listening is the active ability or intention to focus on sounds we want and tune out those we don't want. Hearing is passive while listening involves effort. He spoke of three overlapping actions: hearing, listening, and integration.

Poor listening can begin at any age, including in the womb, for any number of reasons. The person starts to shut out certain sounds. The muscles of the middle ear relax, and over time lose their tonicity. Listening is impeded.

Based on results of testing, one listens through a tape to the sounds of music and voice that have been electronically trimmed by significantly attenuating the lower frequencies. This opens up the auditory diaphragm and enables the person to perceive sound with less distortion over the range from fundamental frequencies to the highest harmonics.

Tomatis talked about the ear as being more than an organ for hearing and listening, or for maintaining equilibrium. It is intended to effect a cortical charge, to increase the electrical potential of the brain, which is then distributed through the body by the nerves. He called those sounds that are rich in high harmonics the sounds that increase this cortical charge. He pointed out the difference between the vitality of opera singers who can produce these sounds, and depressed people with dull, toneless voices with very little high frequency content.

173

The vagus nerve, which connects first with the eardrum, and then to all the organs in the body, is stimulated by sound. The sounds develop new pathways in the brain, which create more options and flexibility in perception. The vagus nerve is a main part of our parasympathetic nervous system, which is often deficient in people who are ill.

This approach has been used successfully with people with:

1. Attention Deficit Disorder
2. Learning Disabilities
3. Depression and low energy
4. Speech, voice, and language problems.

There are now many additional approaches to sound and healing. Auditory Enhancement Training, or AET, is the therapeutic use of sound in the form of electronically altered music. It is a proven therapeutic process in such disorders as autism, autistic-like behaviors, developmental disorders, attention deficit disorders, dyslexia, learning disabilities, and hearing sensitivities. People with the above disorders often have deficiencies in processing sensory input. AET helps to correct these deficiencies by enhancing aspects of hearing perception.

Auditory Enhancement Training, with its ever-changing and deliberately unpredictable modulation of music, influences specific areas of the brain that involve processing incoming sensory input. More specifically, these are areas that concern both auditory (hearing) and vestibular (balance). These areas of the brain contain the neurotransmitter norepinephrine, which is involved in alertness and motivation. As a result, in addition to improvement in sensory integration, one often observes improvements in behavior. These are due to a change in the brain neurotransmitters.

The success of this therapy has been documented through behavioral observations by clinicians and parents. In addition, there have been more objective measurements of the changes in brain function after therapy by using what are called positron emission tomography, or PET scans, at university settings. This procedure provides a radiological measurement of chemical changes in blood flow to the cerebral cortex, thereby indicating when an area of the brain is being utilized differently than before. The changes that are observed in behavior have been verified by measuring changes in the functioning of different areas of the brain that are over- or under-functioning.

There are many other ways that practitioners are working with sound. Some have machines that record the voice and then show the color that corresponds to tones in the voice that a person is deficient in. The patient then views these colors for a certain amount of time per day in order to correct internal biological imbalances.

Others, such as Mary Bolles in Boulder, Colorado, combine color, sound, and movement to help many people improve brain function. Still others work primarily with musical instruments that are individualized according to the needs of the patient. Also, therapeutic eurythmy, an anthroposophical therapy discussed in Chapter 13, involves prescribing movements that correspond to either vowels or consonants. Rudolf Steiner called eurythmy visible speech. The Dorian School of Music is an anthroposophical music therapy school in Kimberton, Pennsylvania.

Sound in Healing has previously been considered "New Age," and has been relegated to the category of "way out there." The modern research now being done by many competent practitioners, using scientific principles and documenting results, are providing us with a valuable tool for healing.

Part of the problem today is that therapies with sound and color are not patentable. They are part of the general field of energy medicine that was growing and showing results one hundred years ago, before they were suppressed by conventional medicine. This must not happen again. When these approaches become mainstream, and are used early in diagnostic and therapeutic programs, then we will be approaching the type of health care system that will help people to heal and be affordable and available to all.

INFRARED AND FAR-INFRARED LIGHT THERAPY

Infrared energy is a form of heat, transmitted by light. This wavelength of light is not visible to human eyes. Far-infrared is a wavelength next to infrared, slightly farther from the visible red. We feel this form of light as heat. There is evidence that when used for 30 minutes daily, infrared light therapy can improve eyesight, treat ringing in the ears, eliminate skin tags, and improve joint function, among numerous other effects.

Studies have also shown that red/infrared lights applied locally to the jaw can help heal cavitations or hidden infections in the jawbone.

Infrared energy is useful in therapeutic saunas. It warms objects without having to heat the air between, as in a regular sauna. Infrared heat penetrates one and a half inches below the skin surface, and can therefore cause the body to sweat when the temperature is only 120°F. The temperature in a regular sauna often reaches 180 °F.

The far-infrared sauna is a medical application of sauna principles that enhance the body's capacity to detoxify. In a regular sauna, perspiration is primarily water and salt. Perspiration in a far-infrared sauna has up to 15 percent of what are called particulates—chemicals, heavy metals, and other toxins that are seldom eliminated in a regular sauna. In addition, the body's enzymes work up to 5,000 times better when using this type of sauna.

We need to detoxify as a necessary part of healing. These toxins also affect the brain. Some toxins live in the fatty tissue of our bodies and our brains. Over the years we have been exposed to many insecticides and other chemicals. The far-infrared sauna allows these toxins to be carried out through the skin.

A far-infrared sauna is much more effective than regular saunas in helping the healing process along. The far-infrared sauna has a wide variety of applications, from heavy metal and chemical detoxification to weight loss and the relief of pain to treatment of high blood pressure. Mercury, for example, is eliminated from the body through the sweating induced by a far infrared sauna and then evaporates from the skin. This takes pressure off the kidneys to do this work of detoxification. Under the far infrared heat, the skin becomes a third kidney. This is a much safer way of eliminating mercury, which can damage the kidneys.

It is optimal to exercise for 15 minutes before the sauna, but not absolutely necessary. Three towels are required: one to sit on, one under the feet, and a third to wipe the perspiration. This last towel is very important for the beneficial effects of the sauna. Wipe off perspiration as soon as it appears on the skin. Also, throughout the sauna sip from a glass of alkaline water or a glass of water with electrolytes. The typical far-infrared sauna session is 30 minutes at 120°F. After the sauna, take a shower. Sit in the sauna daily for maximum benefit, although even once a week is helpful. For more information, see *The Manual of Sauna Therapy*, by Dr. Larry Wilson (www.drlwilson.com).

MATRIX REGENERATION THERAPY (MRT)

According to the MRT manual, the matrix of the human body is the primordial sea that survives inside us and out of which our human cells are nurtured into development. The body is the collective mass of our connec-tive tissue, which contains water, protein networks, and fibrocytes. Our immune, endocrine, and nervous systems, which extend throughout the body, depend on a clean matrix for healthy function. Because of pollution and many by-products of present civilization, our matrix has become toxic. It can no longer function as a regulatory mechanism for our organs and cells; it can no longer help us to keep a balance between buildup and breakdown. This is when disease occurs. Because this matrix connects all areas of the body to everywhere else through its electro-biochemical nature, disease can be communicated from one area of the body to another.

Nerves, hormones, and immune cells all have receptors for each other on their cell membranes. There is constant communication between all areas of the body. With ongoing toxic exposure, parts of our matrix become hyper-reactive. This leads to the symptoms of illness we experience. The functional state of our matrix is directly related to the course of a disease. Examples of toxicities are free radicals, excess acids, heavy metals, by-products of chronic infectious microorganisms, and environmental pollutants. The adrenaline and cortisol we produce when we are under prolonged low-level stress for many years leads to restructuring and hardening of our connective matrix, in other words, premature aging.

Matrix Regeneration Therapy is a mechanical way to detoxify and improve the function of this matrix. With this therapy, a negative pressure is produced on the tissue of the back or other area with a suction rod in a manner similar to cupping. (Cupping is a technique used in acupuncture in which a vacuum is created with a glass cup placed on the skin, which is then moved along a meridian, most often the Bladder meridian on each side of the spine.) Treatment is initially over the entire back. Due to the suction effects, deep red stripes appear on the skin. This may initially be uncomfortable, but the effect lessens with progressive treatments.

Through a roller electrode in the suction rod, MRT is able to repolarize and return our cells to their normal electrical potential. Waste material is then removed from the body, our tissue is depolarized from negative to positive, and our metabolism can switch more easily from depending on fermentation, which is disease producing, to the healthy metabolism of carbohydrates, which is energy producing.

CHI MACHINE

The Chi machine, another from of energy medicine, relaxes the entire body, gently and rhythmically moving the body from side to side. This massages the internal organs. As Dr. Klinghardt has explained, the gentle rocking motion of the Chi machine milks the chain of nerve ganglia on either side of the spine. The result is to relax the sympathetic nervous system. Because most people have an overactive sympathetic nervous system (see "Autonomic Nervous System Assessment" in Chapter 12), and because this over-activity impairs nutrient and oxygen delivery to our cells, any therapy that relaxes the sympathetic nervous system, such as the Chi machine, is beneficial. It has been estimated that 15 minutes on this machine gives oxygenation of body tissues equivalent to 90 minutes of walking.

The major benefits of using this machine are cellular activation, spinal balancing, improving the immune system, exercising the internal organs, and restoring a balance to the autonomic or automatic/unconscious nervous system, which regulates our internal organ function.

This therapy is helpful for many health problems: tiredness, sore muscles, arthritis, poor functioning of internal organs, asthma, obesity, and other chronic conditions. Its gentle rhythmic movement of the spine is therapeutic for many chronic back problems.

For those older than 55 years of age, initially it is best to limit sessions to two to five minutes daily. If no discomfort is experienced, then the sessions can be extended to five to ten minutes the second week, and then to 15-minute sessions in the third week. For those who are younger than 55, initial sessions of five minutes twice daily, increased to 15 minutes per session, if no discomfort is experienced, is a good protocol.

The Chi machine is contraindicated immediately after an operation, in cases of serious heart disease, during pregnancy, and within 30 minutes after eating. If extreme pain occurs during use of the machine, stop and consult with a physician. People who have had brain injuries and still have symptoms, such as dizziness or vertigo, need to consult with their physician before using a Chi machine.

C. ENERGY PSYCHOLOGY

Energy psychology applies the principles of energy medicine to working with the psyche to bring about healing at another level. The types of energy psychology covered here are Tapping and Applied Psycho-Neurobiology.

TAPPING

Tapping, or Mental Field Therapy, is considered an energy therapy. Tapping performs the therapy in specific ways at specifically prescribed points on the body. Patients can learn how to do this tapping for themselves. The points tapped correspond to acupuncture points. Tapping is done to repair the disruptions at more subtle energetic acupuncture points that result from emotional traumas and deep conflicts. Although the roots of tapping go back two thousand years in Chinese medicine, tapping as we know it today comes from the work of Roger Callahan's Thought Field Therapy (TFT). This was then followed by Gary Craig's Emotional Freedom Technique (EFT), and then by Dietrich Klinghardt's Mental Field Therapy (MFT).

Tapping could be the most important of all energy therapies. This is because tapping specifically repairs energetic tears in the meridians that occur because of our beliefs and thoughts, which exert a powerful effect on our electromagnetic fields and our biochemistry.

Tapping specific energy meridian points on the body begins the process of disengaging from negative, destructive emotional and thought patterns that weaken our energy, and restoring life-affirming connections.

A special application of tapping includes tapping while taking a medication, vitamin, or herb. This helps the body welcome the substance and metabolize it properly, and prevents the body from developing an allergy to it. Tapping can also help desensitize the body to substances that cause an allergic reaction. Holding a hand over an organ area, tooth, or other body part while tapping can reestablish normal energy flow through the area. Tapping can help ease aches and pain.

APPLIED PSYCHO-NEUROBIOLOGY

Applied Psycho-Neurobiology is a powerful and effective energy-based psychotherapy. Many people who have developed chronic disease have unresolved psycho-emotional imbalances and traumas from earlier in life. Though they may have been forgotten, the effects of these traumas remain in our organs, tissues, and cellular structures. Specifically, they affect the function of our autonomic nervous system, the part of our nervous system that directly regulates all of the functions in our body. These traumas that are stored our organs, tissues, and cellular structures make us vulnerable to storing heavy metals or developing infections in those areas.

With Applied Psycho-neurobiology, the source of unresolved emotional issues and how they are affecting us at this time can be identified in the body. Often, these stored issues and the diseases that develop from them are connected to one or more of our family relationships. Practitioner and patient review a family genogram, or family tree that spans at least three generations of our family heritage. The treatment then uses colored glasses, EMDR (Eye Movement Desensitization and Reprocessing), tapping (Mental Field Therapy), and other physiological/psychological processes that help to access and lessen the harmful effects of subconscious and unconscious stored memories. More information on this is available from the American Academy of Neural Therapy (www.neuraltherapy.com).

D. SOUL HEALING

Soul healing is a term used to describe levels of healing that goes deeper than physical, energetic, emotional, and mental. Much illness today arises from the soul level, and then manifests at the chemical, physiological, and psychological levels. Our society today is deeply ill on a soul level so most of us suffer from this.

There are an increasing number of good practitioners who work on this level. However, they are often not valued or recognized because conventional medicine, and even much integrative medicine, becomes too focused on products and techniques.

In the area of soul healing, we have practitioners of systemic family therapy, shamans, and medical intuitives who can work from a distance. Some healers, who work from a distance, use radionic devices, pendulums and

179

dowsing. Others are more direct and do not use intermediary devices. Here I cover systemic family constellation therapy, which is an extension and more in-depth experience of Applied Psycho-Neurobiology.

SYSTEMIC FAMILY CONSTELLATION THERAPY

We are all part of a family, and that family goes back many generations through the maternal and paternal lines. Our culture has long acknowledged that future generations carry the hopes and dreams of the generations that came before. What is less understood is that future generations also carry the unfinished business of previous generations, and that this unfinished business can affect our physical as well as our psycho-emotional health. As older generations expect the newer generations to carry on, it may come as a surprise to them and to us, too, that we do carry on. Out of love for our ancestors, we unconsciously adopt their unfinished stories, and live out these stories in our present-day lives, making the same mistakes and suffering the same type of fate they did. This is called an entanglement. We become entangled unconsciously out of love for our family. In comprehensive medicine, it is important to explore these unconscious family ties, or entanglements, because physical healing will not be successful if we do not restore health to our family soul.

Systems theory views the world in terms of interconnectedness. In systems theory the whole is greater than the sum of its parts and therefore cannot be reduced to its parts without losing its identity. Each part of the system contributes to the whole, and whatever affects a part, also affects the whole. Families are systems, and each member of the family plays a role in the homeostasis, or equilibrium, of that system. In other words, each family member will do whatever he or she can to maintain the family equilibrium. One of the ways that balance is maintained is through "rules" that are implicit in the family structure and unconsciously carried out by family members. An example of a rule is "Anger is not allowed in this family." Another example of a rule is "We do not show our feelings." Still another example is the "Don't talk" rule, the tacit agreement in a family never to speak of a family member who died in childhood or a family member who disappointed the family in some way, thus effectively excluding them from the family (which has negative effects and creates an unresolved issue even when the person is deceased). When rules do not contribute to the wholeness of life and inhibit our natural forces, illness may occur.

Because the whole is greater than the sum of its parts, natural forces in family systems push the family toward health. This may take the form of an angry child in a family where anger is not allowed, or a creative, imaginative family member in a family of intellectuals. Out of fear, the family tries to subdue that person to keep its equilibrium when, in fact, that child is a messenger and a teacher for the family. The consequence for the singled-out child is enormous. The child's natural tendencies are thwarted and the child may become a scapegoat for the family and suffer feelings of inadequacy that persist into adulthood. These feelings of inadequacy play out in the form of physical illness, anxiety, depression, phobias, and so on. Because conventional psychotherapy in the United States focuses on the individual, we may not get to the core of the problem and release the internal blame, shame, and self-centered focus that many people carry, because the core of the problem is not the individual's alone.

To keep the family equilibrium, a family member often becomes a diversion and a center of negative attention in the family. An example is the adolescent who acts out so no one has to look at the workaholism of the father and the passivity of the mother. That adolescent grows into adulthood full of blame and shame, not realizing that she adopted that role out of love for her family system. When the family system is rebalanced to a more healthy equilibrium, she no longer has to carry that role. The results can be quite freeing for the entire family.

Thanks to Bert Hellinger, world-renowned family psychologist, we now recognize that the balance in family systems goes back many generations and that present generations unconsciously continue the equilibrium that has kept the family in balance. By restoring what Hellinger calls "orders of love" to families over generations, the present generation is freed from unconscious binds in a way that brings the family to a new, healthy homeostasis. Somewhere in that family tree the love stopped flowing, and to restore homeostasis, we must rebalance the family and restore the love.

According to Hellinger, the fundamental relationship in a family is the relationship between husband and wife. When this relationship is healthy, love then flows from the mother and father to the children, and the children feel secure. The child, says Hellinger, was brought into this world by the parents and owes the parents nothing. It is the responsibility of the parents to take care of the children. When the flow of love is reversed, children grow into adulthood unconsciously carrying a heavy burden. This burden may take the form of stress overload, depression, or anxiety, for example, and/or the physical form of chronic illness, food allergies, obesity, and so on.

Let's examine a patient in Family X where the unconscious rule is that the children take care of the parents. The patient does not realize that her physical pain is related to the burden of the responsibility she had always felt for her parents. Conventional psychology would look at her childhood issues and keep the focus on the patient. Systemic family therapy recognizes a much broader view. The person is a member of a family system, and to effect change for the person, the entire system must accommodate a change.

In Family X, it turns out that the mother of this patient did not feel loved by her mother. The patient's mother had an older sister who died in infancy, a loss from which the patient's grandmother never recovered. The family never talked about the baby again. The grandmother (the mother of the baby that died) had no outlet to grieve the great loss of her baby. She shut down and was unable to show love to her other children, including the patient's mother.

Family constellation therapy, Hellinger style, is conducted in a room with participants acting as representatives of the family members. When representatives are chosen and placed in their roles, they actually take on the energy of these family members and react and respond as family members would have done. This has been shown to occur over and over again in thousands of constellations in countries all over the world. The constellation facilitator looks for where the love stopped flowing in the family constellation and helps to rebalance that love over generations. He does this by repositioning representatives and suggesting sentences to be spoken that help to restore a flow of love.

In the case of Family X, mother and dead baby were reunited energetically and psychologically, through the representatives of the constellation. Love spontaneously returned for her other children, which included the patient's mother. Now the recipient of love, the patient's mother was able to tell her child that she was the mother and it was her responsibility to take care of her daughter and not the other way around. The patient felt a tremendous weight lifted from her body. She saw the larger picture of how she had unconsciously been carrying the unfinished business of her grandmother. She had been providing the love for her mother that should have been coming from her grandmother to her mother, and then down to her. Now the patient is able to continue the process of her own healing minus the burden of her mother. It is not only the patient who receives this healing. As simple as it is to access the energies of family members by representatives, so is the healing extended to the entire family system. Psychiatrist Carl Jung has been quoted as saying that as we heal ourselves, we heal those that have come before, and those that are yet to come.

Applied Psycho-Neurobiology (APN) is a form of Hellinger systemic family therapy developed by Dr. Klinghardt. As part of an office visit, autonomic response testing (ART) is used to engage the autonomic nervous system (the part of our nervous system that carries our unconscious). Organs with specific emotional issues are targeted. ART helps to determine emotional issues connected to unfinished family member issues, which the patient may unconsciously be carrying. The patient is then encouraged to close his eyes and the practitioner suggests specific sentences for the patient to speak in a dialogue with family members, dead or alive. Color therapy and mental field therapy, or tapping, are also often included in the work to aid in integrating the changes on multiple levels.

The comprehensive medicine practitioner is then able to integrate systemic family constellation work into a patient's therapeutic process along with homeopathy, energy medicine, IV therapies, nutrition, and so on, completing a picture of a whole healing process. In this way, the therapeutic program supports the energetic shifts that occur in the patient's psyche and soul as a result of the deep family work.

SOUL HEALING: OTHER EXAMPLES

What really is soul healing? This has become even more dissociated from medicine than has prayer and meditation, both of which now have considerable university-supervised studies that demonstrate their therapeutic qualities even by biochemical and physiological parameters.

This question we are really asking is: what is the soul? And what is soul illness? This is much too large an area to discuss in this book on Comprehensive Medicine. Yet the soul is generally thought of as a part of us that is more eternal.

If we look at areas like homeopathy and anthroposophical medicine, these are, in addition to being energy medicine therapies, also forms of soul healing. For example, when we take a homeopathic remedy or remedies and our arthritis improves, this is homeopathy working on an energy medicine level. But when we prescribe a homeopathic remedy that addresses what we have taken on from our ancestors as predispositions to illness, this is also working on a soul level. As we are unburdened of these predispositions from our heritage, then we become freer to express our deeper soul impulses in our daily lives. The Hellinger constellation work described previously also works on this level.

Anthroposophical medicine is similar. For example, anthroposophical physicians look at the element of warmth in a patient. By addressing and correcting deficiencies in warmth, the physician is helping the patient create an internal environment that is more supportive of soul and spiritual forces living in a healthy way in the body. Most chronic illnesses today are what are called cold diseases. In other words, they represent a process of hardening. This is seen in the hardening of our habits of personal lifestyle. This can be seen as a rigidity in our souls.

Anthroposophical medicine does not perceive the soul as separate from the body. Rather, the anthroposophical physician, in his diagnostic evaluation, learns to perceive how the person's soul is interacting with the bodily organs. Correct prescribing may permit the soul to better interrelate with the body. Therapeutic eurythmy, therapeutic painting, and other artistic exercises, are prescribed to help the person better integrate his or her soul into the body and into daily life. This is soul healing.

In addition, there are many books and teachers that are addressing soul healing. These range from Don Miguel Ruiz to the Dalai Lama to Thomas Moore and others like Jacqueline Small who support patients in reintegrating parts of themselves that have become separated off. These split off parts are what are called obsessive entities that can possess a person's soul life. This reintegration work is also a part of the realm of soul healing, also referred to as Transpersonal healing.

The realm of soul healing must once again become part of restoring the realms of healing in a new health care system. These approaches need to be valued, researched and observed. Many people are already doing this, though they are not reported much in the media. The movie *What the !#*? Do We Know?* addresses the issue of the soul healing by taking us into the area of quantum physics (see Dr. Klinghardt's Level 4: The Intuitive Body)

For 21st century medicine to be truly effective, work on the soul level must be opened up, expanded and valued for what it offers us: an opportunity to do effective deep healing work at a fraction of the cost of today's medical care.

One final note: soul healing goes beyond bodily survival. I am reminded of the phrase that Sam said to Molly at the end of the movie *Ghost*, as he prepared to cross the threshold into the world beyond this life: "The love inside, you take it with you." This is soul healing. If we can move our attention more to this realm of soul healing, then we can support people in doing deep healing work. This sometimes involves the death of the body. Sometimes, when our suffering takes on more meaning, it leads to a resurrected life in the body a person has healed through his or her illness. The person continues to stay alive. Think of what more of such people could contribute to all of us.

E. A CURRENT WORKING MODEL OF COMPREHENSIVE HEALTH CARE

The following diagram, constructed and taught by Dietrich Klinghardt, M.D., Ph.D., is a good illustration of a model of Comprehensive Medicine that is very similar to the one presented in this book. You may want to refer to this diagram while reading through this chapter, in order to give yourself a reference point for a particular therapy. The full diagram may be obtained from The American Academy of Neural Therapy in Bellevue, Washington, at phone number 425-822-2509, or at their web site www.neural-therapy.com.

You will discover that there are some differences in the levels of healing as they are described. Dr. Klinghardt refers to these levels as physical body, energy body, mental body, intuitive body, and spiritual body. In this book, the names are a little different:

- Nutritional and Physical Medicine,

- Energy Medicine (part of Dr. Klinghardt's energy body level),

- Energy Psychology (part of Dr. Klinghardt's mental body level),

- Soul Healing, the examples of which are part of Dr. Klinghardt's intuitive body level.

Dr. Klinghardt has created a very thorough model of medicine that he calls *Holistic Integrated Map (Model) to Health and Healing.*

Chapter 13 is not an attempt to replace his model, but rather to see the material in the context of other areas of this book, like health care reform, how integrative medicine is perceived today, and the psycho-physiological relationships in illness.

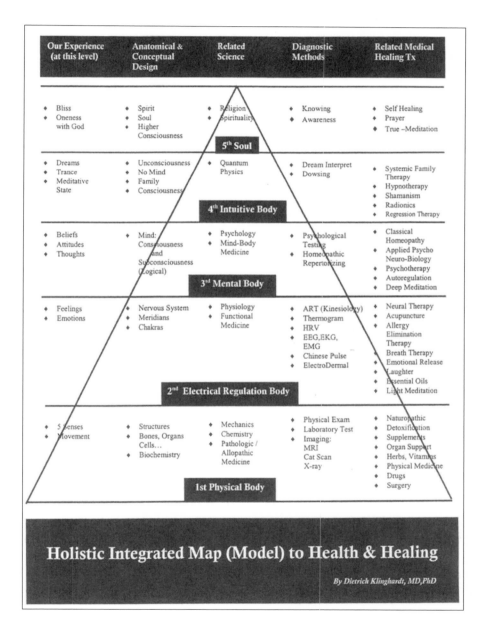

Our Experience (at this level)	Anatomical & Conceptual Design	Related Science	Diagnostic Methods	Related Medical Healing Tx
◆ Bliss ◆ Oneness with God	◆ Spirit ◆ Soul ◆ Higher Consciousness	◆ Religion ◆ Spirituality	◆ Knowing ◆ Awareness	◆ Self Healing ◆ Prayer ◆ True –Meditation
		5th Soul		
◆ Dreams ◆ Trance ◆ Meditative State	◆ Unconsciousness ◆ No Mind ◆ Family ◆ Consciousness	◆ Quantum Physics	◆ Dream Interpret ◆ Dowsing	◆ Systemic Family Therapy ◆ Hypnotherapy ◆ Shamanism ◆ Radionics ◆ Regression Therapy
		4th Intuitive Body		
◆ Beliefs ◆ Attitudes ◆ Thoughts	◆ Mind: Consciousness and Subconsciousness (Logical)	◆ Psychology ◆ Mind-Body Medicine	◆ Psychological Testing ◆ Homeopathic Repertorizing	◆ Classical Homeopathy ◆ Applied Psycho Neuro-Biology ◆ Psychotherapy ◆ Autoregulation ◆ Deep Meditation
		3rd Mental Body		
◆ Feelings ◆ Emotions	◆ Nervous System ◆ Meridians ◆ Chakras	◆ Physiology ◆ Functional Medicine	◆ ART (Kinesiology) ◆ Thermogram ◆ HRV ◆ EEG,EKG, EMG ◆ Chinese Pulse ◆ ElectroDermal	◆ Neural Therapy ◆ Acupuncture ◆ Allergy Elimination Therapy ◆ Breath Therapy ◆ Emotional Release ◆ Laughter ◆ Essential Oils ◆ Light Meditation
		2nd Electrical Regulation Body		
◆ 5 Senses ◆ Movement	◆ Structures ◆ Bones, Organs ◆ Cells... ◆ Biochemistry	◆ Mechanics ◆ Chemistry ◆ Pathologic / Allopathic Medicine	◆ Physical Exam ◆ Laboratory Test ◆ Imaging: MRI Cat Scan X-ray	◆ Naturopathic ◆ Detoxification ◆ Supplements ◆ Organ Support ◆ Herbs, Vitamins ◆ Physical Medicine ◆ Drugs ◆ Surgery
		1st Physical Body		

Holistic Integrated Map (Model) to Health & Healing

By Dietrich Klinghardt, MD,PhD

PART III:

WHY WE BECOME ILL
AND
HOW WE CAN HEAL

CHAPTER 14

UNDERLYING CAUSES OF ILLNESS

I llness takes a long time to develop. It is interwoven with our particular temperaments, characters, and types of lifestyle. The seeds of illness may have accompanied us at birth, originating from heredity as dormant tendencies. Through some event later in life, these tendencies were activated and then manifested as symptoms of illness.

The traumatic assault on the human constitution often begins at birth and continues through infancy and beyond for many years of life. This assault comes in the form of bad foods, over-stimulation of the senses, dysfunctional family environments, over-intellectual education, immunizations, multiple chemical exposures, and/or overuse of drugs, both legal and illegal. These traumas often plant themselves in our internal biochemistry and physiology. As we grow, they gradually make themselves visible to us in the form of illness, accidents, and other crises.

These and other assaults lead to what is called impaired regulation of the system. This means that our capacities to adapt to changing conditions are weakened, eventually resulting in fixed patterns of behavior that affect our internal biochemical environments or milieus and our mental and emotional natures. This internal milieu gradually becomes unable to react and adapt to various illness-generating stimuli.

As a result, multiple enzyme systems in our bodies become blocked. Our fluidity and adaptability to change is impaired both in outward daily life and in the internal biochemistry. The particular fluidity that exists as a supportive matrix between all our body cells becomes impaired. The ability is impaired for nutrients and oxygen to enter the cells, and waste products of metabolisms to leave the cells and be excreted. The internal biochemistry becomes thickened with debris, and is less able to transmit the electro-biochemical impulses that are necessary for a healthy mind and body.

When our internal milieus and our capacities to express ourselves through thoughts, feelings, and actions become inflexible, this means that chronic illness is deepening its hold on our bodies and our lives. Chronic illness is a rigidifying process of hardening prematurely.

The process of healing, then, involves first identifying where we are becoming too rigid and lacking adaptability. Then we need to make the necessary changes to dissolve these areas of rigidity and again permit adaptable movement and communication between our cells and between the different parts of our characters. The rigidity that occurs in the internal bio-chemistry affects our capacities to think clearly, to take responsibility for our feelings instead of reacting emotionally, and to act with intention in response to real needs rather than in response to instinctively driven wants and desires.

SYMPTOMS VERSUS ILLNESS: THE GREAT ERROR IN MEDICAL THINKING

It is no longer enough to say that an illness is due to some bacteria or vi-rus. For more than one hundred years, we have been under the spell of this delusion. And it is superficial to attribute all our symptoms to stress, the big buzzword today. People respond differently to stress. While one person may handle a type of stress with no ill effects, another person's internal milieu may create symptoms in response to similar stress.

Illness is not the same as symptoms. Symptoms are often what lead us to seek help. But the disappearance of symptoms—whether effected through antibiotics, antidepressants, or surgery—does not mean that the illness is gone. This is the great error in our modern medical thinking. Symptoms need to be explored and defined with more depth and commitment if there is to be true healing. If conventional medicine is how we choose to have our illnesses treated, then we remain passive recipients of health care. There is no deep healing in this approach.

The result of an individualized comprehensive medicine health care pro-gram, with its focus on education, is also often the relief of symptoms. However, symptom relief is achieved in such a way that we grow and become stronger in the process, rather than just having something done to us or for us.

In comprehensive medicine, the relief of symptoms may take longer than we have come to expect with conventional medicine. But when relief does occur, we will find ourselves different people, more alive and aware. In addition, assuming we have made the necessary lifestyle adjustments, the symptoms will not keep recurring because the illness has been healed and not just covered over. And we will recognize that this illness that we feared and had wanted to disappear quickly has in truth helped uncover our authentic selves.

In today's health care, both in mainstream medicine and not uncommonly in alternative medicine, we often put the cart before the horse. In other words, we place the elimination of symptoms at the top of our priorities. Our money goes to achieve this priority and we place the relief of our symptoms before the process of healing. As long as we do things this way, we will become weaker in body, soul, and spirit. The process of healing needs to be the prior-ity, and the relief of symptoms is the positive by-product.

We need to value our illnesses and what they can teach us about our-selves. Then we need to have patience and perseverance in staying the course and the determination to awaken dormant forces of self-healing within.

Awakening these forces comes through honest, clear thinking and objective observation about our lives and our purpose, our reason for being, and a willingness to do what is necessary to bring about healing. Working through an illness has the potential to bring one much closer to these goals and living a more meaningful life.

Healing involves disciplining ourselves to take certain homeopathic remedies, herbs, vitamins, and minerals on a daily basis for months, even years. It also involves basic dietary changes so we eat to live rather than live to eat. Furthermore, healing entails a continual and ongoing self-education as we learn to live introspectively, allowing intentional choices to replace impulsive behavior.

The relief of symptoms becomes of primary importance when we are too focused on bodily or physical comforts. By placing emphasis only on our physical symptoms, we rob ourselves of the opportunity for individual growth and service to others. When the relief of symptoms comes about through working with a comprehensive medicine practitioner, we have engaged our inherent capacities for self-healing and we attain a sense of fulfillment at having accomplished deep healing.

The process of healing is a soul/spiritual effort. Illness is an attempt to bring forth our authentic selves from beneath the layers that our personality has created in response to family, community, workplace, and other societal demands. One of the major illnesses of our time is valuing the material over the spiritual. Seen another way, this is the same as placing the elimination of symptoms before the process of healing.

For societal healing, we must build a bridge between these two, the material and the spiritual. Then, through the principles of healing that we awaken in our lives, we can make good use of money, remedies, CAT scans, and operations. Out of these efforts can grow a true sense of well-being that supports our abilities to be economically supported while developing a more enriching and fulfilling life.

In order to heal and prevent future disease, we need to know the more specific underlying causes of illness.

PHASES IN THE DEVELOPMENT OF CHRONIC DISEASE

Chronic disease takes years to develop. According to European Biological Medicine, based on the work of Hans Heinrich Reckewig, there are six phases in the development of chronic disease: excretion, reaction, deposition, impregnation, degeneration, and neoplasm.

1. **Excretion:** healthy excretion of toxins through normal eliminatory organs.

2. **Reaction:** also called the inflammation phase. When the self-healing and self-regulatory capacities of our bodies become compromised and we are unable to eliminate toxins by normal channels, we develop an inflammation. In other words, the body eliminates toxins through inflammation and infections. When we suppress these inflammations and infections and the accompanying fevers with the overuse of antibiotics, steroids, and antipyretics, we lead the body toward the development of chronic disease.

3. **Deposition:** This phase, which often continues for decades, involves the depositing of toxins in various areas of the body. These are toxins that neither normal excretion pathways nor inflammations have been able to eliminate. The toxins deposit in fatty tissues, joints, the lining of blood vessels, and other areas. People who are in this phase develop rheumatism, hypertension, gallstones, obesity, and many other modern illnesses.

4. **Impregnation:** This phase occurs when a person develops fatigue along with the illnesses from the previous phase. Now the functioning of the energy factories inside the cells has been compromised, whereas in the earlier phases the toxins were primarily deposited outside cells. Autoimmune diseases are seen in this phase.

5. **Degeneration:** When over time the body is unable to eliminate toxins adequately from the tissue and from inside the cells, we see the development of pathological diseases such as heart disease, osteoarthritis, and other chronic degenerative diseases of today.

6. **Neoplasm:** Finally, after the previous phases have developed for some time, cancer takes root in an area of the body. This means that the loss of regulatory function in an area has become so severe that the metabolism becomes chaotic

THE FUNCTION OF FEVER

Just as each epoch in human history has been characterized by the development of certain human capacities and gifts, so the various phases in the life of a human being unfold through demonstrating certain strengths and weaknesses. This panorama of birth, growth, maturation, decline, and death will at times be punctuated by illness. Each period of life differs in both the types of illnesses that predominate as well as the capacities of the individual to respond to illness.

On viewing the two poles of chronological life, one notices in youth a picture of mobility and change, which is in contrast to the image of hardening and decreased movement that too often sets into the body and soul with aging. Young children respond to illness with fever and inflammation, the signs of a healthy immune system. As the body grows older and life develops various fixed patterns, the capacity to develop fevers diminishes.

This ability of our bodies to develop fever in illness is an important phenomenon. Why? This is the organism's response to a threat to its integrity from foreign elements, such as bacteria and viruses. Fever means that the immune system is strong and active. Indeed, when a child develops an ear infection and yet has no fever, as is often the case after several courses of antibiotic treatment, homeopathic physicians recommend hot baths as a means of encouraging a fever to develop.

Actually, the "foreign elements" are always present in our bodies. They are not outside invaders. And they are not the causes of illness. Rather, infection is the manifestation of an imbalanced inner dynamic that results in an inflammatory response. Whether the source of the febrile illness is hereditary, psychological, dietary, resulting from toxic exposure, or other, a growing consensus of practitioners believe that if the illness is approached in a positive way and healed through baths, remedies, and the like, the child will grow up with a stronger immune system and perhaps be better protected against those societal forces that collectively weaken the immune response in many adults.

Early on, the inner life of a person attempts to mold the form of the body and the personality as a fitting outward instrument of expression. Often, however, resistance is encountered, sometimes owing to past hereditary influences in the body of the child. Fever assists in burning away these obstructions, and therefore serves a very useful purpose.

With its four constituent elements—calor (heat), dolor (pain), tumor (swelling), and rubor (redness)—the inflammatory response brings into active expression that which lies dormant and hidden and which might later in life prevent the full expression of the individual inner life through a suitable outer form or body. Often, parents notice that a child is somehow different after having been permitted to pass through an inflammatory febrile illness without fear or suppression from the parents.

Febrile convulsions occur mostly when there is a rapid rise in temperature in a short period of time. Many parents do not permit a fever to develop in the child out of fear of a seizure. Where does this fear originate?

The fear may represent a collectively subconscious lingering of older attitudes of civilization toward those who had seizures—namely, that they were possessed by demons.

The fear may also be a manifestation of our contemporary thinking, which is anything that appears to deviate from the normal, healthy child is not permitted to exist. Thus a fever needs to be treated, and the fear of convulsions may provide a rationale for suppression of the healthy febrile response in illness.

Many parents fear that a febrile seizure will leave the child with some permanent impairment. This, however, is quite rare, and needs to be weighed against the harm that can be done to a young person's immune system by not permitting the inflammatory response to flower.

It is generally advisable to permit a fever to exist unless it becomes too high; there is any evidence of dehydration (dry mouth, lethargy, no tears, significantly reduced urination); or the child has demonstrated a susceptibility to having febrile seizures. These tendencies can be addressed with homeopathic constitutional remedies.

Remember, the capacity to develop a fever is nature's gift to a sick person. Fever is the fire that burns out impurities, the signpost of a healthy immune system. Just as the individual with a fiery temperament permits no obstacles to block his or her path, so the healthy body responds with fever in situations that are a threat to its integrity. By appreciating the positive role of inflammatory fever illness in childhood and throughout life, we can better provide a stage for the free unfolding of our true individuality.

THE CHRONIC DISEASE PICTURE

Symptoms begin long after the disease has begun consolidating in your body. The following are the major biological causes of chronic disease in most people:

- Over-acidity
- Toxins and detoxification
- Metabolic causes
- Meridian disturbances
- Focal disturbances
- Dental disturbances
- Chronic, long-term stress
- Diathesis Disturbances

While genetics play a role in the development of disease through the awakening of latent predispositions, it is the imbalances of our internal environments that create the soil for disease to manifest. These imbalances are caused by unhealthy diets, compulsive habits, unexpressed emotions, addictions, and other similar problems of modern life. The internal imbalances present in chronic disease are overacidity of body tissues and damaged metabolic pathways. All chronic disease involves disturbances in the autonomic or subconscious nervous system. In chronic disease the brain has lost control over the autonomic nervous system and the body. The realm of comprehensive medicine is perceiving the imbalances in this system, and helping a patient to restore the inherent order of the autonomic nervous system.

Addressing these underlying issues is the key to allowing our bodies to repair themselves on a cellular level, which our bodies know how to do.

OVERACIDITY UNDERLIES CHRONIC ILLNESS

Where once there was a symbiotic relationship between body cells and simple microorganisms, now there exists what is called a dysbiotic relationship. Harmful diets and lifestyle imbalances have resulted in a growth of even more complex and pathogenic microorganisms within. Dysbiosis occurs in an internal environment that has been changed from a healthy, slightly alkaline state to a state of over-acidity of many body tissues.

The dietary factors that most often contribute to this hyperacidity are:

1. Excessive intake of refined sugars, which generate lactic acids

2. Toxicity from animal protein, especially from red meat

3. Excessive intake of trans-fatty acids, found in solid vegetable shortening

We all have alkaline reserves that exist in the form of certain base combinations with minerals such as calcium, magnesium, and potassium. Eventually, these reserves become depleted. Once the reserves are depleted, the body cannot neutralize all the acids that accumulate during each day's activities. This permits the excess of non-neutralized acid, which clogs arteries, causes red blood cells to stick together in microcirculation, and thickens the interstitial body fluid (the fluid that surrounds all body cells outside of blood vessels). When this thickening occurs, it is more difficult for subtle energy therapies such as homeopathy and acupuncture to work effectively. These subtle energy therapies act on the physical body through the interstitial fluid that moves between our cells and organs.

The increased thickening and decreased permeability of the interstitial fluids do not permit the cells of our bodily tissues to breathe correctly, take in nutrients, and eliminate waste products of metabolism. This leads to fermentation within the cells and excess lactic acid production. (Because there is less oxygen available in cells that are in acid media, lactic acid is produced by our energy-generating metabolism.) The circle of dysbiosis is complete as the lactic and other acids permit even more pathogenic microorganisms to develop.

195

When we remain in or frequently gravitate to states of anger, fear, irritability, or anxiety, we internally generate more acidity in our tissues. This impairs digestion and leads to other unpleasant symptoms.

The underlying factor in chronic diseases is continuous over-acidity—the consequence of imbalanced lifestyles. Improving emotional states and diet need to be part of a therapeutic program. Learning how to live consciously can smooth our emotional waters and help us develop healthy patterns of eating.

THE ROLE OF TOXINS IN CHRONIC ILLNESS

With the growing exposure to information from many different sources today, it is difficult not to be aware that we are full of toxins. Indeed, we may be toxic from so much information. The word "toxin" has become well used. But do we really understand what being full of toxins means in our lives?

Toxins are most often understood as chemicals that we take into our bodies through what we eat, drink, and do each day. Toxins interfere with cellular biochemical reactions that are essential to life. There are chemicals in many foods that disrupt vital enzyme systems in the body. There are heavy metals in the air or in the fillings of our teeth that damage nerve cells. The foods and beverages we crave and love to indulge in, especially sweets, alcohol, and caffeine, poison our body chemistry and alter our capacity to think clearly. The number one poison in most Americans is insulin. When we eat too many refined carbohydrates, our insulin levels go too high. This leads to excess fat storage, decreased immune function, and other problems. And the pharmaceuticals that we have taken for years generate many toxins that the body must labor to eliminate. Other toxins include electromagnetic fields, radiation from multiple sources, pesticide residues, dietary stimulants, tap water, and hidden infections. Tap water is especially a concern regarding aluminum toxicity, which plays a big role in the development of Alzheimer's disease. Tap water can also be contaminated with toxic microorganisms and gasoline additives. Dr. Mercola states that Aqua MD Laboratories (telephone: 866-278-2634) is a good laboratory through which to get an accurate test of your tap water.

The main physical toxins fall into four categories:

1. Chemicals, from food, water, and the environment

2. Heavy metals, such as lead, aluminum, and mercury

3. Microorganisms that have become chronic infections or remained dormant for years and then been reactivated. The metabolism of these microorganisms produces by-products that are toxic to our system

196

4. Pharmaceutical drugs, which have widespread use, and may actually be the most significant source of toxins today. Examples are steroids, antibiotics, vaccinations, and chemotherapy in current massive doses.

Microorganism infections include chronic viral infections. There may also be endotoxins from other microorganisms such as bacteria and parasites, which because of an imbalanced internal biochemistry are able to proliferate in the body. There are many infections that have been created or enhanced because of the overuse of antibiotics. Chlamydial and mycoplasma infections and Lyme Disease are examples. Many people unknowingly have these infections. In the same way that people fear talking about money, people fear talking about chronic infections. There is a fine line between being able to recognize and observe our illnesses and start changing our lives and being able at the same time to remain internally relaxed.

In many of our chronic illnesses there are overgrowths of specific microorganisms. For example, in coronary artery disease there is often a Chlamydia infection. In multiple sclerosis or facial neuralgia, there often is Lyme disease. Rheumatoid arthritis often has a hidden mycoplasma infection. Addressing these underlying infections with specific agents may be helpful, but it is important never to lose the focus of the big picture, of changing the terrain that permitted these infections to develop in the first place.

The whole focus of allopathic medicine, and unfortunately also increasingly of alternative medicine, is to rid ourselves of the microorganism viewed as causing an illness. This is ludicrous. We have 200,000 times more microorganisms in our bodies than our own cells. Healing happens when we change the terrain so that we coexist with the bugs in our body instead of them wreaking havoc and destroying our own cells and tissues.

To combat the onslaught of out-of-control microorganisms and toxic invaders, our bodies utilize organs of detoxification: the liver, intestines, kidneys, skin, and lymphatic system.

The liver is the main organ of detoxification. In its biochemical function, the liver combines parts of its own substances with toxins from foods, chemicals from the environment, and poisons from bacteria and other microorganisms. After combining, or conjugating, these products are excreted through the intestines. If the liver is not functioning correctly, acute illnesses may develop.

If the intestines are not moving well, toxins are reabsorbed and create more problems. In a sluggish bowel situation, harmful bacteria can create new toxins. Even with one to two bowel movements per day, the intestines may still be toxic.

The kidney is another primary detoxification organ. It filters toxins from the blood in order for them to be excreted from the body through the urine. Yet many people have kidneys that are not doing this work well, although the blood tests or X rays that provide gross measurements of kidney function are often normal. These tests are read as normal because those who read them are only looking for severe disease states with pathological destruction of tissue.

The skin is the largest organ in the body. It is the safest way to eliminate toxins, as Dr. Wilson describes in his *Manual of Sauna Therapy*. Too often, rashes are suppressed with drugs. The lymph is our slow-moving circulation. It flows in channels that knead our tissues and draw toxins out, carries them to the larger veins, through which these toxins can then be eliminated through intestines via bile ducts and through urine.

A goal of all natural therapies, whatever the particular form (homeopathy, acupuncture, chiropractic, and so on), is support and improvement of detoxification.

Chemicals, heavy metals, proliferation of unfriendly microorganisms, and pharmaceutical drugs are the commonly known toxins. There are also more subtle toxins we ingest but do not physically digest and assimilate. These enter us through advertising, for example, which is deliberately designed to kindle our subconscious wants and fears. Or they enter us through people we associate with who are raging or exercising less obvious out-of-control behaviors. These subtle toxins combine with the physical toxins and collectively alter the biochemistry and distort the way we live.

It's very important to ask the question, "How am I going to detoxify, on all levels?" This includes thoughts, emotions, metals, chemicals, and residues of drugs. Then, the question becomes "How am I going to protect myself?" The more you can use the skin and the bowels to detoxify, the better off you are going to be because heavy metals such as mercury damage the kidneys more than any other eliminatory organ.

THE METABOLIC BASIS OF ILLNESS

Illness usually involves disorders in metabolism. These disorders can be attributed to a variety of causes in addition to toxicity: genetic, environmental, psychological, and nutritional, among others. There are many chemical reactions occurring continuously, both day and night, in our metabolism. When some of these become damaged, due to a combination of the influences noted, our cycles of regulation are disrupted from their particular rhythms.

The body's resistance to infection then becomes compromised. We permit silent focal infections to develop from what are called opportunistic organisms. The toxins produced by these infections suppress the immune system even further. In addition, the toxins block metabolic pathways of energy production throughout the body's cells. This generates functional weaknesses of internal organs, which then impairs their metabolic functions. The result is fatigue and an alteration of biological terrain, resulting in an alteration of the life cycles of the millions of microorganisms that inhabit our bodies. Once harmless microbes with which we lived in symbiosis or harmony mutate into dysbiotic or disease-producing organisms.

It is very important to strengthen the functionally weakened organs and glands with nutrition, biological remedies, supplements, herbs, and homeopathic remedies and other energetic therapies. These help to unblock our damaged metabolic pathways, which must occur before we attempt to eliminate underlying infections. If we do not unblock our damaged metabolic pathways, our organs will be overwhelmed with infectious microorganisms and toxins that are released from body cells and tissues, which we will have no way to eliminate.

MERIDIAN DISTURBANCES

Through the efforts of Thomas Rau, M.D., director of Paracelsus Klinik of Biological Medicine in Lustmühle, Switzerland, we have deepened our understanding of the relationship of acupuncture meridians to the causes of illness. According to Dr. Rau, each of the meridians has certain life themes, psychological traits, corresponding physical characteristics, and patterns of illness. By improving the function of a particular meridian with homeopathic and anthroposophical remedies, the practitioner can build up a deficient meridian system or alleviate congestion in a meridian system.

For example, people who are in leadership positions, who like to direct others and be in charge, may develop imbalance characteristics of the Liver meridian, such as irritability, sluggishness after meals, or hemorrhoids. By using remedies at specific acupuncture points, the practitioner can improve the function of the Liver meridian system.

Another example that is very common today, especially among women, is imbalances in the Stomach meridian. This meridian runs through the tonsils and the thyroid. Many women have low thyroid function, which is partially due to a weakness in this meridian system. The psychological themes that often accompany these weaknesses are the assumption of a peacemaker role in the family, even from childhood, having to grow up emotionally too soon by taking care of a parent early in life, and finding oneself in codependent-enabler relationships. When these emotional energies become stuck in the subconscious and affect autonomic nervous system function, certain organ functions become weaker, regardless of how much psychotherapy one has. The breasts are part of the Stomach meridian system.

Often, the homeopathic and biological remedies appropriate for the individual patient address the meridians where these imbalances reside.

FOCAL DISTURBANCES

Blockages to healing often occur in areas of the body distant from the area where symptoms are manifesting, particularly in the case of chronic illness. These blockages to healing are called focal disturbances. The most common areas where focal disturbances occur in chronic illnesses are:

- Teeth
- Tonsils
- Sinuses
- Gastrointestinal tract (food allergies, chronic yeast or bacterial overgrowth)
- Pelvis
- Emotions

Focal disturbances are like islands in the body that are cut off from normal nerve and blood flow. Hidden focal infections may develop in these areas, especially in the jaw and teeth. The microorganisms in these infections are actually able to travel to other areas of the body and cause problems. When focal problems are present, regular supplement programs often fall short. This is one reason why a person who takes many supplements and is one of the few who actually eat a healthy diet remains ill.

Other areas of focal disturbances are old surgical scars and areas of chronic intermittent infections.

We can identify areas of focal disturbances through the following methods (see Chapter 12):

- History and physical examination
- Computerized thermography
- Autonomic response testing, a type of kinesiology that determines imbalances in your autonomic or subconscious nervous system, and reveals focal disturbances
- Heart rate variability testing

DIATHESIS DISTURBANCES

Diathesis means hereditary predisposition. In homeopathic terms, diathesis means miasm. Each of us is born with a particular hereditary predisposition to specific patterns of illness. Each pattern includes physical, energetic, and psychological aspects. Good homeopathic prescribing can help a patient to balance this tendency. We do not want to eliminate these diatheses because they also contain good characteristics that can help us grow.

In addition to inherited diatheses/predispositions, we can also acquire a diathesis during life. Overuse of antibiotics and reactions to vaccinations are two ongoing causes of this. Again, good homeopathic prescribing can help correct this.

BASIC TRUTHS ABOUT DENTAL HEALTH

Dentistry is a critical component of comprehensive medicine's overall approach. Tooth problems are often at the root of a wide variety of acute and chronic health conditions. Dental foci account for a large proportion of regulatory blockages and obstructions to healing. Each tooth lies on one of the meridian lines of the body, and problem teeth can create havoc farther up or down the line.

Five areas of dental foci include:

- Periodontal and gum disease
- Mercury fillings
- Root canals
- Impacted wisdom teeth
- Dental cavitations

A common problem found on dental examinations is a mouth full of amalgam fillings. Amalgam literally means, "mixed with mercury." Mercury accounts for 50 percent of the metal material used in dental fillings. Except for plutonium, mercury is probably the most toxic element known.

While mercury has been used in dental fillings for more than 160 years, its use has always been controversial. Beginning in the 1830s when it was first introduced, and then again in the 1920s and most recently in the 1970s, many dentists, doctors, and scientists argued that mercury leaches out of the filling material and accumulates in body tissue. The most common sites of detrimental influences are the nervous system, brain, and kidneys. The book *Toxic Metal Syndrome*, by Dr. Richard H. Casdorph, tells us that after people have their mercury fillings removed, their thinking often becomes clearer. While there have always been dentists who have known that mercury is toxic and refused to put it in their patients' mouths, there are, unfortunately, many dentists who still use mercury.

201

Many research studies now confirm amalgam-filling leaching. This leaching occurs in part through drinking hot liquids and chewing, and also through electrical currents that are produced by metal fillings and other metallic dental appliances in the conductive salt-water environment of the mouth. The mercury vapor and particles change into methyl mercury, a highly poisonous chemical that can travel anywhere in the body.

While the American Dental Association argues that the amount of mercury released by fillings is insignificant, it is becoming increasingly clear that even a small amount, perhaps as little as a few micrograms, can severely disrupt cellular function. Recent research shows that the average mouthful of amalgam fillings releases up to 150 micrograms of mercury per day. This means ongoing poisoning, especially for those individuals who are particularly sensitive or allergic to mercury.

Having mercury present in the body seriously weakens the immune system by inactivating the ability of white blood cells to process waste. This makes us much more vulnerable to developing chronic infections and autoimmune reactions. Mercury is also a neurotoxin that crosses the blood-brain barrier. It also depletes kidney function. Mercury toxicity has been linked to neurological problems, depression, gastrointestinal symptoms, sleep disturbances, gum and mouth disorders, and many other illnesses and disorders. Mercury crosses the placental barrier and can be transferred to infants via breast milk. Interestingly enough, the only legal place to put mercury, which is an EPA-regulated hazardous waste, is in the mouth.

If you have not had your mercury fillings replaced, it is important to consider doing this, especially if you have symptoms of chronic illness. Research and decide how to protect yourself. Much of the work with mercury toxicity comes from such doctors as Hal Huggins, D.D.S, author of *It's All In Your Head*, and Boyd Haley, Ph.D., at the University of Kentucky. There are protocols and guidelines that can make the process of heavy metal detoxification less rocky.

When you have the mercury removed from your mouth, for example, it is important to make sure that you have regular bowel movements so that metals can be eliminated via the bile ducts and into the intestines. It is also important that you take a good supply of minerals, such as MSM or sulfur-based amino acids such as methionine or cysteine. Many people are selenium deficient due to diet and soil problems. So the body will hold onto mercury and other toxic metals in order to run metabolic reactions that require these amino acids. Selenium is important because it protects you during mercury detoxification.

Root canal–treated teeth present another common dental problem. Studies conducted in the 1930s by Dr. Weston Price, a well-known dental research scientist, showed that root canal–treated teeth were always infected, even if the infection was asymptomatic. Dr. Price performed a series of experiments in which he placed the root canal–treated teeth removed from his patients who had degenerative diseases under the skin of laboratory animals, usually rabbits. In almost every case, the animal came down with the very same disease as the patient. When he placed a healthy, non-root-canal-treated tooth under the skin of other rabbits, the animals remained healthy.

Dr. Price's studies revealed that highly toxic bacterial forms are associated with root canal–treated teeth. Furthermore, these bacterial proteins targeted organs or areas of the body that were already compromised or weak. Once the tooth was removed and the infection cleared up, those areas tended to recover fairly quickly. Dr. Price noticed that around 30 percent of his patients had immune systems strong enough to handle their own root canal–treated teeth. That is, they did not show symptoms of illness until their "disease barrel" received some additional load. An example of this was a trauma, a case of the flu, or some mental/emotional stress that overwhelmed their system and allowed the root canal–treated tooth bacteria to compromise their immunity and initiate a serious degenerative disease. In reference to the 30 percent of patients that could handle a root canal–treated tooth, keep in mind that this was 70 years ago. Most people's immune systems were stronger at that time, unless there were sanitary problems that overwhelmed them with infections. Today, with a more polluted environment and a much higher dietary intake of refined sugar, which weakens the immune system, along with many other immune system stresses unknown then, the situation is different.

The problem with dead and infected teeth may begin with dental decay and progress to bone infection. These infections, which are often painless, have direct access to veins in the jaw and can spread from there into the brain. Dr. Price's research showed that dental decay was a systemic problem, not just a tooth and mouth problem. Biological physicians have found that root canal–treated teeth and dead teeth are associated with a wide range of serious diseases, including cancer. Of the many breast cancer patients Dr. Thomas Rau at Paracelsus Klinik in Switzerland has treated, almost all have had a root canal–treated tooth in a premolar or molar that is on the Stomach meridian, which travels through the breasts.

Impacted wisdom teeth are also associated with chronic conditions, especially small intestine impairment, heart problems, migraines, and emotional disturbances such as depression. Impacted wisdom teeth are almost always considered foci.

Additional common dental foci are dental cavitations, which are areas of improperly healed bone from previous tooth extractions. Mainly, these are caused when the dentist who removed the tooth left the periodontal ligament in place. This is the structure that unites bone and tooth, and contains the toxic material from the dead or dying tooth. Leaving this ligament in the socket prevents the bone from healing properly. The toxic material is then sealed in place and chronically seeps into the body thereafter. Cavitations remain dental foci unless they can be cleaned out with a special dental "burr." This is a process that allows the bone to heal firmly and the toxic material to be suctioned away. The bone can also be injected with homeopathic remedies to promote healing. Recent research shows that daily local infrared treatment may also help.

Mixed metals in the mouth can generate electrical currents that can be disruptive to nerve function. This is especially so when there is a silver-mercury amalgam filling next to a gold crown.

It is important to find a good dentist to work with, not only for mercury removal and other dental procedures, but also for your bite, or occlusion. The bite affects the brain. If your bite is off, your nervous system cannot function correctly and your craniosacral rhythms become locked. As a result, the way you think, your nervous system, hypothalamus, pituitary glands, and many of your organs will be affected.

Dentistry in the early 21st century is where alternative medicine was in the 1970s. In other words, in the 1970s, acupuncture and nutrition were looked down upon by conventional medicine, just as today, root canals and mercury fillings are not perceived as problems by conventional dentistry.

As numerous dental problems can affect a person's health, biological dentistry must be incorporated in any overall treatment regime. By so doing, comprehensive medicine makes a truly holistic commitment to a person's health. No longer is the mouth divorced from the medical arena. All parts of the body remain integral to the whole body as one biological system, energetically connected and dynamically regulated to adapt, react, respond, and be able to make healthy interchanges with the living world around us.

To summarize points to consider regarding dental factors:

1. Anything done in the mouth has an effect on the total body. Tooth decay and periodontal disease are not local problems. The booklet "Natural Mercury Detoxification," by William Rasmussen, is a good informative guide to mercury detoxification. The American Academy of Neural Therapy (www.neuraltherapy.com) gives excellent workshops in heavy metal detoxification

2. Mercury is poisonous. Other heavy metals used in dental work are also often toxic. So are the chemical resins used to bind both metals and composites in fillings

3. Mixing metallic restorations, combining metals like gold and aluminum in crowns and bridges, always creates bioelectrical imbalances

4. All root canal–treated teeth are infected. These infections can have effects elsewhere in the body.

5. Jawbone infections are very common and can adversely affect general health

6. Doctor and dentist working together serve our health.

THE STRESS CASCADE

Much has been written today about stress. When we ask people why they are not doing well, they will often say they are under too much stress. This response has become somewhat of a prefabricated answer. It is actually a way not to look at one's problems. In other words, "I am stressed out, so leave me alone."

There are always more complex problems behind the stress. Sometimes, stress comes from the habitual lifestyles we manifest because we have withdrawn from our inner creativity. The feeling of stress is a reminder of this loss and rather than making it go away, we need to pay attention to its message. Stress is not merely a psychological problem separate from our bodies. What we experience as stress has definite effects on the body, emotions, and mind.

- Chronic long-term stress leads to increases in cortisol secretion from the adrenals. These glands become weakened. This has far-reaching effects, including the following:

- The adrenals are our energy glands. Many people with chronic fatigue and tiredness have weak adrenals

- High cortisol levels weaken the immune system, so we are more susceptible to the common cold and flu

High cortisol levels also cause an increase in insulin insensitivity. This means that our cells require more insulin from the pancreas to maintain the same blood sugar level. Over time, the pancreas becomes weakened. The result is diabetes and other chronic problems. Our cells do not receive as much glucose as they need for necessary chemical reactions, so our metabolism suffers. Also, when the pancreas secretes more insulin to compensate for this increase in insulin insensitivity, we store more fat, because insulin is our main fat storage hormone.

An increase in cortisol has been shown to damage areas of the brain that are vital to our ability to think clearly.

These are just a few of the ramifications of high cortisol levels that develop in our blood and tissues as a result of chronic stress. The high cortisol levels keep us in a chronic fight-or-flight mode, always ready to strike back or run away. So how we store stress in our bodies can give us some understanding of what changes we need to make. If we do not make these changes, then these stresses become focal points for the development of chronic disease.

What is important to realize is that the state of chronic stress evolves as a result of stored psychological traumas, economic stress, devitalized foods, chemicals, and other insults to the body. When the cumulative effects become ingrained enough in our psyches and biochemistries, we continue to generate stressful situations. Like attracts like. The healing of all illnesses (except those that are only genetically related) must involve bringing these stress points to light, making ourselves consciously aware of them, and making changes in our lifestyles and ways of thinking to alter the stress patterns.

THE WORK OF CONSCIOUSNESS

Stress and the stresses we have participated in generating for years are not negative, nor are they the causes of our illnesses. They are trapped energies that cannot be destroyed or suppressed. If we ignore stress, it will show itself in other ways that may not be positive for our health and development. Stress challenges us to change and grow. Accepting this challenge awakens the process of consciousness that is necessary for healing to take place in our lives. Accepting this challenge is the process of becoming a mature individual.

Be mindful that when we do this work of consciousness, of changing habits and unconscious patterns, it may be necessary to go through some unpleasant symptoms. In homeopathy, these are called healing crises. In psychology, they are called catharses. Being well does not mean that we feel comfortable and have no unpleasant symptoms. It also does not mean that we experience no effects from stress. Being well means that we choose to recognize discomfort and unpleasant symptoms as signs of complacency and as new opportunities for growth.

It has taken years for the effects of the accumulated stresses that are based on the denial of life on some level to accumulate in our bodies. It will take some time for these irritated areas to gradually transform. It is important to put new rhythms in place in our daily lives. Transformation will come. Be patient.

Many people today have chronic illness. Being ill is not necessarily having a pathologic disease. There is a continuum or a process to the development of illness in our lives today, especially because of the society in which we live. From birth, we are affected by various factors that lead to the development of illness. As noted previously, often these illnesses do not occur until decades after the initiating causes. Many people in their thirties, forties, and fifties have overcome acute infectious diseases in ways that have compromised the body, especially with the overuse of antibiotics. As a result, we are now witnessing an epidemic of chronic illness. We live in a culture of

206

suppression, over-stimulation, devitalized food, and toxicity from pesticides and herbicides. As a result, clear thinking and depth of real feeling—necessary ingredients to healing—are difficult to experience.

When any illness occurs, acute or chronic, it often represents channels of unfinished business or trapped energies tied to the past. Examples are stored emotional traumas, past acute illnesses suppressed with drugs, or the inability to transform anger and forgive. Illness, then, is often a sign that we are still too tied to the past. The working through of our present illnesses offers the opportunity to transform the past into something that awakens dormant forces, rather than allows them to hide.

Many people say they are healthy because they have no symptoms of illness. Yet the seeds of illness are growing, and will at some time appear as symptoms. Again, these seeds are often our connections to unfinished business from the past, fed by our unhealthy present-day choices.

What does it means to have unfinished business from the past? In our daily lives, we tend to choose behaviors that are familiar, even if those choices are not the best options for us. When we look closely, we discover that much of our daily behaviors are motivated by habit, passion, impulse, and suppressed emotions from the past. These suppressed emotions have been hiding out in our bodies. They may show up years later in a totally unrelated area of the body and in a toxic way. Exploring our present symptoms and illnesses to uncover their origins and hidden emotions requires effort, and is the purpose of the biography. In the biography, we work to bring what is unconscious to consciousness. Without consciousness, there is no healing.

The habits and instincts that drive so much of our daily lives reside in our subconscious and unconscious. The unconscious is what lies dormant, repressed, and beyond our awareness. The subconscious is that great storehouse of energy that represents what we have been aware of, yet have denied and suppressed.

After years, these subconscious and unconscious habits and instincts become automatic. They take on a life of their own that is separate from our conscious life. They still reside in our body, often in the autonomic nervous system and endocrine glands. Herein lies the problem. When these independent, unexpressed emotions become strong enough, they lead us into illnesses and/or accidents. Taken to the extreme of independence, they become focal cells for cancer, a disease that represents organisms inside us that are independent of us and which feed on our own cells.

These habits that subconsciously drive our daily behaviors are what lead to illness. By recognizing how illness is formed, illness can then become a positive opportunity in our lives. Without illness, we probably would not have the motivation to undergo change. We are generally comfortable with our subconscious habits and instincts. When life is lived in this way, however, the internal biochemistry organizes around what we are denying and repressing. Our thinking processes become distorted, our feelings become numbed, and our lives of purposeful and self-directed activities wither.

We rehash and repeat the same habits and ways of thinking and doing. Life becomes a series of mechanistic routines. Illness is then seen as something that threatens this life of routines. We go to see a doctor, who writes a prescription that is based on these same mechanistic ways of thinking. Our symptoms disappear, and we are well again, able to return to our habitual, uncreative lives. Millions of health care dollars depend on this continuing cycle.

In this routine life our creative capacities, our abilities to originate ideas and acts, our abilities to imagine and daydream, our creative expressions for life in all its awe and wonder, remain dormant and unused. Unused creative capacities become blocked and restless, and they often make themselves known to us through disease. If we can overcome our fear of disease, change our attitude from one that believes that disease is bad, to more enlightened perspectives of disease as a process that can motivate us to change our lives for the better, we have the potential to unleash our creativity for the betterment of society and ourselves. This can happen with the correct support, with effort and with patience.

To heal, we must be willing to become aware of what motivates our behavior. Then we must take steps to change the fixed patterns with which we have become comfortable, and to get in touch with and learn how to express the feelings that lie behind our fixed patterns. The idea, then, is to gradually dissolve our habitual behavior and replace it with flexible behavior, imaginative thinking, and creative expression of life in all its awe and wonder.

Remember that our consumer-driven society relies on us to continue our present habitually driven lifestyle and suppressed feelings, in order to purchase more of what we are driven to want, rather than purposefully buying what we need. We will need to be persistent and understand that the road to change society is harder and requires more perseverance than the road to conform.

So in addition to working with physical symptoms and our history and predisposition toward illness, our healing process can give us the tools to make healthy lifestyle changes. Healing our emotional imbalances has a therapeutic effect on our physical bodies. An inner sense of spiritual connectedness helps us to relax and let go. This has the effect of dilating the blood vessels to organs and tissues and they receive increased oxygenation and nutrients. Then our cells and tissues detoxify. We need to have a process in place in which the spiritual, the emotional/psychological, and the energetic/vitality parts of ourselves are brought into a deeper resonant relationship.

Just as it takes years for illness to develop, the healing of illness is an ongoing daily process of working with the spiritual, emotional/psychological, and the physical parts of ourselves, changing our daily lives, persevering, and developing new habits.

Too often we do not treat our bodies like temples, the house of our living eternal spirits. Many things in our society attempt to tear that temple down.

Stores are filled with doughnuts, candy bars, and colas, prominently displayed to greet us as we walk in. Every time you eat a doughnut, you deplete your nervous system of B vitamins. Every time you eat a doughnut with its concentrated sugar, your T-cell count goes down and your immune system is weakened. If you do this repeatedly, depletion and toxicity occur.

This book is an invitation to explore the concept of wellness and the basics of good health. Many of us lack awareness that the ways in which we have been living and the choices we have made actually promote illness. In these pages you can learn how to make healthy choices, and how to begin the process of making healthy changes in your life and in the lives of your family members. Start with one thing, add another, make it a part of life, then add another change, and make that a part of life. Step by step. Don't get overwhelmed with the big picture of where you are now and where you need to go.

CHAPTER 15

LIFESTYLE CHANGES
YOU CAN MAKE NOW

Healing will become more effective and efficient when we apply certain basics in our daily lives. It is like a basic training, without which it becomes much more difficult to achieve good health. In addition, doing these things regularly will decrease our financial costs of care.

What can each of us do to enhance the process of healing? To heal, we need first to enter into an internal dialogue with ourselves and understand our illnesses. Then we can learn certain basic priorities and lifestyle changes that when applied will set us on the path of healing.

Most people become ill without knowing why. They then go to practitioners to relieve their symptoms. If this is accomplished, the therapy is considered successful. However, the elimination of symptoms is not the same as the healing of illness, as repeatedly discussed in this book. Often symptoms are temporarily relieved, only to return later. Parents of children who have been on antibiotics for ear infections can testify to this. The same is true for people with symptoms of chronic disease. When symptoms are relieved without awakening capacities to heal that lie dormant within us, the illness often deepens its hold and shows up again in another form at another time.

To prevent illness from deepening its hold requires work to support our inherent capacities of self-healing.

Conventional medicine typically asks the patient to be the passive recipient of care. Questions are asked, procedures are undertaken, and medicines are given. Yet most people remain relatively unaware of their illness. In true comprehensive medicine, the patient is actively involved. As a matter of fact, without active involvement, healing will not occur.

Active involvement requires education. The process of healing is an educational journey that gives insight into and understanding of illness and its relationship to both lifestyle and the way we think, feel, and act.

Many people discover that interviews with an integrative physician are much more extensive than other medical interviews they have undergone. For practitioners to prescribe correctly, it is necessary to perceive clearly the relationship between the patient's thoughts, feelings, and physical symptoms. The interview is also necessary to help all involved see the connecting threads between seemingly separate events and illnesses that have led to the present crisis. The fullness of this exploration is what gives the practitioner the information required to bring about deep healing.

A therapeutic program is highly individualized. Though there may be a name for a disease, names are not as important as we may believe. Five different people with the same illness often require five different treatment programs that involve different medicines and therapies.

To heal involves becoming conscious of what has heretofore worked unconsciously in our minds, emotions, and bodies. Healing involves recovering the lost memories that are stored in the body. This allows the redirection of energies that have become trapped and fixed. Healing requires work. However, this is work that will bring a clear mind and a greater sense of freedom to our lives.

Working with a comprehensive practitioner is a healing partnership. This means that both patient and practitioner have responsibilities in the relationship.

Practitioner responsibilities are:

- Using his/her resources, observations, and experiences to put together an individualized therapeutic program

- Continuing to reevaluate and refine this program as healing progresses

Patient responsibilities include:

- Educating oneself as to the particulars of the illness

- Observing what lifestyle aspects are contributing to illness

- Making the necessary lifestyle changes

- Being consistent and persistent in taking what is prescribed

Keep the following in mind:

1. There is no healing without education.

2. Lifestyle imbalances with toxicities and deficiencies are the main causes of illnesses today.

3. Changing lifestyle imbalances is the main doorway to healing.

212

Education is only partly about the accumulation of information. It also includes an enhanced knowledge of ourselves and what motivates our behavior, thinking, and habits. The emotional, mental, and spiritual components of healing are as important as the physical. Ultimately, we will not heal without doing the work on all these levels. We may get relief of symptoms, but this is not the same as healing.

This chapter includes information of interest as well as suggestions for self-improvement. Study these closely and begin to apply them in daily life. Remember that change must be consistent, rhythmic, and daily to be effective. A new foundation for life is being built, one that will support healing. Our illnesses have imbalanced our current constitutions so it is important that we implement changes to correct the imbalances.

To restate a basic principle: the condition of the internal biochemistry and physiology, which is the internal milieu, affects thinking, feeling, and the capacity to act. The internal milieu determines adaptability to change and the capacity to self-regulate. The process of healing involves making necessary changes in this internal milieu as well as making necessary lifestyle changes in such areas as nutrition, diet, and exercise and becoming aware of unconscious patterns.

A good therapeutic program will, over time, help restructure internal biochemistry and make necessary life changes. The program will help us become more adaptable and strengthen our internal capacities of self-regulation. Treatment programs often contain remedies, supplements, herbs, and other modalities that, to be effective, need to be taken every day, creating a rhythm that will be in synchronization with our internal processes.

This is what the process of healing is about. Healing is not necessarily a comfortable or an easy process. Healing requires time, patience, and perseverance. It also requires educating ourselves by becoming informed, asking questions, and being more observant about thoughts, feelings, and actions. This is self-discovery. It awaits us, and can be an exciting adventure. Our illnesses can become our greatest teachers.

As noted, the primary goal of comprehensive medicine is not to make our symptoms go away but to help awaken our inherent capacities for self-healing. This requires work by both physician and patient. The practitioner must probe and discover the deeper causes of illness that lie within the fabric of the patient's life history. The practitioner must then be able to perceive what natural forces may be drawn on in order to awaken a process of healing within the patient. This requires much more individualized care than is offered or reimbursed in today's environment of managed care, with its statistical measurements of costs and benefits.

As patients, we are likewise asked to look at things differently. We must ask certain questions of ourselves, such as: How has this illness changed my life? Is there a relationship between my illness and the way I live my life? How does this illness offer me opportunities to grow and change? How do I react to my symptoms, and what does this reveal about imbalances in my temperament and character? It is our responsibility as active patients to ask these and other questions as part of a self-educative healing process.

ILLNESS PRESENTS CHALLENGE

Coming to terms with illness is not an easy process. Tendencies to illness are a part of life. They accompany us like shadows waiting to emerge. Illness is an opportunity to lay to rest a part of ourselves that may no longer be necessary, or to which we can no longer afford to continue giving energy. This involves recognizing illness as a waking-up process and becoming more alive through permitting something to die within us. Does simply removing a gallbladder assist a person in coming to terms with the suppressed anger, faulty diet, or hereditary tendencies that may have been involved in the formation of the problem? By looking at illness as an opportunity for self-exploration, we wake up parts of ourselves that help us to become more vital, more alive.

A central aspect of healing is focusing on the elements of our biographies. As the rhythms of our lives are revealed, it becomes clear that illnesses occurring in one time of life may differ in meaning and treatment from the same illness at another time. Illness asks us to become consciously aware of the cyclic unfolding of life through the day, week, month, and year.

Waking up through illness offers us the possibility of more in-depth social relationships. We become more vulnerable in times of illness and need the help of others. Many of us resist illness because of a fear of asking for help. It is interesting to note how two extremes manifest in our society. On the one hand, we have greater dependence on the doctor and the medical complex of drugs and technology to act on us and make us better without us as patients actually becoming involved in the process. On the other hand, there is the excessive growth of the self-help movement, in which, as its name proclaims, many do not seek the aid of others at all. Though money may be given as a reason, the choice not to seek help may be entangled in a denial of relationship and an unwillingness to be vulnerable.

Lifestyle changes, such as using only bottled water or eliminating processed foods from one's diet, involve self-education. They also involve a willingness to become more aware of the illness-generating elements in our social economy and to act on this awareness as an individual and as a member of a community. Waking up to certain realities that one may have previously chosen to ignore has the potential to promote social action if enough people can be awakened. For example, many food and other consumer items that are convenient, easy, and inexpensive are the very items that promote illness and keep people in a state of overstimulation and addiction. By making healthy choices we encourage manufacturers to meet our demands for health-promoting products.

214

The questions may be put: How many people are at work in occupations that are consistent with an inner calling or vocational aspiration? To what degree do people apply themselves to uncover what would constitute a vocation supportive of the development of an inner life of integrity? To what degree do they balance this inner life with outer physical needs? Striving for such a balance between the economic and spiritual spheres of our beings requires diligent and persistent efforts in coming to terms with individual or group (social, racial, religious, national, and so on) imbalances. Out of these efforts, however, will grow a true sense of well-being, which will be reflected in individual ability to be economically supported by the fulfillment of life's purpose.

Many of today's illnesses have grown out of an increasing inability of people to cope with the psychosocial stresses manifested by the chaos of contemporary life. Bodies are breaking down because they are unable to deal with this inner chaos. The barriers to the subconscious realms, protected in earlier times through religious and cultural rituals of right and wrong, are breaking down. A new social system of openness and exploration is emerging, which we must learn how to put into practice. The transition from the old protected and guarded tribal system to a more individualized creative and open system is often unsettling and this can generate stress and resultant illness.

THE DAILY WORK OF HEALING

The following sections detail the basics of health and healing, with guidelines that can be easily applied every day.

Conscious Eating

There is no healing without adjusting the foods you ingest and your emotions and attitudes associated with food. For example, if we eat quickly as a result of feeling angry, we do not digest and assimilate well. Barring certain types of illnesses, you can best support internal healing and regeneration with the Basic Dietary Guidelines detailed later in this chapter. What you eat is important. If you do not carefully choose the foods you eat, all the other elements of healing are jeopardized.

You benefit best from your biggest meal of the day being lunch, your second biggest meal of the day breakfast, and your smallest meal of the day being dinner, preferably before six o'clock. This permits the liver, which is the primary organ of metabolism and detoxification, to do its work for you. Eating late at night presents problems.

215

Water

Most people are dehydrated. Drink water! Drink as much water as you can. Don't drown yourself, but drink a lot of water. Dr. Mercola suggests one quart of healthy water daily per 50 pounds of body weight. Water means water, not juice or tea. Drink water at room temperature. It is also best to drink fluids separate from meals, so that digestion is not impaired.

The best water is actually from a clean stream, but that is hard to find. There are some companies that supply cleaned spring water. Tap water is often toxic with microorganisms and heavy metals. Well water may be contaminated by pesticide runoff and needs to be tested every year because its condition can change.

Research shows that over time distilled water as the source of drinking water leads to a deficiency of minerals in the body. Distilled water is dead water. This issue goes beyond the question of pH and nutrient levels in the water. Whether water is alive or dead refers to whether there is a vital force in the water. That's why fresh and clean stream water is best to drink. That water has what is called etheric or vital forces.

A flow form is a device that is structured to enable water to flow down in vortexes. When you stand by a stream and watch the water going over the stones, you see that vortexes are created. This is healthy water. Nature creates vitality in the water. Flow forms are created in such a way that the water flows through the vortexes similarly to the way blood flows through the human heart. When these flow forms are used in farming, and no other factors change, there is a significant improvement in the nutrient content and the growth of vegetables. We cannot all purchase a flow form to treat our drinking water, but it is important to know the difference between live water and dead water.

Try to find the most alive water you can. If you can't find spring water, consider purchasing an alkaline water machine. Other options are reverse osmosis water. Do not use distilled water except occasionally and with other reverse osmosis water. Also, try to avoid drinking most of the bottled water sold in stores. The plastic of the containers is not of good quality and the water is often not regulated.

Certain brands of commercial water are advertised as having less clusters of water molecules (sold in many health food stores). This makes the water more vital to the living processes in your body, and better able to enter through the cell membranes and hydrate the internal environment of the cells.

Salt

Excessive intake of sodium stimulates the sympathetic nervous system and creates tension in the body. Celtic salt is much healthier than standard table salt.

Glycemic Index and Vegetable Juices

The glycemic index rates high glycemic, middle glycemic, and low glycemic foods. Low glycemic foods are the best to eat. They are the foods that are slow burning and do not increase your sugar level. Breads, rice, bananas, sweets, and root vegetables are all of high glycemic value. People may think that 65 to 75 percent of their diet can be grains, but when we run tests and look at their protein and their clotting factor studies, it is clear to see how blood improves when they go off a high carbohydrate diet. Drinking pure carrot juice quickly brings a large amount of sugar into the body. Good juices contain celery, cucumbers, and greens. Add a little bit of carrot juice or a little bit of apple juice as a sweetener. Juicing exclusively with carrot, apple, and beet is like eating a candy bar with nutrients. For the most part, ingest juice from aboveground green vegetables.

Eat primarily low glycemic foods. These include most vegetables. Fructose is the only low glycemic sugar. Cook oatmeal (stone ground oatmeal, not instant oatmeal) slowly. Instant oatmeal is much more rapidly converted to simple sugars in the body. Remember that simple sugars the body cannot immediately turn into energy will be converted to fat.

Supplements and Herbs (if you are not already on a program)

Supplements are generally prescribed on an individual basis. Some brands are better absorbed or recognized by the body, and therefore more bioavailable. The basics include the following:

- Multivitamin and mineral combination

- Minerals (often deficient in the diet)

- Fatty acids, such as flax, evening primrose, and fish oils

- Digestive pancreatic enzymes, and dilute HCl (hydrochloric acid) as needed

- Other supplements as needed or prescribed for individual requirements

When used correctly, herbs can help strengthen, add tone, and detoxify internal organs. There can be side effects with wrong dosages or combinations, so make sure you are taking a safe amount and combination.

217

Blood Clotting and Supplements

Blood clots too easily in most people with chronic illness. Garry Gordon, M.D., and others have documented this. The result is strokes, heart attacks, and cancer. The chronic infections and metals that we all have as a result of living in our society put toxins in our blood. This leads to blood that clots too quickly. As a result, we slow down and our brain slows down. This is why many people benefit from taking fish oil, garlic, ginkgo, and vitamin E, all of which thin the blood a little bit and dilate the blood vessels. Some people benefit from taking these supplements for a year or two.

At the same time, the underlying dynamic of our lifestyles needs to change. Start with changing one habit, then changing another habit. Build networks so that you call each other, work together, and address changes with each other. Healing is not just the doctor-patient relationship. Healing needs to be built into a community effort. Out of these efforts, healing associations can form.

Digestive Aids

Most people do not manufacture enough hydrochloric acid for digestion, and do not adequately digest protein. Taking organic apple cider vinegar before each meal enhances the stomach's production of hydrochloric acid.

When you wake up in the morning, drink a glass of hot water with a fresh lemon squeezed in it. Lemon is an astringent that stimulates the liver and bile ducts to excrete toxins through the bowels that it has been trying excrete during the night. Drink this in the morning to aid gallbladder activity as well.

As noted previously, minimize fluid intake with meals. Too much fluid with meals dilutes your digestive enzymes and slows digestion. Drink your water between meals, or half an hour before meals.

Intestinal Cleansing

Regular bowel movements are very important. Moving your bowels after every meal is the body's natural way of eliminating. If you have lost this natural reflex, then it needs to be recovered. It is helpful to move your bowels at least daily, preferably twice or three times a day. When healthy, your bowels are the boundary between you and the world. You take the outside (food) into you, absorb it selectively, and make what you need a part of you, while keeping out (not absorbing) what will harm you. Protect your boundaries and help them stay healthy.

Most people's large intestines are toxic and not functioning well. Even if your bowels are moving twice daily, they may still be toxic and dysfunctional. Intestinal cleansing with supplements and colonics is very helpful. There are also relatively inexpensive home colonic machines.

Exercise

Endurance training improves our metabolism. Aerobic exercise is the single best exercise to detoxify the body, but even regular walking is very helpful. For more information on exercise, see Chapter 16.

Lymphatic Cleansing

Dry brush massage: Do this every day before bathing. Use a natural bristle brush from a health food store. Brush up the arms and legs, in circular motions, so the drainage of toxins from cells and tissues into the lymph fluid goes toward the heart, into the circulation, and to the kidneys for elimination.

- Trampoline: Use a rebounder or mini-trampoline, under the advisement of a physician.

- Massage: Get a massage, especially a lymphatic massage.

- Castor oil packs on the abdomen: More than 70 percent of the lymph fluid in the body is found in the abdomen. Daily castor oil packs can improve the function of the lymphatic system.

Most people are sick because their lymph fluid is not moving. Using these methods helps get the lymph circulating. Note that lymphatic massage is different from conventional massage. Work with a good lymphatic drainage massage therapist.

Edgar Cayce recognized the importance of castor oil about 60 years ago. He wrote a book about castor oil called the Palma Christi, or the oil of Christ. It has been found that applying castor oil packs on the abdomen five days a week, along with mild heat for at least 20 minutes, helps to get the bowels moving and helps lymphatic circulation. Use castor oil packs five days a week for four weeks.

Seventy percent of the lymphocytes (white blood cells involved in immunity) in the body are in the intestines. By applying castor oil packs, you improve both immune function and the function of your intestines. Most of us have chronic viral and fungal infections. Using castor oil packs and a re-bounder help strengthen the lymphatic and immune systems. These methods are inexpensive and easy to use.

To make a castor oil packs, heat a little bit of castor oil in a pan until the oil is warm but not hot. Soak plain flannel, not colored, without synthetic dyes, in the warm castor oil. Lie down and put the warm pack on your abdomen. Put some plastic wrap on top of the flannel and put a pre-pared half-filled hot water bottle on top of that. A heating pad also works but a hot water bottle is better. Rest for half an hour. Listen to music. Fall asleep.

Sleep

Most people do not get enough sleep. The body needs to be asleep especially between 11 p.m. and 1 a.m. and it needs to get a good eight or nine hours of sleep, especially in the darker months of the year. This helps the adrenal glands to regenerate and the liver to detoxify.

There are people who only get five hours of sleep a night and are still energetic. But how will they be in five years? Deficient sleep makes us fat, hungry, impotent, hyperactive, and cancerous.

A bear forages in the summer months to eat and bulk up for the winter, because when the light becomes darkness he must live with what he has stored in his body. What we have created, mostly since 1900, is permanent summer. An excellent book called *Lights Out*, by T. S. Wiley with Bent Formby, Ph.D., describes this and more about how deficient sleep affects us. When there is light all the time, and when we stay up late and get up early, our melatonin, prolactin hormones, and neurotransmitters all change. We are constantly on.

One of the problems we have in modern society is that we separate ourselves from nature. Most people do not have a connection with natural forces and with the life cycle of plants and the life cycles and rhythms of development of the foods we buy in the supermarket.

Just like the bear, if you are always storing fats with carbohydrates like the bear does in the warm weather, and if you are staying up late with extended indoor light, like the bear in the long days of summer, then you are living a permanent summer. This means you are storing fat. And in the fat you store chemicals, drug residues, heavy metals, and other toxins that are slowly released into your system.

If you live this way, you will crave refined carbohydrates and it will be very difficult to stop eating them. Many people say, "I can't stop craving carbs," while they deplete their adrenal glands. Adrenal supplements, fish oil, electrolyte combinations, and goat's whey minerals are excellent ways of getting minerals. The mineral chromium helps us correctly metabolize sugars and zinc helps us make insulin and be calm, among other functions. Most people are deficient in chromium and zinc. There are also supplemental minerals you can take. To heal, you need to go beyond supplements, however, and change the pattern of how you live.

It is important to sleep with the lights out. If you have difficulty relaxing, are stressed out, and have trouble going to sleep, lavender oil at night is helpful. There are also many good essential oils that can be used in the bath to help you relax.

Drugs

Healing is not suppressive, but expressive. Allopathic medicine and drugs are very suppressive to healing. Avoid drugs unless necessary. Alternative medicine, as some practice it, is not free of this problem. For example, natural hormones such as growth hormones can pump people up. While there is a place for hormone replacement, internal decay may still be occurring, covered up by the hormonal stimulation. The underlying decay is eventually going to show up.

Warmth

Most people don't have enough warmth in their life. Wearing a wool sash around the waist to keep the kidneys warm can be helpful. Putting a little cayenne pepper in your socks warms your whole body. If people do not have warmth, this is an indication that their thyroid function may be low, among other conditions. Take warm baths and do saunas.

Sun

People who do not get enough sun have more of a chance of developing colon and pelvic cancers. The sun is a nutrient. Start trying to be out in the sun a little bit more, preferably between 11 a.m. and 1 p.m. for 20 to 30 minutes. There is such a fear of melanoma that many people are not receiving enough healthy sun. To prevent sunburns after being in the sun, sunscreens with an SPF of higher than 15 can be put on after coming inside in addition to before going out into the sun. The idea is to prevent a burn after exposure. The fear of the sun has led to a deficiency of vitamin D in many people. Vitamin D is made in the skin when we are exposed to sun.

Sauna

The skin is the third kidney, so it is an important eliminatory organ. Eliminating more toxins through the skin protects the kidneys from having to process them. Metals and chemicals can be detoxified from the body in a far-infrared sauna, which is much more effective than a traditional sauna (see Chapter 13).

Electromagnetic and Geopathic Stress

These disturbances, from transformers, cell phone towers, and underground water, affect many of us without our knowledge. Jewelry, watches, and electronic gadgets, especially beepers, pagers, and cell phones, energetically drain us. EEG testing of brain waves reveals that EEGs change after people use a cell phone. Scientists assure us that cell phones do not cause an increase in brain tumors, as was originally suspected, and the conclusion is that cell phones are not dangerous. It may be true that cell phones do not cause brain tumors. But cell phones have a myriad of other effects on the body and on the nervous system because of the change in the EEG brain wave frequency. Cell phones affect all the organs in the body. They affect thinking. Some researchers believe that 900 megahertz cordless phones have an even greater detrimental effect on us. It is best to use standard telephones.

There are practitioners in environmental medicine who, upon invitation, enter people's homes and observe the position of beds and where the electromagnetic forces are concentrated. A practitioner who had learned how to detect subtle disturbances in electromagnetic and geopathic fields in homes helped a child with chronic insomnia. He noticed that the child's bedroom was above the garage and that the garage door opener was under the bed. When the garage door opener was disconnected, the child immediately started sleeping.

Ask yourself: Do you have a clock at the head of your bed? Are you sleeping with the lights out? Is there a computer in your bedroom? Sometimes changing the position of your bed can help you feel better, as it may remove you from patterns of electromagnetic or geopathic stress that are affecting you. We are highly sensitive, much more than many of us like to admit.

Here are some suggestions for your bedroom that can be effective in improving your health. First of all, sleep with the lights out and do not have computers on. Let your system regenerate, let the melatonin build up. If this doesn't help, turn off the fuse box and turn off the electricity in the room. There are constant electromagnetic fields being generated around our beds. Sleeping on unidirectional magnetic beds can help our systems renew. Where you sleep is extremely important. Where you sit at work is important, too. If you are working with a computer, use the liquid thin screens. The bigger and deeper screens put out much more harmful electromagnetic energy.

Some people are able to sleep with the lights on and not worry about damaging their constitutions. There are also people who can live to be a hundred years old with a mouth full of mercury fillings. Such people are fewer and fewer in number. Within the last ten years, we have seen more people in their twenties, thirties, and forties with significant chronic diseases.

The assault on the human constitution is getting stronger. With more radiation, more psychological conflicts, and genetically modified foods that are altering the DNA structure, we need to start thinking about how to make these necessary changes in our lives and in our community. Yet at the same time, it is important to do this not in a state of fear, but in a state of relaxed knowingness that these changes are for the better of all.

Toxic Exposure

Eliminate exposure to heavy metals, chemicals, and other toxins. This includes toxic exposure from foods, dental work, and the workplace and other areas.

Women and babies are more affected by pesticides and herbicides than men are. Herbicides and pesticides simulate estrogen-producing receptors on cells in the body so that the body produces more estrogen relative to progesterone. They confuse the body's estrogen metabolism. Women have more estrogen than men. Herbicides and pesticides are a significant contributor to many hormonal imbalances, a category that includes breast cancer. Modern lawns and golf courses are manicured with pesticides and herbicides. A golf course is one of the most toxic places to live near. Limit your exposure to these chemicals. Use cleaning products and body treatments from health food stores.

Television

The amount of time we spend watching television is not healthy. Television changes our brain waves in ways that are not beneficial. Television takes away time that could be spent doing other things, such as nurturing intimate relationships and creative endeavors. Also, television advertising subconsciously feeds into our fears and constantly brings up things from the past that live in our autonomic nervous systems.

Psycho-Emotional Imbalances

One person will be more susceptible than another in developing an illness because of the various imbalances in our psycho-emotional natures. Internal psycho-emotional conflicts that have been with us from the first few years of life, even if they have been worked on cognitively with a psychotherapist,

223

often remain within our autonomic nervous systems. More and more research is showing that internal psycho-emotional conflicts lodge in our thoughts, our emotions, and in our bodies, and that talk therapy is not sufficient to release them. Each of us is part of a family constellation. As noted previously, we often unconsciously carry energy from our ancestors. Unless these patterns are discovered and transformed, they may contribute to the development of illness.

Also as noted previously, there are two aspects of the automatic nervous system: sympathetic and parasympathetic. Sympathetic is fight or flight, ready to move, be aware, get things done, execute, and move through obstacles. Parasympathetic is relaxing so that nutrients get through to tissues and the body eliminates. This happens more at night and when we rest. When we are able to, as author David Deida says in his book *Intimate Communion*, "relax into our true nature," then the parasympathetic healing part of us becomes more active. This is good.

Stress Management

Stress is neither good nor bad. Go beneath the surface. The idea is not to eliminate stress, but to understand its presence in our lives, and to begin certain disciplines and exercises that focus the mind and change the emotions. Disciplines include relaxation exercises, yoga and tai chi, prayer and meditation, journal writing, mindfulness, and imagery. It may also be necessary to engage in counseling to gain insight into subconscious behavioral patterns and develop more healthy patterns of living.

Mindfulness is important. This includes learning how to relax and how to develop a focused mind. It is important to be able to observe yourself, observe your actions, observe your gestures, observe your thinking, and act intentionally, without self-judgment.

In a very good book called *The Four Agreements*, author Don Miguel Ruiz says that much of the time we unconsciously form agreements with society in ways that harm us. Developing a quality of mindfulness, a focus of internal relaxation, being able to be present, helps us to discern truth from falsehood, reality from illusion. The art and practice of healing need to be addressed simultaneously on physical, mental, emotional, and spiritual levels. There is more on this in the next chapter.

Being Present

Most of us are either living in the past or having anxieties about where things are going in the future. To be able to heal, it is important to spend more time in the present. Ways to bring yourself into the present are through breathing, mindfulness, chewing well when you eat, and being aware of how you are walking. Otherwise you are running from the past, or you are running into the future, and the future has to be built on a solid foundation in the present.

Breathing

Many of us breathe shallowly, from our chests. When you breathe primarily by expanding and lifting your chest, you are cut off at the diaphragm. There are many reasons why most adults are cut off at the diaphragm. When as children we acquired fear, we began to hold our breath and breathe shallowly. Shallow breathing then became a habit. When we learned to stuff our feelings, we began to use our breath to hold our feelings inside. Shallow breathing ensured our feelings would stay stuffed.

If you breathe mostly with your chest, then you are not oxygenating your tissues well enough. It is simple to start to bring your breath down to your diaphragm. Place your hands on your abdomen, breathe out, and breathe in. Use your hands as a guide. When you are breathing deeply, your abdomen should expand with the in-breath, and your hands should lift up. When you breathe out, you should be able to feel your hands drop as your abdomen contracts.

Practicing deep breathing will change many things in your life. First, more oxygen will be getting to your brain and tissues, so you will start thinking more clearly. Second, your bowels will start moving better. When you incorporate your diaphragm in your breathing, your bowels are constantly massaged. And third, you will relax. Deep breathing brings you into the present and reminds you subconsciously of the trust in the world you felt as an innocent baby.

Emotional Intelligence

In *Molecules of Emotion*, author and scientist Candace Pert talks about how our emotional content comes from all over the body, not just our brains. This is also true of plant life. When you brush by a plant, that plant, or that tree, or that flower, sends out a communication to the other plants so that they know you are coming. They do this to protect themselves.

There is intelligence everywhere. In our bodies that intelligence gets communicated every second, all the time, instantaneously. This does not necessarily happen through nerve impulses but by feel. In the book *The Four Agreements*, the first agreement is to "Be impeccable with your word." Our word immediately affects everybody else and it affects the space we move in, either in a positive or a negative way. This depends not only on how we speak, but also on the motive behind how we speak and what we say, our clarity, our intent, and our compassion.

225

Prayer

In the book *Prayer Is Good Medicine,* author Larry Dossey, M.D., documents a double-blind study in which people who were three thousand miles away prayed for a group of people in an intensive care unit. The people who prayed had no idea for whom they were praying, and the people who were being prayed for did not know about the prayers. There were significant differences in recovery time for the people who were prayed for versus the control group.

We know that thoughts are real. And the focus and intent of our thoughts is very important. Dr. Klinghardt points out that there are two levels of prayer. One level is this type of prayer: "Help our team win." For this to happen, another team must lose. This is selfish prayer. The higher aspect of prayer is to ask for divine guidance in service.

Reverence

Live with reverence for what we have been given. Recall what Gandalf said to Frodo in the movie *The Fellowship of the Ring*: "The only thing we have to decide is what to do with the time that is given to us." We also need to protect what we revere and honor, so that we and everyone else will have free space to be able to blossom as people.

That is how society grows, develops, and heals. And this is how healing becomes a social impulse. Healing is not just about getting well, although that is part of it. Healing is about bringing a healing impulse to the social and cultural milieu of which we are a part.

Letting Go

Have fun. Fun means have a feeling of joy, laughing, relaxing, a feeling of connectedness, and mindfulness.

Be good to yourself. Lighten up. Recognize the reality of the areas in your life that make relaxing into your deepest self more difficult, and make the necessary changes, step by step. It's that easy.

BACK TO BASICS

Incorporating changes will bring about a change in lifestyle. Thinking more clearly, clearing your emotional life, trusting more in love and letting go, and becoming more energetic will bring about changes. Many people get depressed and angry because they do not have energy. Get more sleep, do less, make changes in your lifestyle. Everything is related. If you are going to a therapist and you start sleeping more, your therapy sessions will become more effective. If you stop eating high glycemic foods, you are not going to get irritated as much and you will have more energy. And if you are not irritated as much, you will want to be around people and you will want to be able to think clearly. Everything is connected. Your life will begin to shift in a positive way.

So the basics of healing include: becoming more mindful, more prayerful, and more relaxed; working through emotional imbalances; drinking good water, exercising well, and eating a healthy diet; changing lifestyle; building community; and teaching and supporting each other in making lifestyle changes. That's how healthy social initiatives start in communities. All of these things change our inner terrains and enable us to get along with the multiplicity of microorganisms in our body, to achieve symbiosis.

Make a list of the areas in your life that you need to address, and start doing something step by step. Make them simple things that you can apply. One by one, step by step. If you make one change, you will set something into motion. If you simply practice breathing and do that for a week, you will feel a change. The rest of this chapter gives you more detailed information on some of the basic guidelines. In the next chapters, you will receive further guidance in the process of making changes step by step.

BASIC DIETARY GUIDELINES

These are basic dietary guidelines to help in a process of healing. They will help the body eliminate fatigue, headaches, mental sluggishness, nervousness, irritability and worry, gastrointestinal complaints, and many other problems. A dietary program needs to be individualized, but the suggestions that follow provide a basic framework.

- Eat adequate good protein and good fats, with moderate complex carbohydrates that emphasize vegetables. Good protein sources are wild and low-mercury risk fish or free-range chicken, or fermented soy (i.e., miso and tempeh) for vegetarians. Other good sources of protein are nuts, seeds, beans, free-range eggs, goat's whey protein, and goat cheese.

- Eat vegetables that are especially alkaline and contain a good amount of water and fiber. More than anything else, they will help to cleanse the body. Eat them steamed or raw, at least two to three times a day. This includes a salad per day.

- Buy organic or biodynamic whenever possible. The vitality of this food is much greater than regular supermarket food. Many of the vegetables in regular groceries today are genetically engineered, exposed to radiation, or low in mineral and vitamin content due to soil depletion.

- Avoid cow's milk and all cow's milk products. Suggested reading: *Don't Drink Your Milk*, a book written by Frank Oski, a past chairman of the Department of Pediatrics at Johns Hopkins.

Cow's milk protein is one of the most toxic foods you can eat today. Foods to avoid include commercial cow's milk, cheese, ice cream, and yogurt. If you live on a farm where cows are not given hormones, pesticides, and antibiotics, and graze on fields that have not been sprayed, you may eat the products from that milk. A carton of milk at the store, however, contains the milk of many toxic cows. This is very different from drinking the milk from one cow on your farm. If you have any kind of intestinal problem or allergy, it is advisable to stop ingesting cow's milk products. If you have any problem with your mucous membranes, it is important to stop eating cow's milk products.

Don't worry about the calcium. There is calcium in kale and other green vegetables, and if you do not want to eat those, you can take supplements. In many illnesses, such as osteoporosis, calcium is not the primary deficiency. If your connective tissue is hyperacid from too many refined carbohydrates, your body will pull out calcium from the bones to balance the tissue chemistry.

- Goat's milk protein, even if it's pasteurized, is much closer to human protein. People generally do not react allergically to it, and it is a great source of protein.

- Be careful about eating too many refined soy products. This includes soy cheese, soy-milk, and soy yogurt. Research is showing that soy may be neurodegenerative. Also, soy is an estrogen simulator. Soy needs to be kept to a minimum, especially in young girls and in women who have too much estrogen or estrogen-mimicking chemicals relative to progesterone. Many women have problems because they become hyperestrogenic due to a relative or absolute deficiency of progesterone.

- Some fruits are acceptable, but too much can imbalance. The best time to eat fruit is in the morning. Do not eat fruit in the evening.

- Avoid trans-fats/solid fats, refined carbohydrates, red meats, and stimulants such as caffeine.

- Eat only high quality oils. Butter is preferable to margarine (which is a trans-fat). Avoid canola oil.

- Buy fresh produce instead of processed or canned.

- Avoid microwaving foods, as this changes their molecular structure.

- Drink six or more glasses of water per day, preferably before 6 p.m.

- Take minimal fluids during a meal in order not to dilute gastric juices.

- Eat consciously: chew well, relax, and enjoy!

- The biggest meal of the day should be lunch; second biggest meal, breakfast; smallest meal, dinner.

- Do not eat late at night. This interferes with the optimal function of eliminatory organs, especially the liver and kidneys, which work hard at night to help us stay balanced by eliminating excess toxic metabolic waste products.

HEALING WITH FOOD

Maximize:
- High water-content vegetables and salads

- Dark green leafies: kale, spinach, romaine, beet greens, Swiss chard

- Cabbage family

- Yellow, red, and orange veggies (see Glycemic Index)

- Raw nuts and seeds

- Grains as tolerated, but not in large amounts. Best to avoid wheat/gluten

- Any herbs for seasoning

- Vegetable juice daily

- Free-range poultry and lamb

Moderate use:
- Fruits: apples, berries, cherries, melon, grapes, pears, pineapple, peaches, plums

- Good oils for salads

- Beans and legumes

- Ocean fish: best are sea bass, halibut, mackerel and salmon

- Herbal tea, non-caffeinated

- Apple cider vinegar

- Eggs (boiled or poached only)

- Nightshade vegetables (tomatoes, potatoes, peppers)

Avoid or Eliminate:
- White flour pasta and breads

- Refined sugars and artificial sweeteners

- Cow's milk products

- Cream and ice cream

- Beef, pork, and any processed meats

- Poultry and lamb, unless free range

- Peanuts

- Dried fruits (they contain molds, sulfites, and concentrated sugar) and commercial, bottled fruit juices (they may contain mold)

- Wheat products

- Shellfish

- Processed soy (soy milk and tofu); tempeh and miso are acceptable

- Hydrogenated oils and margarine

These are suggestions drawn largely from the excellent food program of Dr. Joseph Mercola (www.mercola.com).

GLYCEMIC INDEX

An important part of metabolism is the level of insulin in the blood. Insulin causes the body to store fat, so too much insulin causes weight gain. Whether the foods we eat are high, medium, or low glycemic foods determines how much insulin we have circulating. The high glycemic foods lead to a higher insulin level and more glucose being stored as fat. Middle and low glycemic foods stimulate less insulin release, and therefore are less stressful to our adrenal glands.

Excessive insulin is our number one poison. Too high insulin levels are very common today. Insulin is secreted by the pancreas to lower blood sugar. When we overeat refined carbohydrates, over time we may develop insulin resistance. To be very clear, refined carbohydrates means cakes, cookies, candy bars, colas, pastas, white rice, unrefined rice, and sometimes even potatoes. Many people cannot handle potatoes until their system starts to get balanced. Refined carbohydrates become simple sugar quickly after ingestion. When the body cannot use sugar for immediate energy, and when the energy is not needed in the moment, the sugar is stored as fat. In this process, the body does not want more insulin, so the cells communicate that they have enough. In response to the excess sugar, the pancreas secretes more insulin to do the same job of storage it was able to do before with less insulin. The blood sugar drops in response to insulin. The adrenals then must act to stimulate the liver to raise the blood sugar to an adequate level, so the adrenals and liver become chronically overworked.

Insulin stores magnesium, so when too many refined carbohydrates are ingested, the cells of our body have difficulty absorbing magnesium. Magnesium is then lost during urination, and we become deficient in magnesium. It is not uncommon for our diets to be deficient in magnesium. This is a key reason many people develop insulin resistance, which in turn makes magnesium absorption inside cells, where it is really needed, more difficult. Magnesium helps our nerves to relax. Many people benefit from being on magnesium supplementation. The supplements are a band-aid, however. Without changing the way you sleep, the way you eat, and the way you breathe, you become dependent on the supplement. It's better than a drug, but the underlying dynamic does not change. It is much better to change the underlying dynamic.

High Glycemic Foods (minimize)

1. Bread (any bread, even whole wheat), pastries, cookies, crackers, pretzels, pancakes, i.e., anything made with flour, except pasta

2. Rice (both white and brown), corn, millet, barley, chips, cold breakfast cereals (including muesli), cooked cereals, except slow cooked oatmeal

3. Bananas, pineapple, raisins, melons, mango, papaya, pumpkin

4. All sweets. This means literally anything that tastes sweet. This includes sugar, honey, fruit juices (canned and bottled fruit juices are also loaded with mold), corn syrup, maple syrup, high fructose corn syrup, maltose, barley malt, maltodexrin, and molasses. Always check the ingredient labels for sugars. Anything that ends in "ose" is a sugar, except pure fructose and artificial sweeteners.

5. All root vegetables, including potatoes, carrots, sweet potatoes, and beets. The exception is yams.

6. Beer and wine (even the low alcohol kind)

Middle Glycemic Foods (moderate use)

1. Oranges, peaches, plums, pears, and apples

2. High protein pasta, yams, and 100% pumpernickel bread

3. Peas, pinto beans, garbanzo beans, canned kidney beans, navy beans

Low Glycemic Foods (emphasize in diet)

1. Kidney beans, lentils, black-eyed peas, chick peas, lima beans

2. Soya beans and soy products such as tempeh and miso

3. Nuts and nut milk

4. Apricots, grapes, grapefruit, cherries, and berries

5. Slow-cooked oatmeal and 100% whole grain rye bread

6. Fructose. This is the only low glycemic sugar. It is very sweet.

Protein

The preferred protein sources are (not necessarily in order of importance):

*   Beans, including tempeh and miso

*   Nuts and seeds

*   Free-range eggs and goat's milk products as tolerated

*   Seaweed products

*   Healthy meat (grass-fed cows and buffalo)

*   Fish, especially wild

*   Fowl, free-range

233

Try to rotate these foods and not have the same ones every day. Raw sunflower, pumpkin, or sesame seeds are good. Raw nuts like pecans, walnuts, or almonds are fine but should be limited if trying to lose weight or lower cholesterol. Peanuts should be organic and used with caution as many people are allergic to them. Soaking seeds and nuts overnight improves digestion of them. Refrigerate or freeze these items, as they are perishable. It is advisable to avoid soy unless fermented or soaked for several days (rinse every 12 hours) and cooked until soft like regular beans. Non-meat protein sources include pumpkin, sesame, and sunflower seeds, fish, lentils, pinto, adzuki, and great northern beans, eggs, tempeh, bee pollen, chlorella, and spirulina. Raw Brazil nuts and cashews are also acceptable.

Healthy Fats

Become an efficient burner of fat. The primary focus of calories needs to come from good fats and good proteins. Eat low saturated fats, especially frozen northern salmon, good nuts, animal foods if not fed grain, and good oils. All fish has mercury in it. Some are better than others. Farm-raised fish, which comprises most fish sold today, has less fish oil than frozen northern fish.

Most people do not get enough good oils and fats from the food we eat. The brain and the nervous system are comprised of about 60 percent fat. A good portion of that is cholesterol. Cholesterol is necessary. Low cholesterol is not healthy for women because if a woman does not have high enough cholesterol she is not going to be able to make female hormones and adrenal hormones, and she is not going to have enough cortisone in her system. Research is showing that because of the over-ingestion of refined carbohydrates, most people have too many omega 6 essential fatty acids (EFAs) in relationship to omega 3 EFAs. That's why we are seeing an emphasis on taking more fish oil.

Yet we still need good omega 6 oils, like evening primrose oil or borage oil. These omega 6 oils can help us lower cholesterol, enhance vision, and, for women, balance hormones, especially if taken between ovulation and menstruation. Many people do not tolerate flax oil (a source of omega 3 EFAs) well. It can go rancid quickly, even when refrigerated. But whole flaxseed, run through a coffee grinder, and used immediately or within 24 hours of refrigerated storage, is good. Mix it with a salad or vegetables. Raw sunflower and pumpkin seeds are also good sources of these fats. Many people benefit from fish oil capsules. Consult with a practitioner.

According to Drs. Mercola, Klinghardt and many others, fish oil is an essential nutrient. Studies in Europe have shown that almost everyone is deficient in EPA and DHA, the main omega-3 constituents of fish oil. Fish oil is protective and therapeutic in cancer, chronic viral infections, nervous system and psychological healing, and arteriosclerotic vascular disease. Interestingly, salmon does not provide adequate EPA and DHA oils.

There are five grades of oils. The worst are the trans-fatty acids in margarine and solid oils (except coconut, which is very healthy). There are some brands of fish oil sold in health food that are good. Coconut oil is a very good antiviral oil. It may be used in frying, and also on the skin as a lotion. Coconut oil and olive oil are the only oils that do not go rancid when cooked. It is best to keep all oils in the refrigerator, and to take them between meals for better absorption.

For those who are vegan and do not eat any animal products, there are good EPA/DHA oils from plant sources that are available in supplements. Be aware that the human body does not convert most of the flax omega 3 oil into adequate quantities of EPA and DHA.

Eat More Vegetables

ALL vegetables promote health, unless you are allergic to them or they cause gas or intestinal problems. It is best to eat them uncooked, but it is acceptable to steam them lightly. Not all vegetables are created equal. Avoid iceberg lettuce as it has minimal nutritional value. Swiss chard, kale, collards, and spinach are better options. Other good choices are dandelion greens, green and red cabbage, red and green leaf lettuce, romaine lettuce, endive, Chinese cabbage, bok choy, celery, cucumbers, cauliflower, escarole, zucchini, Brussel sprouts, and parsley.

Buy organic or biodynamic vegetables if possible. These will decrease exposure to pesticides, and increase nutrient value by two to five times over non-organic vegetables, which are also increasingly genetically engineered. Most of the vegetables in standard groceries today have been exposed to radiation and are low in mineral and vitamin content due to soil depletion. If you buy non-organic, rinse the vegetables in a sink full of water with 4 to 8 ounces of distilled vinegar for 30 minutes. Be sure to rinse in a salad spinner and squeeze out most of the air in the bag before storing them in the refrigerator. This will double or triple the normal storage life of the vegetables. Remember to replace grains where possible with vegetables.

Beans and Legumes

These are generally excellent foods and should be consumed. Remember that beans are slowly digested carbohydrates and are a source of good, but not complete, proteins. Use some additional proteins with them if they are the primary protein source of a meal. Also soak beans (not lentils) for 48 to 72 hours, rinsing every 12 hours, before cooking. Cook them for 8 to 12 hours in a crock pot and the protein will be more easily digested.

IMPROVING INTESTINAL HEALTH

As discussed previously, symbiosis means a balanced and mutually beneficial relationship between the cells of our bodies and the microorganisms that live in our bodies. Nowhere is this relationship more important than in our intestines. Through our food habits, antibiotic and other drug overuse, stress, ingested toxins, and other lifestyle imbalances, this symbiotic relationship has been severely upset. For example, antibiotics both from treatment of acute illnesses and from hidden sources such as animal meat and dairy destroy healthful intestinal bacteria.

Improving intestinal health is vital to healing. We do this with what are called "probiotics" and by having good eliminations.

1. Healthful Bacteria/Probiotics

Probiotics are substances that help to repopulate the intestines with healthful bacteria. The two main strains of these bacteria are Lactobacillus acidophilus and Bifidobacteria. Both protect against pathogenic toxic-producing bacteria and Candida overgrowth in the intestines. These friendly bacteria work by producing organic acids. These acids, especially acetic acid, inhibit the growth of undesirable bacteria, which are often acid-sensitive.

1. Lactobacillus: Produces lactic acid and hydrogen peroxide and other substances that kill pathogenic bacteria.

2. Bifidobacteria: Produce short chain fatty acids (SCFAs), especially acetic acid. These SCFAs increase colonic blood flow, increase pancreatic enzyme flow, and enhance intestinal mucosal growth.

2. Fiber

Fiber significantly reduces certain toxic bacteria in the intestines. Because our digestive enzymes do not act upon fiber, it serves as food supply for healthful microorganisms in the intestines. The best fibrous foods are vegetables and to a lesser extent fruits. Vegetables are both complex carbohydrate and high fiber. Rice and other grains are complex carbohydrate, which is good, but they are relatively low in fiber.

3. Improving Eliminations

Every cell has a metabolic process with waste products. These waste products must be able to leave the body, or we have symptoms of illness. Improving eliminations is critical to healing. It also minimizes reactions to therapies. In a healthy gastrointestinal system, we have what is called a gastrocolic reflex. This means that each time our stomach fills with food we ought to have an urge to have a bowel movement soon after. If we do not have this, or if we suppress the urge because we become too busy, then our intestines and our health suffer.

The following can help improve gastrointestinal function:

- Probiotics
- Whole foods/diet
- Exercise
- Water
- Enzymes
- Flax: 1-2 tbsp/day of ground flax
- Breathing
- Colonics
- Lymphatics
- Castor oil packs
- Yoga

The following can help improve kidney function:

- Water
- Minerals
- Yoga
- Epsom salt baths
- Hydrotherapy
- Hot and cold showers
- Cranberry extract

THE BASICS: A REVIEW

Read this material daily for two weeks as a reminder of what it will take to turn the corner and regain health. The suggested lifestyle changes may seem overwhelming at first, but with persistence will soon become habit. This material derives from the work of Dr. Dickson Thom, N.D., of Portland, Oregon, who is an instructor with Seroyal USA. Much of it has already been covered, but there are some additional points.

Have Fun

- Do something fun, something enjoyable, every day.

Food

- Practice conscious eating.

- Do not drink when eating.

- Chew your food well.

- Make lunch the largest meal, breakfast the second largest, and dinner the smallest of the three daily meals.

- Leave the table before you are overfull.

- Emphasize plenty of vegetables and some fruits.

- Choose organic or biodynamic whenever possible.

Greens

- Green drinks help detoxify; start every morning with a green drink, mixed into water or juice.

- Eat green vegetables.

Water

- Drink 6-8 glasses per day, room temperature. This is water, not juice or tea.

- Minimize fluid intake with meals.

- The best is alkaline water, reverse osmosis water, or a good spring water.

- Do not use distilled water except occasionally.

- Avoid drinking most bottled water sold in stores, due to the poor quality of the plastic containers.

- Do water therapy with baths containing good oils, or showers with telescopic heads. Hot and cold showers, 3 minutes hot and 30 seconds cold. Avoid this if you have a heart problem.

Digestive Aids

- Take organic apple cider vinegar and 1-2 teaspoonfuls in pure maple syrup or honey in a glass of water 15 minutes before meals. This stimulates cells in stomach to produce more HCl for digestion.

- Use ground flax seeds. Buy a coffee grinder and grind the seeds. Use 1-4 tablespoonfuls per day on food. This is an excellent way to obtain fiber.

- Castor Oil packs: Use these every day for one month initially, especially with bowel irregularities, or at least five days a week for four weeks. With children, rub in warm oil on the abdomen. Everyone benefits from this therapy.

Directions:

- Take some flannel, fold it three times, and saturate in castor oil that has been slowly heated to warm, not hot.

- Cover the abdomen with this wrap (you may also put smaller wraps on joints that hurt). Then cover the pack with plastic wrap, which will prevent stains.

- Cover this with a hot water bottle, and leave on for at least 20 minutes.

- Rest during this time and do abdominal breathing exercises.

- Modification #1: if too oily, put on and wear ace bandage (not the best).

- Modification #2: rub castor oil on abdomen and leave on.

- Use the same pack for 30 days

- Use old flannel and sheets, because of stains.

- Between applications, put the wrap in a zip-lock or other plastic bag and keep moisturized.

Cookware

- Avoid ALL uncoated metal cookware. Avoid aluminum. Stainless steel is not as ideal as porcelain, enamel coated metal, or glassware, which is inert and will not add toxic metal to your food.

- Teflon-coated cookware is less than optimal, but acceptable unless chipped.

Bowels

- Allow time for a bowel movement every morning.

- Ensure adequate fiber by adding 1-2 tbsp of freshly ground flaxseed to breakfast daily.

- Take a good form of acidophilus daily.

- Sauna

- Find a place to sauna as often as possible.

- Infrared and far infrared saunas are better than standard saunas.

Movement

- Do some form of exercise daily.

- Spend time in sunlight and fresh air.

- Walk, do yoga, tai chi, or qi gong, or whatever form of movement attracts you.

- Be consistent.

Breathing

Practice conscious breathing. This means breathing primarily with the diaphragm rather than shallowly in the chest.

Sun

- Sunlight is a nutrient. Try to get 1 hour/day.

- The best time is from 11 a.m. to 1 p.m.

- Install full-spectrum lights indoors if you are affected by lack of light.

Dry Skin Brushing

- Loufah or natural sponges have tiny hairs that reach into pores, and so are good to use to promote detoxifying through the skin.

- Proceed from feet up and from hands to heart.

- Takes less than one minute

- Improves circulation

- Removes dead cells

- Improves oil-producing cells that keep skin moist

- Helps nervous system

- Improves detoxification

Water Therapy

- Baths, with suggested oils

- Use a telescoping showerhead, 3 minutes hot and 30 seconds cold, or with help put hot and cold towels around the chest, again 3 minutes hot and 30 seconds cold.

Sleep

- Get 8-9 hours of sleep per night, especially in dark time of year.
- Go to sleep no later than 9:30 p.m. to keep your adrenals strong

- Prepare for sleep by reviewing the day in reverse order to the sequence that things happened. Practice this observation as if watching a movie of your day

- Avoid any violent television in the two hours before sleep.

- Sleep in complete darkness to ensure good melatonin production.

Electromagnetic Radiation

- Cell phones are dangerous to hold to the head. It has been demonstrated via EEGs that cell phones disrupt brain waves. This affects thinking and emotions. Purchase an inexpensive ($20-$40) small device to attach to a cell phone to make it less dangerous to the brain. You can look on the Internet for such devices, or consult www.neuraltherapy.com.

- Avoid sleeping with your head near an electric outlet or against a wall that has pipes behind it.

- Do not microwave to cook or heat food.

- Avoid electric blankets and waterbed heaters.

- Minimize the unnecessary use of drugs and seek safe alternatives whenever possible.

Dental Care

- Be cautious of having a root canal.

- Try to have mercury amalgam fillings removed by a dentist who is experienced in this removal. And certainly do not have any new mercury fillings put in. Consult a physician about a plan and timing for amalgam replacement.

- Brush and floss daily.

- Avoid fluoride.

Chemicals

- Do not use conventional antiperspirants, as they contain aluminum.

- Use nontoxic toiletries and cosmetics.

- Avoid synthetic chemical sprays in house and garden, as these are harmful to people (they imbalance estrogens, among other toxic effects) and the environment.

- Use a nontoxic cleaner for kitchen and other household cleaning

Remember, chronic disease took years to develop, and will require months, maybe years to heal. Be patient, persistent, and willing to change. Illness is not something separate from life that can be surgically removed or driven away with drugs. There is a reason illness exists. Discover this reason. There is no healing without education. Education is not just information. It is becoming informed about oneself.

Sources: Joseph Mercola, D.O., of Chicago, and Dickson Thom, N.D., of Portland, Oregon.

CHAPTER 16

CREATING A FOUNDATION OF WELLNESS

Now that you understand the basics of good health and the lifestyle changes you can make now, and have begun to make some of these changes in your life, let us go deeper. When you apply these changes, they need to have a fertile soil in which to take root and help you heal and regenerate. This fertile soil is a living new foundation, one that is strong enough to withstand the changes that are inevitably part of healing. This foundation ensures that you have the capacity to think clearly, the willingness to feel, and the energy to act during each day.

The words heal and whole come from the same root. Healing begins by examining the weaknesses and the strengths of our foundational structures, and then setting about building a new foundation. Wellness is true preventive medicine, because it means to have insight and to be able to change one's life in a preventative way. Wellness does not mean the absence of physical or emotional imbalances, but rather the use of these imbalances as a tool to make positive changes.

One result of making foundational changes is building a new internal biological terrain. Terrain is like the soil in agriculture. If the terrain is low in toxins and high in available energy, then the plants will generally be stronger and contain more nutrients. The same principle applies to the human body. Most therapeutic programs put medicines first and the mental, emotional, and spiritual aspects of healing are secondary. This is even true of many practitioners of alternative medicine, who too often focus on supplements and chelation, for example. When medicines are put first, we never really heal. And we remain dependent on whatever therapist we are seeing.

The process of wellness involves developing common sense. There are volumes of information available to people on how to lose weight and how to exercise. The problem is not a lack of information. The problem is our lack of motivation to change, and our deficiency of common sense.

The three big areas commonly covered in wellness are eating, exercise, and stress reduction. Wellness is actually quite a bit more than just these three areas. Wellness is not restricted to getting your cholesterol checked, or exercising. Wellness is not something you have done to you. Our society encourages passivity and dependence, and this in turn generates illness. The sleeping will needs to be awakened.

245

WELLNESS AS A PROCESS

In the story of Sleeping Beauty, the prince arrived at the castle that had become overgrown with thorns. These thorns are metaphors for the negative emotions that surround the purity of the human soul. The prince is the force of spiritual presence that awakens the sleeping will, so that the individual can begin to recognize his or her purpose and direction in life. It is never too late to do this. The princess is the feminine aspect of every man and woman that awakens. This feminine quality is the active receptivity and openness to life, the willingness to respond to need instead of being driven by wants. The prince is the positive masculine archetype that penetrates a situation to clear things up.

Wellness involves creating a new foundation for daily life, one that has the strength to support us in efforts at self-healing and becoming fulfilled. This is a process of self-discovery. A foundation is the beginning of a structure. So wellness is initiating into life a new beginning and new birth. Many aspects of wellness involve things that we normally do every day. We eat, walk, dress, breathe, experience stress, and so on. The first step is to become conscious of what we are already doing.

A child is constantly engaged in discovery. At first this discovery is of his mother, and then of hands and feet, and then of objects in the environment. A child will adapt to any situation in order to discover. At some point in our lives, we allow thorns to grow around us and we lose our sense of spontaneity. Part of the process of wellness is reawaking that sense of awe, wonder, and self-discovery. Wellness is a daily discipline that will make us feel better about ourselves.

In our society, the finished product has become more important than the process. Everybody has creativity within. We judge ourselves, however, and do not give ourselves the space and permission to become involved in a process of creativity. The process of wellness and of healing is a lifelong creative process.

Life is about being on a continuum between illness and healing as dynamic processes that we are attempting to bring into balance, every day. This is wellness. For example, every time a person loses focus during the day, that person is in a state of illness. If in the midst of an argument with another person, an agitated person leaves and drives away, he may have an accident. Insurance companies, hospital emergency rooms, lawyers, and insurance adjusters enter the picture. Lack of physical symptoms does not mean that we are healthy.

Likewise, a fit body does not mean health. Many people work out, bringing definition to their muscles, and believe they are practicing wellness. Most do not look further. Exercising is often driven by an egotistic desire to look good or by the fear of gaining weight. We do not define what has deeper value for us, and then create the circumstances for manifesting these values.

We have an illness-generating society. When a patient's heart stops beating, a throng of health professionals will surround that patient. This is the backward health care system we have, which has to change. We pay physicians to give people attention when they are in crisis, not to support them in developing wellness. Wellness is not technology dependent, whereas treating illness is technology driven in our society.

Wellness is simple and practical. Practical means practice, every day. Wake up with an attitude that "Today I will make a difference." The past affects us, and we need to develop an image of where we are going in the future. And all of this revolves around what we do today.

What is well-being? Some say that it is inner peace. Or it is when our relationships with others and ourselves feel right. Well-being is a sense of deeply knowing who we are so that people and events do not draw us out of our center. Instead of reacting, blaming, denying, and rationalizing, wellness means developing a focus of what has meaning and value in life. That is what creates a center.

Become an active, responsible participant in your life. Active does not mean being outwardly busy, constantly on the go. That's hysteria based on denial. Be inwardly active. You can be active inwardly while you are totally still physically and in a deep prayer or meditation. This activity means we are engaged in the moment, instead of being passive.

In illness we are passively habitual. We find ourselves throughout the day doing the same rituals that we are comfortable with, rituals that have lost deeper meaning for us. These are ways that we hide. A big pile of stuff in a corner of our house may be the current reservoir of our "stuff" that is not being dealt with. This big pile of stuff is a metaphor for those parts of ourselves we shove aside so we do not have to deal with them.

Active receptivity is being actively alive inside and asking questions all the time. This results in receptivity, strength, and flexibility in any situation, enabling us to respond in the way we need to respond. That clears the energy, so illness does not find a place to hide in the body. Illness often takes years to manifest as physical disease. It takes years for suppressed anger to create enough of an imbalance to manifest as a heart attack or a stroke, for example. So people do not make the connection between passivity and illness. It is important always to ask what the meaning of a symptom is.

LEVELS OF WELLNESS

Wellness is not about having a perfect physical body. The purpose of having a good physical body is to have the foundation and mental clarity to be able to live our spiritual principles in daily life, working with other people in the course of our service. This is called vocation, our calling. Wellness is not defined by whether we play tennis when we are 80. Wellness is not the absence of symptoms of disease. Wellness is a presence, a state of mind, and a sense of who we are, where we are going, and active participation in our own process. There are people who have physical symptoms and illnesses in their lives who are nevertheless in a state of wellness.

Creating a strong and flexible physical body gives the support, the strengthened vehicle, for what we are building in your lives through our daily practice of spiritual principles and mental focus. Quick weight-loss programs do not work because people most often gain the weight back. This is because they have not built the life structure to regenerate their lives on a daily basis, nor established a support group that constantly supports the self-invoked discipline. Often it is also because people do not drink enough water or do simple lymphatic detoxification work such as ten minutes of jumping on a safe trampoline per day.

In what follows, we will look at creating and maintaining a state of wellness in the deeper foundation. We can look at wellness as having five basic constituents or levels:

1. Spiritual
2. Mental
3. Emotional
4. Energetic
5. Physical

The wellness model starts at the top with the Spiritual and works down through Mental, Emotional, and Energetic to the Physical. Our emotional imbalances can affect the physical body by accelerating or decelerating our nutritional rhythms, like the rhythm of contraction/expansion of our small intestines, for example. As in homeopathy, we do not heal by fighting illness, but rather by turning our attention to developing more love and compassion, more rhythm in daily life, so we may let go of the energies trapped in our habitual patterns of illness and participate in the new life we are building. We have to go over the same path that illness has followed and recreate our life. We go over this same path with a different intent and a more rhythmic process. Like cures like. As we are able to do this, we regenerate our life.

There is reciprocity among the five levels. Having mental focus helps organize our emotional life and build a proper physical body. Also, exercising our body in the correct way and with right timing helps to maintain mental focus. Wellness comes through addressing our spiritual principles, our mental focus, our emotions and feelings, our energies and what in the environment may weaken them, and our physical body through nutrition, metabolism, and observing the correct rhythms of eating. This means we eat when not in a fearful, angry, or hurried state, that we attempt to eat with others in communion, that we give thanks while eating, that we chew well and breathe between each bite of food, that we limit talking while chewing.

In what follows, we will explore each of these five levels of wellness.

- Spiritual Principles

- Mental Focus

- Emotions/Feelings

- Bodily Rhythms

- Physical Structure and Chemistry

LEVEL I: SPIRITUAL PRINCIPLES

What are spiritual principles? How do we make these a part of our daily life? Spiritual principles consist of value and meaning, purpose, service, ceremony and ritual, prayer and meditation, and community.

VALUES AND MEANING

Value is too often is spoken of in terms of money. Every time we make a purchase, we make a decision on how we value something. Most often, this decision is made unconsciously and is based on our habits. This enables us to remain hidden in illness-generating lifestyles. Defining an image of where we are going in our lives can guide us in our purchases and change the nature of our spending. Then what we buy will have value in our lives and contribute to our well-being.

What has value to us? How often do we ask this question? How much do we value ourselves? What is the meaning of what we are doing right now in our lives?

We first invoke the spiritual and mental spheres to support us in ordering our emotional and feeling nature. Otherwise, chaos rules our emotional lives. This chaos in turn creates an imbalance in the way we organize our sub-stance—our nutrition, metabolism, and rhythms. If our emotional life is imbalanced, the body's natural rhythms artificially accelerate or decelerate. This creates more disorder in how and where the ingested substance is deposited in the body. This is why deep meditation or family constellation work to restore emotional balance is essential to healing.

Once we have focused mentally and spiritually, ordered our emotional life, organized our metabolic rhythms, and re-deposited the substance of our bodies, we have recreated our body in a different image of life. This redefined body gives us support to continue in developing and refining the process of spiritual and mental focus. This is the cycle of wellness.

PURPOSE

Each of us has a calling deep within to follow our life's purpose. Our early training, however, may be to follow someone else's wishes for us, such as those of our parents, family, partner, teacher, or minister. Ask: Do I feel a purpose and direction in my life? What did I do today that was purposeful? Did I mostly get caught up in going from one thing to the next, doing what someone else wanted me to do, but not feeling purposeful?

Part of the reason why many people become ill is because they are in jobs that are not suited to their temperament or character. This generates stress. When people try to adapt to lives that are not of their inner choosing, they become imbalanced and prone to having accidents. They may end up in an emergency room where their physical problems are addressed, but there is no real work done on researching why the accident happened in the first place.

Doing something with purpose affects everyone around us. This is healing and it radiates out to others.

SERVICE

How often do we have an attitude of service? Service does not mean that we deny ourselves and let people run our lives out of guilt so we can supposedly serve.

Take stock of different situations you are in during the day and sense how the situation requires a type of service. What we usually do in any given situation is try to read the situation and see what we can get out of it for ourselves. This is a symptom of the selfish individualism prevalent in our culture.

At the end of the day, ask: Was I willing to serve today? It doesn't matter what the circumstances of serving are. If in a corner quick-stop store we sense that the person taking our money is not doing well today, and we make a joke and help the person to laugh and feel humor, this is an act of service. This is being in the moment. Then we feel good about ourselves, and value who we are. And this supports everything else we are doing in wellness.

All spiritual principles are connected to our emotions, nutrition and physical body. Without defining spiritual principles in our lives, we will have a difficult time putting this information into an image of wholeness. Without having established a vision, guiding principles, and clarity of mind, we will begin to feel overwhelmed with all that we have to do.

CEREMONY AND RITUAL

Pay attention to how the seasons of the year have the potential to create meaning in your life. Religious celebrations often connect with the time of year—harvest celebrations in the fall, merriment in the spring after the cold dark winter, and so on. We may feel the need to hibernate in the winter and go to sleep early as the hours of daylight decrease, and then feel bursts of energy in the spring.

The entire body operates through rhythm, observing the rhythmic laws of nature. There is a rhythm to organ functions, glands, and blood. Sleeping and waking is a rhythm. The corticosteroid levels in the blood have maximum and minimum times of the day. The liver's maximum anabolic or constructive time of day is at about three in the morning, which is its best time to synthesize new body constituents. Twelve hours later, at about three in the afternoon, the liver is maximally involved in catabolic or breakdown activities. Following the rhythms in our daily lives is part of creating wellness. The Chinese work with the relationship of the cycles of organ function and different psychological states.

PRAYER AND MEDITATION

Meditation and prayer are cornerstones in many spiritual traditions. Many studies have been done on the efficacy of prayer in healing. Alcoholics Anonymous, the Twelve Step approach to addiction recovery, believes that sobriety is based on the acceptance of a "Higher Power." The Steps encourage prayer and meditation as an important part of the recovery process. When we accept a Higher Power into our life, in essence what we are doing is letting go of believing we are separate from others and that we must be in control. These are the issues that bring us to addiction in the first place. Believing in a Higher Power encourages acceptance and support from something outside ourselves and changes our locus of control from external (if everyone will do as I say, then I will be fine), which is anxiety producing because it is impossible to control other people, to internal (everyone can do whatever they want and I know I am okay). The latter is a more relaxed, self-confident way of living.

Gratitude is an important attribute to bring into our lives. Larry Dossey, M.D., writes in his book *On the Power of Prayer*, "Saying grace or giving thanks before a meal has been a component of many spiritual traditions for centuries. It is a display of gratitude to the creator who has provided for the basic needs."

During the day, it is good to observe our thoughts. Are they our thoughts? Someone else's thoughts? Happy thoughts? Angry thoughts? What do we really want to be thinking?

The other aspect of mental focus is imagination. When we allow ourselves to imagine, and when we pay attention to our dreams, the images we receive help us to understand the deeper aspects of ourselves. Imagination is different from fantasy, which we control. Imagination emerges from letting go of control, as in sleep. Imagination is the language of the soul. When, through meditation or simply being quiet, we clear out the clutter of our thoughts, we can activate our imaginations and our creative juices.

COMMUNITY

There are three basic levels of community: tribal community, intellectual community, and consciousness community.

1. A Tribal Community will circle the wagons to protect itself. When people expressively and blindly identify with their race, religion, or nationality, they are being tribal. The family member who brings attention to the closed nature of the family will be labeled an outcast. In *The Family*, author John Bradshaw writes about the rebellious child who in his or her behavior acts out family secrets. Often, families keep people ill through unconscious family rules that members of the family follow unnecessarily. Staying on this level of community can keep us too bound to the past.

2. An Intellectual Community will sit around talking about things or books that everyone is reading, and focus on information. Intellectual community is the basis of many professional and business groups today.

3. A Consciousness Community includes people who are attempting to integrate, to bring things to light, and to develop a spirit of service with each other and with the larger community of humanity to which we all belong. This type of community, in which individuals come together out of recognition of connectedness to the spirit within another, is the future of healing.

One may, of course, be a member of different communities on these three levels. Healing movements begin to be effective when we combine all three in our lives simultaneously.

There is no healing without community.

SOURCES OF ILLNESS

Addressing the sources of illness is a huge task. Suffice it to say that there are several central areas that represent the common soil out of which illness can grow. Be mindful that these are always in constant interplay.

- Hereditary background, including those common physical and psychological patterns that younger members of a family, race, or nationality often take on as their own in the course of life.

- The efforts of the soul to mold the personality into an effective vehicle for the expression of life's purpose. There is a purpose to being alive, something within each person that strives for fulfillment, and there is a force directing this purpose. In this context, any process or substance which inhibits movement toward this fulfillment must be challenged by one's inner forces. This struggle may often appear as illness, often with symptoms that are uncomfortable reminders of how one's inner life is not being expressed.

- Group illnesses, many and varied. These include environmental poisons and toxins, and the stresses of our shared contemporary psychological and economic life, that grow out of the common materialistic desires of many people. Furthermore, in this mechanistic and materialistic culture, the epidemics of earlier times, which were of infectious and hygienic diseases, have been partly replaced by epidemics of psychological illnesses. These range from neuroses to schizophrenia and other psychoses, suicidal tendencies, and such "popular" illnesses as anorexia nervosa, bulimia, depression, and obsessive fears. Other epidemics of today are AIDS, chronic Epstein-Barr viral infection, and cancer. These should not be viewed as diseases of the individual; they are group ills. People also share racial, religious, economic traumas, and memories. One can view the economic condition of our country as representing elements of a national group illness.

Healing in one's own life, then, must be viewed in a larger context than that of merely going to a doctor and getting a medicine to make it all go away. Healing involves the following:

- Hereditary endowment

- Inner ability to bring forth purpose and reason for being alive

- Involvement in the social fabric and the effects that the decaying aspects of this fabric have on our personal lives and our bodies

Cancer is a group disease, meaning that it that affects millions of people and the causes are common to most. The cancer cell expands and promotes its own interests. Cancer cells are ruthless. Their motive is to establish bases for their own growth. This could obviously be said of many people and corporations in society as well. Cancer is not an individual disease. It is a disease of our culture. The illusion of cancer is: "I can act alone." Most people in our society think this way. Our medical care system reinforces this attitude. Physicians do not look at the multiple causes that can contribute to symptoms, including lifestyle and the unhealed traumas that the family carries. People think that their illnesses are their own. This is illusion.

We need to open our points of view and judgments, look at them, see how we are attached to them, and how they are affecting others. Our attitudes and actions affect the whole. Remember, cancer is a disease in which cancer cells proliferate. The cancerous cell does not care for the whole of your being. If permitted, it will take over the whole and destroy you and itself in the process. Healing and wellness involve the effort to stop being an overly individualistic, separate person on whatever level this is manifested, and recognize the need to participate in community.

Dean Ornish is a well-known cardiologist in San Francisco who is working effectively with people who have heart disease. He educates and supports them to change their lifestyles and thus activate a self-healing process. The success of this approach has been measured with objective tests such as coronary angiograms. By working with diet, stress reduction, exercise, and group work, people are able to reverse pathological changes in the coronary arteries. Dr. Ornish made the statement on Bill Moyers' *Healing and the Mind* that, of all these changes, the most important ingredient was being in group.

People with cancer who participate in cancer support groups increase their chances of survival, and people in grief support groups move through grief more quickly. People in chronic pain support groups that include yoga and meditation have an easier time in managing their pain. Everyone has the seeds of one of these major illnesses in his or her life. The less we shoulder alone and engage in groups that are communities of shared values, the more we increase our wellness.

Community as a Homeopathic Remedy

There is a growing recognition today that involvement in a community-building process is a necessary ingredient for healing. No one gets well without being involved on a greater level of service beyond themselves. Often, however, such communities and groups are limited. They become mere social gatherings or information-accumulating sessions. Or they become too confessional and sympathy-oriented, without enough insight and action. There is a need today for groups and communities that extend beyond these limitations and become conscious and active vehicles of healing. The application of homeopathic principles in daily life supports the development of such communities.

Homeopathy is not just the dispensing of certain bottled remedies. It is the practice of certain defined principles in daily life that support a regenerative process. When these principles are practiced actively in a community or group process, we have the opportunity to bring healing to a level beyond our personal lives. This is service.

The three principles of homeopathy apply to everyone. They are principles of homeopathy and of life.

- The Law of Similars
- The Microdose
- The Totality of Symptoms

The Law of Similars

The first basic principle of homeopathy, the law of similars, states that what can cause an illness also holds within its nature the potential to heal an illness. This is why so many poisons become powerful therapeutic agents of healing when used homeopathically. After a careful and thorough history and physical examination, the homeopathic practitioner prescribes a remedy or combination of remedies for a client that can produce the same picture of illness in another person, but will generate a healing process in the client who is already experiencing the remedy picture.

There are many examples of this in homeopathy. One example is the remedy Sepia. It is made from the juice of the cuttlefish. Just as this fish puts out a dark cloud of ink to cloud up the waters and make it easy to escape, so the person who benefits from Sepia often will put out a dark cloud of moodiness and irritability in order to escape and drive others away. This dark cloud is the shadow or suppressed elements of a person's psyche that he or she attempts to hide behind.

In our daily lives, subconscious agreements and denials are what are called "shadow forces." As discussed previously in this book, there are places in our subconscious where we hide our secret motives and unfulfilled desires about which we are not honest with ourselves or others. We typically project these motives and desires, these shadow forces, onto others so that we do not have to look within ourselves. Our shadows are often revealed to us at some point in life through illnesses, accidents, and crises. (Read more about shadow forces in other sections of this book.)

The type of groups and communities we need today are those in which the individual participants support each other to become conscious of the totality of these shadow forces that, when denied, often lead to illness. We commit to doing the daily work to transform these into forces of regeneration. This is the process of healing.

Such a community becomes a homeopathic remedy. The remedy is the poison that we often habitually keep hidden in ourselves. However, each participant in such a community is committed to bringing this poison into the light of consciousness and transforming individually. The remedy is the suppressed shadow forces that have been redeemed by the conscious efforts of each individual in daily life, and then offered to the whole. This is an act of will and selfless service.

We can only know what course of action is called for as a remedy in a given situation from having observed illness in our own thoughts, words, and deeds. One learns how to take these forces of illness and redirect them into constructive and life-generating actions. These compose the remedy that is then offered to others with similar suffering (homeo means "similar," and pathos means "suffering"). The individual, and consequently the community, becomes the homeopathic remedy.

Participants in such a community practice the principles of self-observation, discernment, honesty, and creative imagination in an artful process of daily life. This enables individuals to bring a conscious focus to the glamour and illusions that exist within everyone's life and which, when denied, lead to illness. By doing this work, we are breaking the habitual bonds of subconscious agreements that are based on denial and rationalizations. These subconscious agreements decay the foundation of most of our relationships, whether these are in the family, religious institutions, business establishments, hospitals, or political institutions.

These agreements have promoted the growth of our individual and collective shadows. And our legal, medical, political, religious, media, and other institutions collude in perpetuating these shadows.

In sum, such a community lives by the homeopathic Law of Similars (like cures like). The same agents (shadows) that provoke illness can, when embraced artfully and by focusing through principles and honest feelings, become curative agents. When the individuals in such a community are willing to work together to transform those shadow elements within themselves, then these communities in the United States become homeopathic antidotes to our major contemporary imbalances (materialism, mechanistic thinking, and selfish individualism).

The Microdose

The second basic principle of homeopathy is the microdose. The smaller and more diluted the original substance, the greater its capacity to invoke a healing response in a person. This is because the process of both diluting and succussing (vigorous rhythmic shaking) releases from the original substance a measurable energy field that resonates with a person's illness. The quantity of original substance has no bearing on the capacity to heal. The more of the original substance that is broken down to release trapped energy, the more healing capacity there is in the remedy.

The same principle applies in the relationship between the principles of community and the central illnesses of America—selfish individualism, materialism, and overintellectual mechanistic thinking. These three are the death forces that are at work in America. They are the forces that trap people in lifestyles in which their spiritual natures and creative genius are not given the opportunity and encouragement to be born and grow, and thus they wither and die.

Just as the capacity of a homeopathic remedy to generate healing has nothing to do with the quantity of substance in the remedy, so the capacity of positive and mature energies of a community to bring about a healing process in the greater social whole has nothing to do with the quantity of people in a curative community. What matters is the focus, quality, and commitment of those involved, not the quantity. A new matrix based on spiritual principles is then generated within the whole.

We may enter such a community with an accumulation of psychological and physical imbalances. As these imbalances are offered up by bringing them into the light of conscious awareness to be observed by everyone on a daily basis and in a nonjudgmental way, new creative forces are awakened in all. These are forces that invigorate our lives and the lives of the whole. These forces are like the essence of a homeopathic remedy that is released when the original form of a substance is changed.

Conventional medicine's central scientific objection to homeopathy (not considering its hidden financial and control motives for objection) is that there is nothing in the remedy bottle but sugar pills. Current medical dogma does not recognize the therapeutic energies that are released in the homeopathic preparation process. This is understandable. Conventional medical thought reflects our culture's fear of dying, of letting go of the form so that the essence can be released and reborn in another way. Conventional medicine also reflects our culture's obsession with quantifying and measuring. Current educational dogma measures success by scores on tests rather than basing it on the awakening of creative genius in practical application. Economists measure our economic health by statistics.

Just as there exists within a plant or mineral an energy that is liberated in the homeopathic process, so there is in every child and every adult a creative energy that we need to help liberate. This benefits the individual and the whole community.

The Totality of Symptoms

As a form of holistic medicine, homeopathy takes into account the whole person. This is the third basic principle of homeopathy. It does not merely treat the parts or just make symptoms disappear, as if the absence of

257

symptoms is the definition of good health. This is one of the major illusions fostered by conventional medicine.

Similarly, in order for a community to do its work effectively, all participants must be continually conscious of the whole. This means being observant of our behavior and motives, and always asking questions. An effective community also means embracing a willingness to serve something or someone outside ourselves or our families. Being aware of and in service to the whole does not mean our individuality is lost. Does the kidney lose its life by serving the whole body in its role as an excretory organ? What we do have to give up are old attachments, old hardened, individualistic lifestyle patterns in order to discover a sense of self, a greater depth of feeling, and a sense of self in service to others.

Just as a homeopathic practitioner creates a whole picture of the physical, emotional, and mental imbalances in a patient, so do participants in a community that consistently does this work of consciousness observe how the death forces or the forces of decay without regeneration are manifesting in their own lives, in the lives of others in the community, and in the nation as a whole. Out of this work, a picture emerges of remedies that will encourage the transformation of the death forces that are trapped in the lives of most Americans and our institutions. These principles apply to all people.

Almost everyone is involved in a group or community on some level, whether through family, church, friends, or work. Unfortunately, these common areas of daily life too often become places where we collude in hiding. This leads to more illness, regardless of what conventional medical technology promises. Anthroposophical medicine and homeopathy are not just the dispensing of bottled remedies. They are the practice of living principles in daily life that support a regenerative process. When these principles are practiced actively in a community or group, there is an opportunity to bring healing both to ourselves and to the greater community.

LEVEL 2: THE MENTAL

Wellness begins with having a spiritual focus, having meaning and purpose, and developing mental clarity—clear thinking. This is a gradual process that starts to build a new momentum toward wellness in an individual's life, even in the midst of illness. Observe your lifestyle imbalances and write about them, talk about them, make a change in those imbalances in the moment, every day. That is how a person starts to develop clarity of mind.

There is a tendency for us to begin each day with a racing mind. Break this by exercising, or by creating a ceremony for the new day. This way we give ourselves permission to discover what the day is about rather than being bombarded with energies that want to pull us in their direction, whether this is advertising or other people's thoughts and desires. If we do not do the work to create our own clarity of mind every day, then we do not have the opportunity to discover ourselves on that day. Then at the end of the day, when we look back, we see all the things we have done; yet we do not feel fulfilled. Without clarity of mind, we are more likely to be driven by habitual thoughts and actions with which we have come to feel comfortable. Then we end up in accidents, illnesses, or bad relationships.

A clear mind invites inner suggestions—to exercise, to call someone. These suggestions are not thinking. They are receptivity. And if we respond to this inner suggestion, then we are opening up a communication to receive the next suggestion. This then carries forth in our relationships with people throughout the day.

The bombardment of others' thoughts and energies weakens us because it encourages the lack of discriminating thought. The healing process involves thinking our own thoughts, and being aware when a thought in our minds at any given moment is another's thought, or is an old habitual thought, or is a thought that arises in us from our vulnerability and feeling in the present. This can be very subtle. It takes work to discern the source of our thoughts. Our family wants us to be a certain way. Our work wants us to think a certain way. So do advertisers on television.

We feel good at the end of the day if we have responded to real need. People admire human-interest stories about people who save other people's lives. Those who are interviewed afterward feel good about themselves because they responded. They were able to emerge from their normal daily routines and respond to someone else's need in an unselfish way. And they felt a deeper sense of self in this selfless act.

By doing these mental clarity exercises and responding to inner communications, we begin to feel good about ourselves. Then we are less likely to travel to the store at 50 mph in a habitually driven way and have the accident that serves to wake us up.

LEVEL 3: EMOTION

It is on the emotional level that much illness today originates and deepens its hold in our lives. Let us look at one emotion: anger. Anger is a healthy emotion when aroused in a situation that calls for it, rather than as a reaction triggered by something in ourselves we don't want to deal with. Anger is not separate from what goes on in our body. Our emotional state has a direct effect on our body. If we are in a constant state of anger, we are producing too much adrenaline. This speeds up and puts chronic stress on our heart. Anger raises our blood pressure and blood sugar. If we are depressed, our immune system is suppressed, and we have decreased T-cell function.

What is the difference between emotions and feelings? Feelings are of the soul. Joy and sorrow are feelings. Emotions generally arise when we deny and suppress what we are feeling. Emotions generally involve attachments. When we live in denial, we build up thoughts that leave us to react with anger, greed, envy, and so on. Feelings are what we experience in the present. Emotions are what drive our words and actions when we are still living in the past, as a result of our denials and rationalizations.

This is where the importance of asking questions enters in. How am I feeling in this moment? Am I feeling inadequate? Superior? Insecure? What is behind the emotion of envy? Feelings involve honesty; emotions are generally a result of our dishonesty with ourselves, and our reactions to what we are denying, yet are feeling.

Whereas there are appropriate times to become angry, it is harmful to react and dump on someone else because we are unwilling to look at what is going on in our own lives. Dispassionate anger is healthy anger expressed in the moment because we care about another. The anger is then expressed because that is what is needed in the moment.

Most of us respond emotionally with anger because we are immediately drawn out of ourselves. There is no centering. We act like victims. Someone else is doing something to us, and we respond with anger. We pour adrenaline, cortisol, and other substances into our bloodstream. Over a long enough time, this takes its toll on the body. A certain process of chronic tension builds up in our lives. This translates into bodily tensions, irritable bowel, or headaches. Or the blood flow to an organ is affected. We often do not make the connection between this chronic anger and organ disease.

In relation to shame and guilt, most people do not want to acknowledge their feelings of shame and unhealthy guilt drives their activities. Guilt can be healthy if it makes us take responsibility for our actions. Shame is the internalization of our faults and can be toxic to our systems. Translating unhealthy shame into constructive guilt helps move us toward wellness. Author John Bradshaw distinguishes guilt as something we have done, whereas shame is about who we are.

Emotions rise up within us from what has been suppressed or repressed. They are like sudden weather changes, as when we suddenly flare up in anger or plunge into fear. Even when emotions subside, the residues accompany us to the next situation we are in. This is true whether we are speaking of parts of the day or periods of our lives. The residue accompanies us—unless we are able to clear our minds. Emotional reactions often arise because of what we are attached to. Therefore one needs to ask: What am I attached to? And what am I suppressing?

Wellness is the process of appreciating the whole picture, which consists of the relationship between our spiritual life, emotional life, and physical body. We referred earlier to clearing the mind and having spiritual purpose. Doing that work on a daily basis provides an order to the emotions, a way that they can be integrated instead of wreaking havoc.

Emotions rise and grip us, take hold of us like an animal that clamps its teeth into your arm and hangs on. The human part of us has the capability for developing clear thinking and objective observation, freeing the feeling part of ourselves from the grip of emotions. Feelings lift us away from being drawn into emotional chaos. The more sensitive we are, the more we will have the tendency to be drawn into other people's chaos. If we are not doing our own work of clearing our mind and enlivening our feeling nature, we will be unbalanced and drawn into the emotional chaos of others. This leads to illness.

The more we do with this work, the more we are able to be an agent of healing wherever we go and with everyone we meet. Healing is not the province of doctors, who are mostly technicians and practitioners. Healing is working on a consistent process in our own lives; doing this work gives us a presence. When we go into any situation, this presence radiates and helps everyone around us. Instead of being passively obsessed by our own emotional attachments, we are able to be actively receptive in whatever situation we are in at the moment. This gives us the capacity to serve in that situation, to be receptive to whatever is called for in order to support each other in our healing processes.

Develop reverence. Feel enthusiastic, and be willing to protect what is being developed so that it cannot be stolen by others or be undermined by what you keep hidden from yourself. Create a wedding between your developing feeling nature and clear mind that is learning to perceive situations clearly without being clouded by emotional attachments. This combination supports us in becoming willful in a positive way so that we can serve what is needed rather than what we think we want.

There is a difference between intellectually analyzing and objectively observing. Intellectual concepts are different from observations in the moment. Write about what is going on within you, or talk with someone. Real communication helps to clear your energy. Observe if you are reacting emotionally in a given situation, be honest instead of veiling it, and write about what you experience. Write objectively rather than subjectively. For example, observe the anger. Write about it. This objectifies the anger. Look at this anger in a detached way as opposed to taking it personally, and perhaps realize that this is part of an intolerant character streak you have. By writing, an inner door is opened. More observations will follow the first one. This is not intellectual. This is not analyzing. Rather, it is honest self-observation that then opens up the feeling nature.

Asking questions opens many doors. How am I driven in this situation? Why am I angry, or envious, or fearful? What am I attached to that blinds me from seeing clearly? If we don't explore these areas, we remain driven. We keep ourselves away from our true feelings, and judge ourselves for having these emotions, or we become angry for being so emotional. Asking the questions in the moment empowers the parts of ourselves that are split off from our center. Asking the questions opens the door for self-knowledge and feelings. If we don't open the door, our suppressed emotions will come out in illness, in an accident, or in toxic relationships.

It is easy in our society to suppress instead of regenerate. We are supported in suppressing emotions from many different directions —advertising, politics, and family. To regenerate requires a depth of feeling and clear thinking. These are mature feminine and mature masculine qualities waiting to emerge. If we are in denial, a part of us is dying without being regenerated. However, if we open up and work with our emotions, we bring what is unconscious into the conscious realm, and the destructive physiological effects on our tissues and organs are reversed.

The daily process of observation and self-honesty takes persistence. There is a part of us that may believe we are above this. We have other more important things to do. This thinking is arrogant, egotistical, and not wise. It takes will to do the work of self-healing. It is not the path of least resistance. Each day that we write, asking questions of ourselves, writing about the resistances and the emotions attached to the resistances, it objectifies our resistance. Clarity will come.

Studies have shown that when we are telling someone about our problems or writing about them, immune function improves and heart rate and blood pressure go down. Research has found that writing about traumas hastens healing; writing even speeds up post-surgical healing. This approach is creating wellness by communication. Notice the common derivation of words: communication, communion, and community.

Writing becomes a daily ceremonial process of clearing the mind. Through writing, we become observant of what habitual thoughts bubble up from our subconscious, and we become aware of what is behind them. This is a process of developing consciousness. In a sense we are researching what our weaknesses and strengths are, and then observing how these manifest during the day. Then we may ask: What do I want in this situation, and is that what I really need? This is the difference between emotions and feelings. When we are in touch with our feelings, we are able to respond to needs. Doing this makes us stronger. When we are driven compulsively and habitually by what we want, we react emotionally when these wants are not met.

Another way of looking at this crucial difference is that feelings are centered in the chest, in the center of our being. Our hearts are open. Emotions usually bring together the worst of the polar aspects of our nature: a cold clever intellect and a ruthless will.

We need to be willing to have that internal sense of dialogue with ourselves, and be honest about what we observe, even if we don't like what we see. What is driving me in this situation? Why do I want this cigarette? Why do I want to run out and buy something? Is my decision to do this a free decision, or is it a compulsively driven and therefore unfree decision? There is an illusion in this country that people are free. We are free to go anywhere we want, but we are often not making a free decision, because our habits and compulsive wants are driving and chaining us to an unhealthy way of living. This is the difference between individualism (selfish wants) and individuality (selfless responding to needs, ours and others').

Before going to sleep at night, write to sum up the day. If you asked yourself a question in the morning, evaluate how well you were able to address that question during the day. Look back and see when you were centered and when you were pulled out of yourself. Observe the weaknesses and the strengths being shown to you through this self-reflection. And be good to yourself in this. This is discernment, not self-judgment.

When I become angry with a slow driver in front of me, sometimes I lose my temper, but more and more I take a deep breath. I ask myself why I am in such a hurry. By asking a question I open up a dialogue with my true self. I laugh at myself. This gives me the strength to stop the destructive behavior.

LEVEL 4: ENERGY

As we have seen, imbalances on the higher levels—spiritual, mental, and especially emotional—can wreak havoc on the physical body. But we have another level that can help protect our physical bodies from these effects. This level is called the energy level. Some have called this the etheric level.

The energy level includes all the physiological functioning in our bodies, and how our physiological rhythms are disrupted by emotional imbalances and by noise, artificial light and sound, electromagnetic field effects from cell phones and their towers, and underground water lines. Much of this was discussed in Chapters 14 and 15. The point to be made here is that if you work on the higher levels, and create as much clarity as you can there, this will reduce interference effects from these higher levels, and permit higher forces to help you in better organizing your physical substance in a more healthy way.

LEVEL 5: PHYSICAL

Finally, we are at the fifth level or grounding point of creating our new foundational structures of healing—the physical body. Nutrition, exercise, and medicaments are discussed in this section.

Nutrition

Without a good diet, and supplements when needed, it is very difficult to heal. This is important for many reasons. The problem today is that most people have come to think that having a good diet is like taking a bad-tasting medicine—no fun. But we only perceive it this way when food has become a substitute for other more important aspects of life. Much of this has been covered previously in the book.

Nutrition involves much more than what we ingest, digest, assimilate, and excrete. Nutrition is not just food. It is everything we take in. Food is simply the most material part of what we take in. What we take in through the following sources can be viewed as ranging from the subtle to the gross.

- Through the brain: what we absorb as thoughts from other sources

- Through the eyes: what we absorb through light and through television

- Through the ears, what we absorb through hearing—conversations, music, chaotic noise—all of which affects us whether or not we are aware of their effects

- Through the nose: what we smell can make us irritable, improve our memory, make us remember certain emotional experiences

- Through the mouth: what we taste and take into our body as food.

How much of what we ingest do we digest? For example, in our destructive consumer economy, television is designed to put us into trance. We are constantly bombarded with clever methods to manipulate our subconscious and unconscious in order to motivate us to buy a product. In a constructive consumer economy, we are encouraged to have the capacity and inner strength to make a conscious decision about what we need to feel fulfilled.

On a physical level, many people, especially as they age, have a deficiency of hydrochloric acid or certain pancreatic enzymes, which makes it difficult to digest foods. Many nutrients that people eat are excreted because they do not have the capacity to digest and assimilate them.

What happens to our experiences that do not get digested? These experiences often remain as part of our emotional or mental life whether we are aware of them or not. They are stored, accumulate, and lead us into difficulties. They are foreign substances that have not been digested by a process of consciousness and made a part of our conscious life. They then feed the unconscious desires that drive our behavior and lead to accidents, illnesses, and bad relationships.

Eating as Ceremony

Is your eating habitual and fast? Do you read while you eat? Do you ingest a doughnut in one or two bites as you walk out the door in the morning? If your answer is yes to these questions, then you are decreasing your digestive enzymes by eating in these ways, and thus impairing your ability to digest and assimilate nutrients. Perhaps you already have a ceremonial activity that you do with eating, such as saying a prayer. Ceremony needs to permeate all aspects of our lives, including the way we eat. Have a cup of tea in the morning and ponder the day. Have some quiet time.

Exercise

Much research has validated the positive effects of exercise on our thinking processes and bodily functions. Aerobic exercise has many positive effects, including the following:

- Increase of blood flow to the brain

- Enhanced growth of brain cells, and more synapses or connections between brain cells

- Burn-off of harmful stress hormones

- Increase of neurotransmitters, thus enhancing memory formation

- Relief of depression

- Relaxing a person for up to four hours after exercise

There are other beneficial forms of exercise besides aerobic. These include:

- Weight training

- Tai chi

- Qi gong

- Yoga

- Dance

- Eurythmy

Some of these forms of exercise require taking classes in order to learn. Define a time frame for learning a form of exercise and start.

The biggest problem people have with exercise and other disciplines does not lie in not knowing how to do it, but in lacking the will to undertake the discipline. Begin small, step by step. Take a 20-minute walk three times a week. Meanwhile, look into swimming, or check into local yoga or tai chi classes.

If you are already exercising, ask yourself first if this has become a routine, a habitual exercise. If it is, ask how you can alter your routine, change the path, or change the pace or time. Be flexible and persevere.

MEDICAMENTS

There are a number of categories of medicaments that may be part of a comprehensive treatment program:

- Homeopathic remedies

- Herbs

- Biological medicines

- Anthroposophical remedies

- Alkalinizing agents to rebalance the hyperacid condition of tissues

- Hormone replacement therapy (plant-based bi-estrogen, progesterone, natural thyroid hormone)

- Pharmacological drugs when needed

Prepare a list of what needs to be done on a daily basis. This includes work, medicament schedule, foods that might need to be prepared, exercises, and other activities related to health. This list can help keep you from becoming overwhelmed with everything that needs to be done. It also helps place your daily needs into a rhythm that you then carry with you and check on and update as necessary. Rhythm is the key to healing. Most of what we do and say, and what we are exposed to throughout the day, generates internal and external chaos. So you need to consciously and creatively develop a rhythm of the day that will work for you for the next month.

STRESS, WELLNESS, AND THE BODY-MIND CONNECTION

From an intellectual perspective, stress is about being overwhelmed by the responsibilities of modern life: work, family, relationships, and lack of time. There are biochemical and physiological stressors. But let's be more imaginative, and not so intellectually confident that we know the reasons for stress and so make stress reduction exercises the solution. What else is involved in creating stress and in making the changes needed to keep stress in balance?

Stress is also self-generated. It comes out of the need to be in control, to protect our false lifestyles of comfort and security, or our "false masculine and feminine shells," according to David Deida. Stress imbalances our autonomic nervous systems as much as mercury does. The stress of the energy we must put out to maintain a false persona, or a mask, is generated internally by holding back our innermost selves every day. When we discipline ourselves to express ourselves outwardly in constructive ways, with moral integrity and loving openness, then we gradually move our centers away from habitual, unconscious, driven lifestyles, and begin to relax.

Let's look at stress from a deeper perspective in relationship to milieu and daily life. When we are living in a driven, habitual, and obsessive-compulsive way, we are constantly being polarized by likes and dislikes, by wants instead of needs. This stress is self-generated by our not being willing to observe our own shadows, the darker side of our natures. This mode of living can be very difficult to shift, and support is helpful, through psychotherapy, color therapy, and even nutrients such as amino acids, which improve neurotransmitter balance. The feeling of being stressed arises when our daily lives are not being lived in a deeply soulful way.

The questions that comprehensive medicine physicians ask when working with patients become: How can we use our objective observations and measurements, and our perceptions of and receptivity to the subtleties of temperament and character, to see how the soul-spiritual nature of this patient may again become a vital part of this person's life? If the patient's soul-spiritual nature is not a vital part of this person's life, why is it not? Physicians need to train themselves to perceive the pneumena, the hidden causative factors behind the phenomena, let both be present, and develop a relationship and a dialogue between these two in their work.

The blood, nervous system, and endocrine or glandular systems, are all interconnected. On the surface of white blood cells are receptor sites that respond to various neurotransmitters, or chemicals that transmit nerve impulses. Examples of these neurotransmitters are epinephrine and serotonin. Manipulating the amounts of these in the body is the focus of millions of dollars of drug research. When we think, a chemical messenger is secreted as the vehicle of a thought. Neurotransmitters not only affect the nervous system, but also affect blood cells and glands. Every time we are depressed or enraged, our blood is being weakened and our glands are being imbalanced. There is no separation. This connection is the foundation of what is called mind-body medicine.

The term "mind-body" reminds us of the interrelationship between the way we think and feel, and the condition of our bodies. People acknowledge this relationship when saying that they are stressed. Stress is often acknowledged with a strong note of resignation, as if a person has no control over what is bringing on stress and how one deals with the stressor. "I'm just stressed out!" Stress becomes the scapegoat for many of our problems.

Psychopharmacology looks at psychological problems and mood changes as caused by chemical imbalances in the nervous system that can be corrected with drugs. Drugs can alter our neurotransmitters. Psychopharmacology believes that the reason we are depressed, for example, is because we have a deficiency of serotonin. Antidepressant drugs such as Prozac are thought to work by increasing serotonin levels in the brain.

Conventional medicine suggests that we take a certain drug and change our mood. But there is no insight and no change in lifestyle. We do not have to talk with anyone about what troubles us. We simply have to take a pill. We are not involved. It is the drug and our biochemistry. Our individuality, our strivings and difficulties, our mental focus, or lack of it, are not taken into account. This is akin to giving a pill—if there were such a pill—to a child to enable that child to know instantly how to ride a tricycle or recite the times tables without any learning required.

As discussed repeatedly, conventional medicine treats us without requiring that we change our lives. If we permit ourselves to be seduced by this pervasive approach, then we are stealing from our own life. Drugs can serve a purpose in the short run. So can amino acids such as 5-hydroxy tryptophan (5-HTP), which can increase serotonin, or L-tyrosine, which can give us energy. Drugs or amino acids can create a bridge to help people change their lives so that the drugs will no longer be needed. Drugs can provide positive support for people until they are able to take over the function of what that particular drug is doing. The problem, however, is that people stay on drugs and sometimes even supplements for the rest of their lives. This supports habitually not looking at what is behind the depression or other disorder. People push this denial down into their bodies instead of working with the issues on the higher levels with focus and questions.

The number one disease in our society is high blood pressure, which is chronic underlying stress that has now become part of the cellular structure. Because stress has not been dealt with consciously, it sinks into the body structure. Adrenaline or epinephrine, one of the major hormones we secrete when emotionally imbalanced, constricts the blood vessels. The walls of a blood vessel are muscles. In high blood pressure, these muscles are chronically tense. This resistance can also show up as arthritis, cancer, or depression, depending on many individual variables.

Everyone has heard of the Type A person, who is angry, time-obsessed, has hypertension, and is always in a fight mode. This type of person has an overactive sympathetic nervous system. The body is producing more adrenal hormones than it needs. This affects blood sugar, energy, thyroid function, and sleep patterns, to name a few. It also alters the number and kind of cells in our immune system. This situation exists in millions of people today, both men and women.

This and many other examples point to the significant interrelationship amongst our endocrine glands (adrenals, thyroid, part of the pancreas, and the reproductive glands), nervous system, and immune system. What occurs in one system almost always has an immediate impact on the other two, and subsequently on every organ, tissue, and cell in the body. So what and how you think and feel is not something that is separate from your body.

People feel stress when their internal life rhythms are out of balance. This refers to the balance of day and night, activity and rest, inspiration and expiration. In our culture people are too awake, too active in the day, take too much in without being able to process it, and have difficulty resting or letting go of what is accumulated.

In other words, our sympathetic nervous system is too active, and our parasympathetic nervous system is too weak. We depend on a healthy sympathetic nervous system to be able to run when there is danger. This is largely due to the adrenaline from our adrenal glands. But the other hormone that is also secreted from the adrenals during stress—cortisol—stays around much longer and wreaks havoc on our hormones, nervous system, heart and blood vessels, and most other bodily tissue. It is ironic that we are afraid to take steroids for diseases, and yet we are producing higher than necessary levels of steroids most of the time because of lifestyle habits we refuse to change.

Cortisol makes it difficult for our brains to use glucose, so we have difficulty thinking clearly. Cortisol also interferes with our neurotransmitters, on which our brains depend. So we take Prozac for depression or Valium for anxiety. These drugs do relax people, but they have side effects, and they do nothing to address why our neurotransmitters have become imbalanced in the first place.

Because of chronic over-stimulation of the sympathetic nervous system, organs become depleted, leaving us in a state of exhaustion. When our sympathetic nervous system is chronically over-stimulated, we have the following:

- enlarged adrenal glands putting out too much cortisol

- increased stomach acid

- decrease in the number of white blood cells, which reduces the ability to fight infection

- change in neurotransmitters in the brain, so more anxiety

- increase in beta waves in brain (uptightness)

When the sympathetic nervous system is always engaged, we feel stress. When the parasympathetic nervous system is engaged, we feel relaxed. These two can be evaluated with a Heart Rate Variability test (see Chapter 12).

Both stress and relaxation must be present for healing to occur. We need to be able to call on either part of our autonomic nervous system as the situation requires, throughout the day. This means being able to respond with energy and clarity of mind in some situations, and then to be able to relax and permit our body-mind to recuperate in the next. We cannot afford to be in a constant state of alert throughout the day. When we are in this over-sympathetic, over-alert state, our body generates acids. And when we are out of balance in this way, we tend to crave those foods and beverages that generate further acidity in the body—refined carbohydrates, fatty foods, meats, chocolate, and coffee. Over a period of time, the organs of elimination become overwhelmed, and are unable to eliminate these acids from body tissues. We then begin to experience physical and psychological symptoms of illness.

In addition, whether we feel stressed depends on what we perceive as stress. Lightning can stress some people and bring great joy to others, as can a cloudy day. Lack of enough money often evokes a stress response, based on the same fear as when we need to run quickly from a lion. Yet this fear may not be life-threatening at all. It may be based on our fear that we will not be able to continue living as comfortable a life as we have become used to living.

Reducing Stress

We often grow through stress. When people at school or work lovingly lean on us to help us move to the next level because they know that we have the capacity to change, that is stress that can help us grow, even though our resistances to needed changes may surface and we feel these resistances are stress.

How do we activate internal self-healing systems? We apply certain practices and disciplines such as yoga, tai chi, meditation, prayer, relaxation, visualization, and therapeutic eurythmy. These produce what is called the relaxation response. Many studies point to increased T-cell and antibody levels and decreased cortisol and catecholamine (adrenaline) levels brought on by the relaxation response.

Our internal imagery affects our body. Negative thoughts produce chemical changes in the body. The doom-and-gloom internal monologue—"I'm no good, I'm never going to make it, people think I'm a jerk."—lead to a decrease in norepinephrine and dopamine neurotransmitters in the brain and to symptoms of depression. Targeted amino acids can greatly help here. However, too often the doctor diagnoses depression and prescribes drugs without addressing the patient's internal imagery. It is not necessarily true, as conventional medicine teaches and many in alternative medicine also believe, that chemical imbalances are the cause of disease. We all have the capacity for changing and redirecting our thinking processes, which then changes our chemical brain function. Sometimes we need support in doing that—homeopathic, nutritional, osteopathic, color, and sound therapies, and even drugs at times. People too often use chemical imbalance as an excuse and take drugs to make the symptoms go away. This is an escape from the real work of changing internally and of detoxifying chemicals and heavy metals and replenishing nutrients.

Positive imagery activates the right hemisphere, and increases serotonin levels, leading to a sense of calmness and well-being. This is the same thing that Prozac does for depression. Patients are often told that they will have to take this drug for the rest of their adult lives. Similar stories are heard regarding anti-hypertensives and other common drugs. This shows the built-in mind set in medicine today: that we are dependent on drugs for good health and there is nothing we can do in our daily lives to improve our health and not take the drugs. People often choose to believe this so that they do not have to be more active in changing their lives. Or they have given over authority in their lives to professionals. This is another example of the collusion in health care between doctors and patients.

By using drugs, we may gradually die inside because we are not activating our own internal self-healing processes. Behaviors and relationships with others all suffer because we are not encouraged to recognize that our own attitudes participate in difficulties with significant others or in the workplace, for example. The will to heal is allowed to sleep, and there is no real healing. When the drug does the work for us, part of us atrophies. The drug makes us feel better with no corresponding change in behavior or perception.

Common sense is an important ingredient in self-healing. All of us know that if we are more caring, experience more beauty, laugh more, we will feel better about ourselves and be more internally relaxed. This permits a healing process to occur daily. This is being confirmed scientifically. When people watched a movie on the life of Mother Teresa, their salivary IgA increased. This immunoglobulin has to do with protection against respiratory illnesses. People who care for pets recover faster from illness than those who do not. The caring quality is healing. Nature scenes increase the amplitude of alpha brain waves, which have to do with relaxation. Beta waves are connected with the left-brain thinking we do daily.

Thus it is to your benefit to make a conscious effort when driving to look at trees and flowers instead of billboards. Observing nature in general opens us to a more relaxed state of mind. Ten minutes of laughter has been found to lower the blood pressure, as biofeedback can also do. Prayer has the capacity to improve immune system function and decrease levels of harmful hormones such as cortisol and adrenaline.

Learn to include some form of a relaxation response in daily life to counter the stress response that is often present. There are a number of ways to do this. And there are many good books, tapes, or classes in the following areas:

- Breathing exercises
- Progressive muscle relaxation
- Meditation
- Prayer
- Voice toning exercises
- Guided imagery
- Humor

All of these produce the following beneficial effects:

- Decrease blood pressure and heart rate
- Decrease cortisol
- Decrease tissue oxygen requirements
- Improve white blood cell count and capacity to fight infection
- Increase blood flow to the brain
- Increase alertness and memory

None of these relaxation approaches are difficult to learn. Some of them require time set aside daily. Most require a change in attitude, a willingness to change habits, and a few minutes. The amount of time these are practiced is not necessarily related to the benefits accrued. A few minutes can bring big results.

Pausing for a few minutes at numerous points throughout the day to breathe abdominally, slowly, and with conscious attention to the breath can often be more helpful than a long period of prayer or meditation. The same holds true for exercise. Dropping down and doing push-ups for a minute, or jumping for five minutes on a small safe trampoline, can be more effective than a 45-minute workout. Of course, how we do the push-ups or the workout will determine its effectiveness.

Through practicing relaxation, we learn that at any given moment of the day, we make a decision as to how we feel. We also learn how to identify the sources of tension that are particular for us, and to change the way we react in those moments. We learn how to switch from reacting, which is instinctive and unconscious, to responding, which is conscious.

- Progressive muscular relaxation is a simple and effective antidote to the fight-or-flight, driven behavior. A common progressive relaxation exercise involves starting at the toes and working up the body to the face by tensing and then relaxing each muscle group. This exercise helps us to recognize physically the difference between tension and relaxation in each muscle group in our body. When we become tense in areas of our body during the course of the day, we understand that we are making that area tight and that we can relax that area, too. Each one of us makes the decision at any given moment to tense or relax. Where do we tense our body? Is it in the upper back, or throat, or solar plexus?

• In biofeedback we learn not only how to relax, but also how to redirect. For example, migraines involve dilation of cerebral blood vessels. Through biofeedback we learn how to redirect our blood flow away from our head and into our hands. Brain-wave biofeedback teaches us how to change the patterns of our brain waves. This directly impacts our autonomic nervous system and can promote healing.

• Guided imagery is a particular way to enter into and awaken parts of you that are normally dormant. Knowing how to breathe in a relaxed way with the diaphragm, and also how to relax the entire body is helpful. In these states, deeper images may appear. Audiotapes are helpful in accessing our internal imagery.

Or, you may also develop your own images. In these situations, relax first, clear your mind, and then consider something that is of concern. Become aware of the images that enter your mind. It may be the image of something from the Bible, a myth, a symbol, or a remembrance of a contact or dialogue with someone earlier in life. Imagery does not mean seeing something like when our eyes are open. Some people see internally, through their mind's eye. And imagery is not always visual. Our internal imagery may be auditory and kinesthetic, too.

The significance of an image or a feeling or a sense may not be immediately understood when in these internal states. Nevertheless, write it down. Its meaning may be revealed some time later. Do not demand to know the answer immediately.

Imagination is not unreal. Imagination is not fantasy. Fantasy is often based on illusory hopes, wishes, and dreams from unfulfilled desires. Imagination derives from our inner spiritual natures and is the language of our soul. Guided imagery is a beginning step toward learning how to differentiate between these two. As we learn how to recognize the inner nature and feeling behind a certain fragrance or visual image in an exercise of guided imagery, the senses gradually change from a tool for experiencing the outer world to a way to open inner doors into one's life story.

These approaches are very effective when practiced persistently over time. They can help to alter positively our internal biological terrain. They also work well together. A relaxation exercise is often followed by guided imagery, for example.

Imagery and many other similar mind-body approaches help us to create a meaningful dialogue, an interface language between what we objectively experience in our body and brain, and what we subjectively sense internally. We need to learn how to create a bridge between these two. This is central to healing, because we need to be able to understand what the illness brings to us. To do this, we need to open all channels of communication between the different parts of ourselves. Most often we block these channels of communication. We ignore insights, dreams (night dreams as well as daydreams), recollections, and other similar, often subtle communications. These are the windows to our inner world.

It is as if through an illness we enter a different country. And this country has different currency. We keep trying to use the same currency we have been used to using in the country in which we live. Yet in order to communicate effectively with the people of this new country, we need to learn how to use its currency. Remember that the use of currency implies value and exchange. So what we are really being called upon to examine is what we value in life, and if our energies have been going into areas that do not create real value for us.

All of these approaches involve taking responsibility for what goes on in our bodies. The stressors we are often exposed to are not always outside us. Suppressed traumas and unresolved psycho-emotional conflicts from decades earlier are stored in our bodies. If we are not doing the active work of becoming conscious and aware of our lifestyles, we may suddenly find our heart racing or our stomach hurting, for no obvious reason. We spend hundreds of dollars on tests that come out normal. And we are told it is our heads. It isn't. It is our whole being—body, mind, emotions, and spirit.

What is stressing me out? What are my habit patterns? Under what circumstances do I go into my habit patterns? When do my addictive obsessive thoughts come in? What are my basic weaknesses, and how can I address them? Examples are intolerance, anger, envy, greed, laziness, gluttony, lust, avarice (wanting to possess what another has earned without doing the work for it), and so on. What stresses us out are elements or people in our external environment that mirror or bring to the surface aspects of ourselves to which we blind ourselves. An excellent way to address these questions and remember observations is to write them down.

- Journal writing is more than keeping a diary. Keeping a daily record of your thoughts and observations may be a key element to healing.

Journal writing is not a record of what happened during the day, whom you met, and so forth. This is mechanical. Carry a small notepad during the day. When an insight or an observation comes up, write it down. Sometimes this is only a few words or sentences. Something that someone says has an impact. Write it down. This makes objective that which is normally experienced subjectively. We often have insights or are affected by things people say, or something we noticed. Typically we let it pass, and it fades into the background of the day. And we never really discover anything about ourselves on that day.

We get so consumed with what we have to do—the meetings, computer work, the fun times ahead, what's for dinner, the family, and so forth. It all becomes external experiences, roles we have learned to play, routines we have built into our lives. Yet behind these routines are parts of ourselves we have disowned. It is these parts of ourselves to which we need to open doors of communication. Without an inner life and growing self-awareness, it will be very difficult for you to heal an illness.

Writing about what touches you during the day is one form of beginning this work. Then at the end of the day, review what you wrote. This is part of a larger review of the day. Look back at events, thoughts, experiences, perceptions that formed the day. Ask questions. These can be: What did that person really want? Why did I react that way? How did I feel about work? Why did I become angry in that situation? What you write provides helpful remembrances that become pathways to reenter the experiences of the day. Do not demand immediate answers to your questions. Answers come in different ways and at different times.

- Conscious breathing. An ancient and effective approach to relaxation and mindfulness is to observe your breathing during the day. In part, this means taking notice of when your breathing pattern changes. And it will. When do you sigh? What was going on when you sighed? Were you feeling resignation? You can make similar observations in other situations, like how you were breathing when you felt anger, frustration, and so on. What were you thinking at those moments? To heal, you need to be able to change the way you think.

Many people are in a chronic state of anxious readiness. This ultimately brings on physiological and physical changes, and eventually chronic disease. Until we are consistently doing the daily work of developing self-awareness, of observing what motivates our behavior, this chronic anxiety will not go away.

It is important to become aware of all the little voices that constantly speak in our heads. "I have to do this." "What will he think of me?" "I'm afraid of losing my job." "I want that." And on and on. This is mind chatter, and it keeps us from being focused on our life in the present moment. The first step in dealing with this chatter is to be aware of its existence. Then begin to write down your thoughts, or look at them when they come up. Do not suppress them or act as if they are not there. The key is to find that balance between not suppressing thoughts and not giving yourself over to them. This takes effort and practice. Mind-body disciplines, journal writing, and conscious breathing can help with this.

- Decide on a particular form of mind/body discipline, and begin to incorporate it daily, even if only for a few minutes. Do this for one month.

- Purchase a journal book and begin to write daily self-observations. Do this at the end of the day. Carry a small pad with you during the day, in case there are any thoughts and observations to record in the moment.

It is important for a process of healing to begin to build this foundation into everyday life. Do the simple things that make life work. I remember the line that Donovan sang at the beginning of the movie Brother Sun, Sister Moon: "If you want your dream to be, build it slow and surely. Small beginnings, greater ends, heartfelt work grows purely."

A healing partnership is based on a balance of self-care and professional care. When we eat well, exercise, do some form of relaxation, engage in a creative art, do journal writing, and become more aware of what motivates our behavior, we are becoming active in our own self-care. We are changing the internal biological terrain of our body, and invoking a process of healing. Then the remedies, supplements, and herbs we take can support us even better.

Remember, self-observation is not intellectual and analytical. Observation is an act of conscious will and open feeling. Observe, be honest about what you observe even if this conflicts with the great person you think you are, and then write about it or communicate in another manner. Follow where the observation takes you, and ask questions. This builds living connections within you. This is self-knowledge. You do not have to read another book in order to engage in active self-observation.

Recent studies illuminate the importance of self-observation and reducing your stress:

- Major life change in the setting of a highly ritualized family—in other words, a family that was overly structured and rigid—appeared to predispose to greater illness severity.

- Bacteria and viruses were present in both highly stressed and low stressed children, but the high stressed children suffered from more prolonged and severe illness. (High stressed means that the family is ignoring the pressures of life so that they build up.)

- Stress was four times more likely to precede an infection, as it was to follow an infection.

Only one-fifth of low stress people (people who are under stress but who are able to deal with it, changing their attitudes or way of life in some way) became physically ill when they had a positive strep throat culture. In other words, in the other four-fifths, the immune system was strong enough to deal with the infection because the stress was being worked with and integrated.

Studies on the effects of behavioral factors on immune measurements have shown how loneliness and expressing the need for power and control decreases the number of natural killer (NK) cells, which is a measurement of healthy immune system function. Also, people who have need for power and control have significantly decreased secretions of IgA in their mouth and upper respiratory areas. IgA is an immune globulin or protein in the saliva that is important in resisting respiratory infections.

These types of studies reveal how negative behavioral patterns are reflected in physical problems. On the other side of the coin, personal sharing, humor and laughter, and group intervention strengthens the immune system.

The media contributes to keeping people ignorant. The media is constantly filled with reports of how people can become ill, from viruses, bacteria, foods, ozone depletion, electromagnetic radiation, and so on. These factors are all important, not to be ignored. But they are usually used to sell us something out of fear. Very infrequently do we see reports that attempt to educate people as to how they may strengthen their immune systems. Many of these methods are very inexpensive, whereas many of the therapies that people will require if their immune systems remain weak and they become physically ill are expensive.

The key word in dealing with stress is adaptability. If we are adaptable, we will have a much greater capacity to constructively work with stress. This means having flexibility. This also involves active self-observation, communicating, writing, and constantly making necessary changes within ourselves.

CLEARING THE MIND

In invoking your purpose, working with community and group, clearing emotions, changing what you eat, how you exercise, and how you sleep, the common denominator is clearing the mind.

A woman was seen in an emergency room. While working in her garden she suddenly developed a severe pain in her right lower back. She received a full evaluation to rule out any serious causes of acute sudden low back pain, and none could be found. Her right lower back was very tender to touch, which suggested that the problem was musculoskeletal. She was angry that her lower back pain was disrupting her day, and wanted her pain relieved.

This is an illustration of a collusive relationship between doctor and patient. The doctor does not want nor have the time to spend inquiring why the patient might have this back pain. The patient does not wish to discover this either. She wants the problem taken care of. The patient does not ask "Why do I have this back pain? Is it related to things that are going on in my life? What does the low back mean in terms of supporting the rest of my body? What have I not been willing to support, or where do I not feel supported? Do I have a kidney weakness?" In Chinese medicine, the kidneys are the organs that have to bear the chaos in our lives. In the same way, the liver has to bear our anger. These kinds of questions need to be asked if we are to clear our minds, become more conscious human beings, and heal our illnesses.

Symptoms of illness present a picture that we need to learn how to read and interpret. It's not just something you "get" that you go to a doctor to get rid of. We have collusively built this approach into our health care system and it is why this system is largely ineffective in deep healing, and is going bankrupt.

Looking at the roots of illness in a person's biography sheds light on current symptoms and helps to understand that immunizations, diet, and exercise may make symptoms go away but do not get to the root of the problem.

The book *Love Your Disease: It's Keeping You Healthy*, by John Harrison, M.D., tells the story of a man who made a decision earlier in life not to express his feelings. As a result, he developed sinusitis. His symptoms were really related to the suppression of feelings, which led to pursuing a career in an intellectual profession. It led to his marrying an accountant, because like attracts like. He had no close friends. He played football. He hated soap operas. He smoked 50 cigarettes per day, and never cried. And then, for some unknown reason, he developed sinusitis and went to a doctor for antibiotics to make his symptoms go away. Only when he began to uncover and express real feelings did the frequency of sinusitis decrease. The sinusitis was the suppressed feelings looking for an outlet.

DISCIPLINE AND RHYTHM

In this chapter, I initially spoke about developing focus through spiritual principles, mental exercises, and being involved in community. Having this focus helps us create natural rhythms that make sense of life. I then spoke about emotions and feelings, nutrition, exercise, and stress reduction.

With new awareness, you may continue to do what you did before, but now you do it in a conscious way instead of unconsciously. Discard what you no longer need. Focus on the present instead of being habitually driven by the past. This present focus will guide you to your next activity. Do conscious research on your daily routines. Ask questions. Note that a ceremony, too, can become a rigid habit when we do not re-invoke it every day, so vary your ceremonies, and do them in different ways. Ask, "Am I placing this object or drinking this tea consciously or habitually?" By making these changes, you have the opportunity to rediscover yourself each day.

We will not be able to change destructive patterns until we ask questions and become aware through observation of what we are doing. The soil for illness in our lives is created by the ways that we do things habitually and subconsciously driven. By changing these habits, we generate wellness.

PART IV:

ILLNESS AND THE PSYCHE

CHAPTER 17

THE PSYCHOLOGY OF ILLNESS

In order to create a new economy of healing that works, we will need to include in our dialogues all the levels discussed in the previous chapter—spiritual, mental, emotional, energetic, and physical. The importance of including all the levels is highlighted by the fact that an estimated 50 percent of illnesses originate from the fears, attitudes, and beliefs that we hold, 20 percent from how we are affected energetically in our daily lives (by electromagnetic fields, for example), and less than 20 percent from causes that are purely physical. Yet it is this latter area where we put almost all of our funds and treatments, even in alternative medicine. This has to change.

This chapter explores the psychology of illness. We need people in our economic medical institutions that understand and integrate these principles in their work.

THE GOOD IN ILLNESS

Almost nothing gets our attention more than illness. Our lives may be moving along smoothly and we are in good health, then we become ill and are not very happy about it. The illness forces us to be in the present. The pain of illness brings us right into the moment. When we stub a toe or have a sore throat, we stop caring much about the past or the future.

The physical symptoms of illness often wake us up from our mesmerized existence, where we have been numb to many parts of ourselves. These parts have been asleep, in a deep freeze in our subconscious. We have learned to repress, deny, or project onto others what we do not wish to see. Most of us do not discipline ourselves to observe what really motivates our daily thoughts, words, and activities. Are we thinking our own thoughts much of the time? Are we open to whatever feeling may arise in any given moment?

Illness is not a pathological process for which we prescribe a drug or surgery in order to be healthy. Illness is an integral part of life. It grows in the soil of our individual and collective lives. It is part of the terrain.

By getting our attention, illness forces us to face ourselves. If we chose to ignore this opportunity and treat only the symptoms, then the part of ourselves that is calling for our attention will again attempt to remind us that it is still there and that we need to embrace it. Unfortunately, the present health care system permits us to continue to deny and go back to sleep. It provides a mechanical escape or release from the lessons of our illnesses.

Physical illness can be very positive. It often occurs after years of denial and habitual living that has become normal and comfortable. During illness, we need constructive therapeutic support on physical, psychological, and spiritual levels. The idea is to give our illness space and time to manifest physically so that it is not suppressed while we receive support. This way the illness will not deepen and produce destruction. This is the middle path through illness. When we tolerate our illnesses and ask for guidance, we learn to work through the hidden residues from past artificial lifestyles in a relatively short period of time. The door opens for new growth and the gradual emergence of our true selves.

ILLNESS AND DEATH

Illness confronts us with death. We fear the death of our physical form. Form means structure, any structure. Our habitual lifestyles take on forms of their own. We come to deny these forms and then attempt to blame or sue others for bringing on or not relieving the unpleasant repercussions of our self-perpetuated denial.

The Native Americans have a phrase, "today is a good day to die." Illness is the opportunity to learn how to die. We permit an old part of ourselves to die by becoming conscious of the way these habitual forms are poisoning our self-evolution.

America is obsessed with death. We go to movies to watch people deal with the imminent reality of death. Yet in our real lives we create elaborate and expensive ways of avoiding death. That which is denied, which we do not permit to die, or let go of, is banished to the subconscious. It then shows up years later as physical illness. Our health care system does not support us in recognizing these denials and in developing the tools to work through them and grow. There is little acknowledgement of the relationship of lifestyle to illness, except on superficial levels with the role of diet, exercise, cigarettes, and alcohol. Think how long it took for even those to be acknowledged. Holistic doctors who practiced by these precepts have until recently been persecuted.

We deny death—the death of the physical body, the death of having to be physically young, the death of habitual patterns of behavior. Denying death sows the seeds of destruction of life. These forces of denied death manifest as a health care industry that devours an increasing portion of the national economy. Our fear of becoming ill is increased by the probability of not being able to afford treatment. And the promise of more expensive endeavors such as genetic therapy and the war on cancer will fall far short of expectations. Programs that deny death in illness are doomed to failure.

284

We need to give ourselves permission to become physically ill. This is not to encourage us to try to become ill. Rather, we need to cultivate an attitude of accepting and understanding the principle that physical illness is sometimes necessary for individual growth.

This attitude has to be cultivated by a reformed health care system that ceases to focus on mechanically fixing people without initiating a process of self-educative healing. No insurance company or other third party can shield us from the need to deal with what illness brings to us. No physician can take away our chemistries of poison and then discharge us back into the world without there being a re-accumulation of these poisons in often deeper and more self-destructive ways. No lawyer who helps someone win money by blaming another can take away our eventual suffering as we taste the bitter fruit of our own denials and rationalizations.

When we accept and work with these realities in our everyday lives, we will evolve a health care system that supports life and the process of healing. This can occur right now.

ILLNESS AND VULNERABILITY

It has been astutely stated in the book *Who Gets Sick*, by Blair Justice that "the more vulnerable we are, the more risk we run at getting sick." It would be helpful to look in some depth at this statement and what it means in our daily lives. There are three significant words in the quotation: vulnerable, risk, and sick.

- **Vulnerable.** To be vulnerable is to be willing to experience life without judgment. It involves developing an active feeling nature that becomes one's source of strength. Vulnerability also implies a trust that serves as an antidote to the epidemic of fear in our society. The problem is that vulnerability is too often perceived as a sign of weakness instead of a means to further growth. Vulnerability enables us to build bridges between an active inner life and an effective and constructive outer life in the world.

- **Risk.** We strive to create a risk-free society. Avoiding risk has become a cultural obsession. We have collectively constructed a medical and legal structure to protect us from risk and from the consequences thereof. Built into this is the scapegoat attitude of blaming others and making them pay for what may in truth often occur as a result of our own imbalanced lifestyles. This attitude is prevalent in our legal structure. It is also paralleled by our medical ideas that there is something out there, such as a bacteria or virus that is making us sick.

Even though the more obvious contributing factors of illness are all around us, in the news daily, and impinging on our so-called secure lives, we continue to act as if we are not involved. This refers to the growth of psychological problems and obsessions, environmental toxicity that grows out of our insensitivities and greed, and hereditary patterns that are unnecessarily permitted to continue from one generation to the next. These are symptoms of our individual and collective denials. In truth, society demands that we deny, and will make people pay who dare to bring denials into the arena of our conscious awareness. Whether or not we ignore them, the effects of this denial of the true "causes" of illness continue to exist and grow in proportion to our denial. And their growth will add further strain to our present method of dispensing medical care in terms of cost, availability, and effectiveness.

Even though most people know that to grow requires risk, our culture attempts to shield people from risk-taking. Risk-taking in our culture shows up in a variety of forms, however. Youths are attracted to gangs in order to prove that they have courage and are willing to take risks, albeit without any constructive purpose and more frequently associated with drugs. Millions of people flock to the latest movie to participate in the life of a regular man or woman who becomes the courageous hero. We collectively participate in this adventure, this willingness to take risks in order to achieve something meaningful. Television talk shows and specials sensationalize violence and draw large Neilson ratings.

All of this is a collective portrayal of our striving to break free from the rigidities of an intellectually oriented and subconscious-denying modern technological culture. This is our unconscious attempt to heal. Movies have become the real place of teaching in America. When we go to the movies, we participate in ancient myths, such as those of Hercules and Odin, redone in modern mythological portraits of good and evil, as in *Star Wars* and *The Lord of the Rings*.

- **Sick.** This is a word that most of us would rather do without, choosing instead to imagine, our family, everyone else and as healthy. We have built a multibillion-dollar medical structure aimed at conquering all disease. This in itself is the true illness, based on a cultural heritage of conquering and subduing. The result today is that sickness is becoming predominant in many lives in more chronic and incapacitating ways.

If sickness is judged to be something bad, as is often the situation, then it is understandable that people will avoid being vulnerable and therefore avoid taking risks. Yet without vulnerability and intelligent risk-taking there can be no growth. Such is the double bind in which we have placed ourselves.

A child takes the risk of trying to master riding a bicycle, even though she knows that a painful fall could be the result. Even after such a fall, with the knowledge and experience of the possible painful outcome of her efforts, the child persists. She is confident of success and of growth in her activities. She is the hero of her own life.

It is the labeling of sickness as bad and something to be avoided that places us in the difficult position of not being able to grow because of a refusal to be vulnerable and to take risks. The way out of this predicament is obvious: change our attitudes about illness.

Why are we at a greater risk of becoming sick when we are more vulnerable? When we are willing to be vulnerable, to keep our hearts open, then what we have suppressed is given permission to resurface, to be seen and named. This may bring on symptoms of illness. Though we often think we are worse off, at these times we are actually closer to breaking through and healing. This is true both personally and culturally. Our epidemic of chronic illness is due to our collective and individual suppression. As we deal with our issues, we may become sick but we are on the way to healing. Illness can be a path to healing.

When we permit our lives to become more vulnerable, we are opening up a breathing process between the dualities in our nature. These are the dualities of consciousness and subconsciousness. We encourage a dialogue between the opposites in our nature. We recognize that light and shadow work together to create a work of art. As efforts at integration intensify, there are often periods when symptoms of illness enter.

The problem is that illness is not often appreciated in a positive way. Our culture of narcissistic self-interest holds contempt for vulnerability. Much energy goes into control and being headstrong. This illusory way of living is supported by the foods we eat, the medical care we seek, and the consumer-oriented advertising culture in which we participate. Because of this, symptoms of illness are not appreciated for what they really are. Instead, we suppress them because we have fear, or we become resigned to them and do not attempt to change. We would rather be ill than change our lives. We would rather die with anger toward a parent than work to open up the flow of love in our heritage.

Acknowledging that we cannot fight our weaknesses is an acknowledgment of vulnerability. We need to understand and respect our weaknesses for the way they have affected our life. And through this daily work of reorienting our entire way of living, we permit the old ways to die. This is a process of expansion and contraction that may take many years.

The healing process is also greatly assisted by learning to live an artful life. Certain myths may be helpful in understanding the deeper meaning of our illnesses. It is important to pick stories that relate to what each of us is experiencing. For example, there is the myth of the Holy Grail and the wounded Fisher King who found the grail through his weakness, and the myth of Perseus who killed the Medusa. While psychological support as well as physical therapies and remedies assist the process, entering into the rich imagery of myth provides us with a framework to develop and nurture the creative imagination. Myths are guides for us to become more vulnerable to life, more tolerant of and accepting of our weaknesses and difficult life situations, and more able to transform our weaknesses into a renewed life of purpose and service. Myths and the creative arts as tools for healing are discussed in the chapters to come.

IMBALANCES OF THE PSYCHE

Our tendencies to illness often appear not only in the obvious physical symptoms, but also in imbalances of the psyche. How well we observe these weaknesses and create antidotes may determine whether we can prevent incapacitating chronic illnesses or accidents in the future. The latter often manifest as a final physical way to bring our attention to imbalances in temperament and character, and to what we bear from our family of origin.

One tendency in illness is to accelerate into the future before we are ready. This occurs when we are not being observant about what is running our lives. Many of us relate to the world through our abstract thoughts and hidden fantasies, rather than through reality. We are always thinking of something rather than focusing on the moment. Thinking becomes an escape from feeling. This type of thinking, combined with our habitual activities, may wreak havoc in our lives. Much illness comes from the extremes of being too much in our heads and simultaneously acting chaotically, without rhythm. The present has been stolen. Our middle, our center, our balancing point of feeling, has been overshadowed by a thinking that is out of place and activity run amok.

This cultural trend toward acceleration begins during the perinatal period of life. Insensitive hospital-based births, the devitalized foods consumed by pregnant mothers and fed to infants, immunizations, overexposure to television, and education that stresses premature stimulation of the intellectual functions in young children are examples of this acceleration.

The process of healing is learning to be in the present. This means observing the many ways we retreat back into the past or lurch too quickly forward into the future, often in just those instances where we need to be in the present. This is illness. We participate in this illness in every phase of the day through such common everyday activities as eating, walking, or sleeping.

How do we develop an antidote to these imbalances? Listen to music, or have dialogue with someone. Observe your breath. As noted previously, practice looking at the trees instead of the billboard signs when you are driving. These are ways of being in the present. It takes vigilance. The illness of staying in the past or escaping into the future always wants to assert its control, because we have for so long given it such a strong position in our lives.

Developing a sense of being is central to the transformative process of regeneration. Without this, we will individually and collectively be hurled into the abyss by the rampant death forces of world chaos.

CHAOS

Chaos occurs when there is no directed purpose that guides our activity.

Each human being is composed of:

1. Physical substance

2. A field of life forces that stir the physical substance into activity and movement

3. A still more evolved field of consciousness that guides the activity of life forces into directed and purposeful activity, which in turn guides how our physical substance manifests.

This composite picture of a human being is the basis of energy medicine and energy psychology.

In the human physical constitution the forces of consciousness are centered in the head and act through the nervous system and the sense organs. The head needs to be still like a quiet pond to function appropriately. At the other polarity, powerful life forces are constantly in movement in our metabolism, with a constant fluctuation between the destruction of ingested food and the creation of new bodily substance that grows out of the process of destruction. As a result of this abdominally centered metabolism, there is fuel for our worldly activity and movement through the limbs.

What does this dual polarity—consciousness and life, stillness and movement—tell us about illness on both the individual and collective levels? Let us view this from the perspective of our system of education, because incorrect education generates illness.

Our educational system stresses the acquisition of information and concrete factual knowledge. We have convinced ourselves that in order to compete as a nation in the world, stay ahead, and maintain our high standard of living, this system of education must continue. To this end, we begin our children on informational learning and computer-oriented linear education very early in life. Many parents fear that if they do not encourage this, their child will not be equipped for success.

Faced with limitations in both funds and in student time spent at school, many schools are placing even more emphasis on intellectual learning at the expense of both the arts and physical education. Over the past hundred years and particularly recently, the central focus of education has become books rather than the arts and the observation of life. As a result, the focus within the human constitution is on the intellectual thinking process through the nervous system in our heads. What does the skull represent on bottles of poison or in various mythologies? The skull portrays Death. The place that the Christ was crucified was called Golgotha, the "place of the skull."

In our masculine-oriented Western culture, knowledge is acquired mostly through head-centered intellectual thinking. Our abstract thinking has been separated from its life-generating imagination. As a result, many people, and especially professionals, often live in their heads and experience the world primarily through intellectual thinking. This has fractured the unity of many people. When intuition, subtlety, and feeling guide our thinking, there is healing.

UNDIGESTED KNOWLEDGE LEADS TO CHAOS

What is the relationship between illness and our information-oriented education? The answer lies in the following principle: Undigested knowledge leads to chaos.

An overtaxed head pole often causes us to be too awake, too engaged in the day, with an overstressed sympathetic nervous system always thinking and worrying. We can see this on such tests as the autonomic nervous system assessment (see Chapter 12). As a result, epidemics of insomnia and headaches affect many people and contribute millions of dollars to the income of pharmaceutical companies. The seeds of these problems often begin in childhood. Witness the growing number of children on antidepressants and stimulants.

In a correct relationship of consciousness and life, our life forces are guided and directed by our forces of consciousness. When our heads are overtaxed with undigested knowledge, this diminishes our capacity to think clearly and be more self-aware. As a result, the inherently chaos-producing life forces that arise in the lower or metabolic pole are free to run rampant. We see this in so-called hysterical people who move every which way, without any reason or direction. Chaos-generating over-activity of our life forces is a key factor in cancer. Cancer pathologically occurs when cells that normally have a regulated and directed pattern of activity through the cycles of birth, growth, maturation, decay, and death begin to proliferate at accelerated rhythms and refuse to die when it is time.

Chaos is our subconscious will gone rampant. It is the manifestation of what may be called the destroying archetype that is predominant in our world at this time. This is especially true since World War II with the entrance of atomic fission onto the world stage. A fission reaction that becomes a bomb of destruction is a reaction out of control and in a state of chaos. Fission is the splitting of the nucleus, the center, which releases energy by fracturing the wholeness of an element, permitting the life forces contained therein to expand and destroy the form.

Just as many of us fear that if we do not expose our children to informational learning earlier in life, they will fall behind in the competition of American culture and economic life, many us have this fear for ourselves, and it weighs on our subconscious. Do I have the intellectual skills to keep my job? Does walking into a bookstore remind me of how much knowledge I do not possess? Do I possess the knowledge or am I possessed by the drive for it? And so the illness continues. Most of us have enough knowledge and information, often too much. The problem is that we too often have not developed the skills to integrate this knowledge into daily life. We live in a time of an intensifying epidemic of fear that is often just below the surface. We are increasingly worried and fearful about our economic and physical security.

Our attempts to create life that is risk-free and our view of illness as a threat rather than a doorway to growth are characteristics of the illness of our time: the chaos in the social fabric. Much of the chaos in our society derives from our collective narcissistic pattern of living, which has accelerated in the past two decades.

THE DYING PROCESS OF ILLNESS

During an illness, the one who is ill needs to ask the question: How do I need to die daily so that I can heal from this illness? The physicians and other practitioners involved need to ask: How do we guide this person in the process of dying, which means letting go of a part of himself that he has become used to defending and investing energy in? By asking this question, health care professionals, in addition to relieving physical suffering, aid in the growth and development of their patients.

Through an illness, the elements of our soul and spiritual nature seek to be expressed and reintegrated, and to guide our life in ways that they were unable to do before the illness. This is the redeeming quality of illness, the reason for its existence. It is why the author of *Blessed by Illness*, L. F. C. Mees, M.D., states that we are blessed by the opportunity to become ill in order to wake up to ourselves. When this becomes the focus of medicine, rather than the alleviation of symptoms and the removal of organs that are mistakenly identified as the cause of the problem, then medicine will fulfill its divine and true purpose in the work of healing.

291

For this to occur requires courage on the part of the health practitioner and the patient to end the current collusive agreement between practitioner and patient. Simply stated, the agreement is as follows: "If you take away my symptoms and make me better, then I or my insurance company or my employer or the government will pay you." In this way of doing things, neither doctor nor patient has to take the risk to become more vulnerable to life or to each other. There may be an improvement in symptoms, but no healing.

This collusive agreement is one of many examples of collusion that are rampant in our society. There is the collusion of big business to fix prices. There is also the parental collusion to keep secrets and not to deal honestly and openly with family problems. The child then acts out these collusions as a subconscious service to the parents, out of loyalty. There are very obvious interrelationships among the way we do business, approach our health care, and live our lives as family members. The days are over when we can keep all of these fragmented parts of our lives separate from each other. Life will not permit this anymore.

We need to apply a psychology of death in disease. This is the death of our isolated identity as a controlled personality with all of our secret ambitions and unfulfilled desires. This death becomes a positive and life-enriching process when we invoke soulfulness and spiritual principles in our daily lives. The soul's urges toward wholeness, development, and expression, are guided by such spiritual principles as truth, beauty, and goodness. The major institutions of today's society—family, education, religion, medicine, government—are not doing this work. As a result, we have people who are psychologically fractured, addicted to materialism and its trappings, isolated, and narcissistically driven.

We need to recognize that physical disease and its particular biochemical imbalances often originate in the psychological imbalances of the mental field. These imbalances often have a multigenerational component both in genetics and family dynamics. They may grow out of inner wounds sustained in early childhood as the child adapted to family dysfunction and his or her body changed accordingly. Physical disease often permits latent multigenerational imbalances that might otherwise have remained dormant to manifest physically. This is the basis of Hellinger's family constellation work.

We need to become attentive to recognizing when these shadow forces are directing a person's life, i.e., when we are being driven and possessed by these forces. Shadow forces sometimes reveal themselves in obvious character changes or temperament imbalances. Other times one must be more observant to notice the subtle changes in lifestyle, body movement, or the look in a person's eyes that indicate the shadow forces are in control. A more obvious example is the crazed look in someone's eyes, or their erratic hand gestures.

Physicians need to go beyond the built-in lazy and narcissistic patterns in the way they approach health care. They will then be able to provide appropriate remedies and other methods to help a patient lift the excessive weight of these shadow forces, thus assisting the person in returning to a sense of self.

After one of my patients with asthma began to take the homeopathic remedies I recommended, his bronchial spasms relaxed. At the same time, he became much more open and less defensive. I could feel a quality of surrender in him. This was a positive surrender, a letting go. It was surrender to the process of healing. His life became more rhythmic as he responded to the urges of his soul rather than to the compulsiveness and habitual patterns of his formerly isolated rigid personality. His story illustrates the relationship between lifestyle and illness. In his case, there was a clear connection between his desire to control his environment and his asthmatic predisposition. The homeopathic remedies aided him in looking honestly at his life and making the necessary changes to support healing.

Many do not make this choice. I recall advising a man in the emergency department of a hospital to stop drinking. He replied that he would have a transplant when the alcohol destroyed his liver. In other words, his view was that drugs and the surgeon's knife would do the work for him so he didn't have to change. One study revealed that when given the choice of changing their diet or having their gallbladder removed, most people choose the latter. This is the attitude that medicine today is fostering.

Such attitudes do not invoke real healing, because healing does not occur without a change in consciousness that is then carried into the activities of our daily lives. Without these changes, people's health will continue to deteriorate in spite of all the great advances in medical technology.

The explosive dependence on pharmaceutical drugs characteristic of the second half of the 20th century has made it possible for too many of us to maintain the view that our illness, symptoms, and our lifestyle imbalances are separate. Even some alternative medicine practitioners collude in this separation. By the time in life that drugs, or other approaches, are no longer effective in providing symptom relief, and chronic diseases are setting in, a person's vitality has often deteriorated to the point where it is more difficult to be actively involved in daily life. This is occurring earlier in many people's lives. It is why more people are developing chronic illnesses in their thirties and forties.

Many people do not awaken to what their lives are about until their forties. From a biographical perspective, the years before this time are a completion of old family matters, school, work, and establishing our place in the world. Then we arrive at the time of life when we need to recognize and become more aware of what the deeper needs of life are and what we must do to enable these deeper needs to be met.

Just at this point, because of the way illnesses have been treated for several decades, what do we see? The person's constitution is often no longer able to summon the vitality to meet what is approaching in the fourth and fifth decades of life: the spirituality we need to incorporate into a plan of regeneration. This is the great robbery of our times, resulting in the resignation, fear, and addictions we see in many people in this age group. Energy medicine and energy psychology are what we need to implement at this stage.

The purpose of medicine should be to guide people to greater energy and self-awareness by helping ensure that their vital forces remain strong enough after the first three or four decades of life to be able to meet the deeper needs of the second half of life.

Having the creative capacity and the will to give back is what characterizes the middle years of life. Our culture puts on a pedestal teenage and childhood prodigies. This becomes a cult for selling products to those who can least afford them, based on talent that derives from heredity. The creative individuality of the second half of life is from the individuality within that is able to emerge from the limitations of heritage. With this we can contribute something new and contemporary to our social and cultural development. These are the guiding principles we need to invoke in caring for ill people seeking help.

WHAT IS SUFFERING?

Every time we turn on the television or read the newspaper, we are constantly reminded of people throughout the world who are suffering. Yet what is suffering?

Illness is not suffering. Illness is an opportunity to overcome an obstacle to growth by striving to activate and unfold our inner healing powers. It calls on us to awaken qualities that are often dormant and unused in our everyday lives.

Aging is not suffering. The process of aging is the opportunity to draw out of our selves the deeper principles of life. We contract into experiencing life primarily through our physical senses. We identify so closely with our physical bodies as the only way to experience life and we interpret aging as suffering because it involves decay of the physical body. We need to prepare for aging for many years by learning how to overcome our imbalances and grow in our humanness, our depth of feeling, our self-awareness, so that as the physical body decays we ascend. This means developing an active inner life that may find expression in daily life through the creative arts, relationships, or new vocational work. If we do not accomplish this to a satisfactory degree, then as we age we hold on to a residue of unfulfilled desires and excessive attachments to a strictly physical sensory experience of the world. In such situations, which are common, the aging process can become a nightmare and a living desolation. We can see this in the faces of many elderly people today.

Death is not suffering. Too many of us see death as suffering because of our fear and ignorance of death. Death becomes the enemy when we have not learned how to die during daily life. Death becomes an ally when we learn to shed aspects of ourselves that need to be permitted to die at timely moments, so that we may enter into a greater and more fulfilling life. Illness offers these opportunities. It points to our weaknesses and challenges us to strive to transform them. Surrendering to death does not mean being passive and resigned. We actively surrender much in the same way as we surrender at night by going to sleep. Letting go is an active act of surrender.

If neither illness nor age nor death is suffering, then what is suffering? Why do we see the picture of suffering on the faces of so many people? It is the picture of a sense of loss, perhaps the loss of missed opportunities. These may be opportunities to go vigorously about doing what we inwardly feel called to do, or opportunities to develop caring and honest relationships. When we consciously respond at certain turning points in life, illness does not have to deepen and become debilitating.

In order to evolve out of our obsessive quest for comfort and happiness, and the avoidance of pain at all costs, let us dissolve the walls that hinder our capacity to experience the depths of life in both joy and suffering. The crises of our times require that we strive to build and maintain the bridges between an active inner life and an outer life of responsibilities and good relationships. We do this through the arts, the workplace, at home, and in every daily opportunity that we are offered.

FAMILY, HEREDITY, AND ILLNESS

There have been two hugely significant developments in science in the past half-century. One was the splitting of the atom by atomic fission. This has led to a release of the forces of the mineral kingdom that can be used either creatively or destructively.

The second development has been in genetics: unlocking the codes of the life of the cell through DNA research. Through this development, humanity has acquired the capacity to manipulate life in various ways, from creating new hybrid species of plants to gene splicing. The result is an assumption that by altering the genetic makeup of people in the laboratory we can cure all disease. This way of thinking is very strong today. It is the contemporary "opiate of the masses", as Karl Marx called religion.

Each person carries the latent imprints of what can be termed, "ancestral genetic weaknesses." On a physical level, these vary from obvious conditions such as Down's syndrome to more subtle genetic traits that affect metabolism. Unfortunately, the prevailing consideration of ancestral weaknesses is limited to the merely physical. If we are to grasp the inner significance of illness, however, and see how we can act on the opportunity that illness offers for growth and transformation, then we must create a bridge between the present mechanistic materialistic approach to one of imagination and depth.

295

Ancestral genetic weaknesses are pictures that are lodged in the memory of our cells. They exist in the collective psyche of humanity. These ancestral memories pour through tribe, race, religion, nationality, and family. Each person is born with a certain combination or coloring of these memories that lead to certain tendencies or susceptibility to illness. In homeopathy, they are called miasms, or hereditary predispositions.

The manner in which modern medicine has addressed genetic problems is first to identify the genes implicated in a particular illness, and then make changes in the gene structure, often with drugs. However, when we focus on a person's biographical life, the following picture emerges. When at certain times in life our temperament becomes imbalanced or we become toxic with metals or deficient in basic nutrients, this activates latent genes in our DNA structure. Out of this, certain symptoms begin to emerge as patterns of illness. This is not taken into account in modern medicine's approach of changing the gene structure.

Let us consider the schoolchild. Schools rarely work constructively with children to help them come to terms with their temperaments and grow stronger as a result. Rather, children are often punished and then rebel, which sets a destructive cycle into motion. Out of the resulting imbalance in the psyche, physical or psychological weaknesses emerge as diagnosable diseases, which are then treated with drugs.

Let's say, for example, that a child has an excessively sanguine temperament. The positive attributes of a sanguine temperament are flexibility, adaptability, and interest in many things. With an excess of this temperament, the child may get stuck in being what we call hyperactive. He is moving all the time, fearful, curious about many things but unable or unwilling to focus on any one area for more than a very short time. This becomes the child's way of life. As his deeper forces of character begin to develop, qualities emerge that continue this weakness of temperament. For example, he moves from relationship to relationship, or place to place, never involving himself to any real depth with anyone.

Out of this pattern, certain psychological complexes may begin to emerge. He develops sexual problems and has relations with many women but intimate relationships with few. He develops symptoms of prostate disease. His father also had prostate problems and eventually had prostate surgery. Temperament imbalances early in life led to this prostate problem by activating latent ancestral weaknesses, or what in homeopathy are called predispositions. The temperament problems may have resulted from vaccination reactions, food allergies, excess television, or a host of other modern-day sources.

The prostate symptoms developed in the young man at about the age of 29. Fortunately, just before that, he entered into new friendships with several individuals for the first time in his life and he let himself feel more supported. Through a multifaceted approach that included homeopathic supplements and meditation, the progression of the prostate problem was halted. The man was able to permit the deeper individuality within him to emerge, instead of having suppressed it for years. The excesses of his sanguine temperament – avoiding intimacy, never staying with one job or one relationship for long – began to lessen. The fear, and the accompanying constriction of blood vessels in his pelvic area, diminished. This helped him to arrest the prostate problem and stop the destructive cycle of the accompanying imbalances.

Psychologists like Bert Hellinger and physicians like Dietrich Klinghardt are showing us that each of us lives within a field similar to a magnetic field. This field is our family of origin. Some of our habitual behavior patterns develop because of our still strong though often unconscious connections to our families of origin. This is further evidence of how connection to our heritage can interfere with the development of true individual expression, and how illness gives us the opportunity to resolve this struggle for the benefit of all.

The two great streams of heritage and individuality that we all carry within us are never separate. The lifelong struggle between these two streams creates the climate for illness and healing. It is the struggle discussed in Chapter 14 to balance our hereditary diathesis. It is the struggle to heal what we may be subconsciously carrying from someone in our family lineage. It is the struggle of the small duckling to emerge from the shell. It is the struggle to emerge from the womb, the comfortable life and become oneself, to be true to one's true calling and self-expression. It is the efforts so well portrayed by Keanu Reeves in the movie, Little Buddha. The particular weaknesses of the excessively sanguine man's ancestral hereditary stream brought to the surface certain inner weaknesses that might have otherwise never been noticed. This is very positive. The ancestral weaknesses gave him the opportunity to heal the weaknesses in his inner nature, his individuality. Out of the symptoms of illness and the relationships he began to form, this person discovered the strengths that he otherwise might not have found. He chose to transform his character and his habits. This transformed character then became the soil that supported him to discover his true vocation or calling in life.

MOTIVATING BEHAVIOR PATTERNS

It is becoming more difficult for us to prevent subconscious and unconscious patterns of behavior, individual and collective, from coming to the surface of our daily lives and appearing as symptoms of illness. Growth in addictive and psychopathic behavior must be seen in this light. Our psychological patterns have a direct influence upon our economic lives. There is no separation. To deny the former can and will destroy the latter.

Many modern illnesses grow out of this process of surfacing subconscious and unconscious patterns of behavior. This is a positive development, although unpleasant for many people. Illness makes it increasingly difficult for people to ignore the realities of their lives. Many of us resist change. In the field of tension that the illness creates, a person migrates to one extreme or the other—fear or resignation, chaos or rigidity—as does society as a whole. Often, there is movement from one pole to the other, without any balance or capacity of being centered and not pulled to the extremes.

The story of Jason and the Argonauts relates how the men were aided by the god Neptune, who represents what Jung called the collective unconscious, in order to guide the boat between the two sides of clashing rocks known as Scylla and Charybdis. The collective unconscious is the part of the unconscious that we collectively share in the form of archetypes that are the underpinnings of our lives. In order to stay focused on fulfilling our purpose, we must become aware of what lies in the collective unconscious. For if we do not follow this path on our own, events may lead us to this path in ways that become more difficult to integrate constructively.

Illness can be one of these difficult events. Let us look, in the context of illness, at what a human being does each day. There is a threefold aspect to the constitution of each person. This may be expressed as the trinity of Head (requiring stillness to function properly), Chest (which rhythmically expands and contracts throughout day and night), and Abdomen-limbs (whose function is normally in movement). These are the opposite poles of stillness and movement.

These three bodily areas have corresponding living relationships with our souls. We think in our heads, feel with our hearts, and carry out our wills with the actions of our limbs, which that get their fuel from healthy metabolism. In our culture especially, these three areas of our being have become separated from each other. Now we must reintegrate them so that we do not just think with our heads, for example. Hence we see such phrases as "Thinking with the heart" or "Intelligence pervades the entire body." When an extreme of either excessive thinking or unbridled will becomes predominant, or when the two extremes combine without a balancing and living center of feeling that gives inner strength, then a person is drawn to live out of the extremes of either resignation or fear. One sees this in the stillness and lack of movement of the person who is resigned to things, or in the continued chaotic out-of-control movements of a person who is obsessed by fear.

We can also view each day in a threefold manner. In general terms, we spend one-third of the day at work, where we are often moving. There is another one-third in sleep, where we are still. In the middle is the other third of the day when we are involved with family, creative endeavors, social contacts, study, or other pursuits. This is the balancing and centering part of the day where we create a bridge between work and sleep, activity and stillness.

298

BODY AND SOUL
QUALITIES

24-HOUR DAY

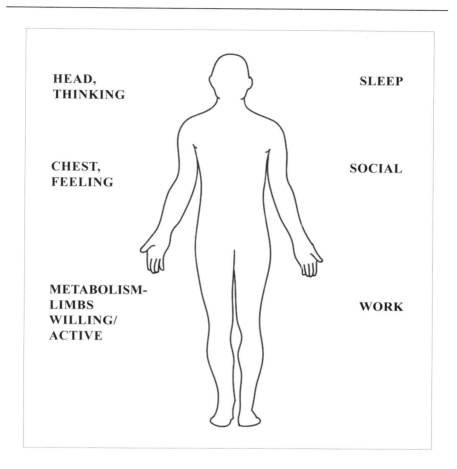

HEAD,
THINKING

SLEEP

CHEST,
FEELING

SOCIAL

METABOLISM-
LIMBS
WILLING/
ACTIVE

WORK

And yet what are we witnessing today? There is an increasing meaning-lessness in many people's work. While more people are employed, they are often in service-related jobs that pay little and involve repetitive work that requires little exercise of the creative imagination.

The inner life is starved and forgotten. Concerning another one-third of the day, we are seeing an epidemic of insomnia and other sleep-related disorders. Many people stay up far too late in the evening and do not surrender to sleep.

It is important to understand that one aspect of the threefold day feeds the other, either in positive or negative ways. The lack of a sense of fulfillment at work during the day creates a sense of uneasiness that often makes going to sleep or staying asleep difficult. This uneasiness often bubbles up because there is a part of everyone that knows when we are not living the life of our potential. This inner life yearns for expression and is the reason we are here.

Being too much in the head during the day makes it difficult to leave the head at night in order to sleep restfully. In addition, many people are experiencing life primarily through over-stimulation of visual and auditory senses and through abstract mechanistic thinking. Television furthers this way of life. So do most of the foods in the diet of many Americans. Advertising stimulates people to experience the world artificially through their heightened physical senses, especially seeing and hearing. This process begins very early in life. And we are at the same time less touched, less held.

To become a success economically and materially involves learning how to function in this too-awake mental environment of intellectual cleverness and manipulation. Our intellect grows at the expense of a starving inner life that is itself relegated to religious institutions where we participate only one day weekly. This sense of being too awake makes it difficult to surrender oneself to the night. The subconscious realms of life, where we hold the residues of our unfinished business, may often rise and create a state of chronic fear and uneasiness. This creates certain imbalances in the internal organs, especially the liver and the kidneys. These imbalances are then seen in conditions of insomnia.

And what do we see in the middle aspect between these two processes, between the economic life of work and the strictly personal life of sleep? In this part of the day, the forces of healing must arise in order to nurture both work and sleep. Yet the traditional institutions of family, church, and school that have dominated this part of the day are crumbling and decaying.

This middle part of the day is eroding in the same way that our feeling nature is not being strengthened. In other words, just as the middle aspect of the day, between work and sleep, too often does not provide a nurturing and creative environment, so the feeling nature that must act as an antidote for an exaggerated intellect and an unbridled will is unable to do so. It is in the context of these realities that contemporary illnesses need to be seen. The extremes of fear and resignation grow, and these precipitate more illnesses that lead people to seek medical care.

In summary, we need at this time to reintegrate an understanding of the psychology of the whole human being with the way we approach health care. A technological and mechanical medicine that denies this necessity will only further deepen the illnesses of our times and continue to create further financial crises.

CHAPTER 18

FREEING THE IMPRISONED PSYCHE: THE ROAD TO TRANSFORMATION

An important principle portrayed in many myths states that as we begin to take account of our lives and make fundamental changes, an opposite force often makes its presence known. When this opposite force acts within us at its own will, we become prone to illness and accidents. In these situations, opposite forces are drawn out of the cave where they hide. These are the dragons in myth and fairy tale that hold the princess captive and will not surrender without a fight.

One aspect of these contrary forces within us is the shadow, as Jung called it and as previous chapters in this book explored. In his short story "The Double," Dostoevsky referred to these contrary forces as doubles. They are elements within our fragmented personalities that we have decided are too negative, so we banish them, or so we think. We turn our back on them, often escaping into intellectual or emotional indulgence, or into a supposedly serene and comfortable social life of family, work, and play. We assume they will disappear much in the same way as we assume people we do not like will leave.

Of course, these unwelcome parts of us do not die. On the contrary, because of our attitude, they have license to live secret lives through us and play tricks on us at most untimely moments. One of our shadow's characters, called the Trickster, is discussed in an earlier chapter.

These banished forces are not merely the stuff of psychology books. They are quite visible every day in various forms of deceit and undermining of our lives. We see examples of them in the theft of billions of dollars from financial institutions and government that were intended to provide a web of so-called security for millions of people. This theft is the shadow of our own attachments to security, and our too ready willingness to sacrifice our souls so that we may be financially secure. These banished shadow forces are nothing more than the forces of our imprisoned psyche that we must embrace if we are to grow.

Psychology describes the shadow as that part of us that we fail to see or know, the traits that we reject because they do not fit into the ideal of who we think we are and how we wish to be perceived by others. We invest much of our precious time and energy in maintaining false images and denying our shadows. To acknowledge and integrate the fragments of our selves involves many hours of conscious effort dedicated to dismantling our hidden patterns. This is something that most of us greatly resist.

Other names used for the shadow are the disowned self, or the darker brother or sister. Though the shadow most often refers to what we consider inferior about ourselves, there is also a positive side. Our shadows are also our hidden treasures, our gifts, which we often also expend much effort to keep hidden.

Everyone has a shadow. When light shines on physical substance, a shadow is thrown on the wall behind it and becomes visible to us. The more we permit the light of consciousness and awareness to shine in our lives, the more we are able to see this shadow that we have kept hidden and which has undermined our lives because we have tried to banish its force. To say that people and institutions do not have shadows is clear denial, a denial that permeates our society from individual and family to corporation and government.

When we deny the presence of the shadow, it gets bigger. Our rationalizations to keep the denial in place take more and more of our precious energy and life forces over the years. In this denial we create our own demons, and these further feed our compulsive habits and negative ritual activities. The problem is that many of these compulsive habits and negative rituals—from gambling and shopping to exercising or going to sporting events too often—become socially acceptable. And our economy becomes dependent for its survival on our continuing these compulsive habits.

The shadow is formed in the first 21 years of life, and especially from birth to three years old. As the shadow forms, we develop a fragmented personality called a persona, a mask that we want everyone to think is our true selves. Our mask is how we want to be seen and is often very different from who we really are. We hide and protect our true selves because of feelings of inadequacy, deficiency, shame, and guilt, or whatever other emotion has become a driving force in our lives, and which we often carry from our family of origin out of love and loyalty.

At some point, we have to take a good look at ourselves and integrate the imprisoned elements of our shadow that have become entrenched in our bodies and our compulsive habits. We must make the commitment to do this, and support each other in this process. Then we create a marriage within us of persona and shadow. For an outer marriage to be successful, the inner marriage must be worked toward. The persona is the positive person we want to be seen as. The shadow is the negative person we do not want to be seen as or see in ourselves.

As we acknowledge our shadow and our false persona, the egocentricity of who we think we are begins to break down. A third or middle force begins to emerge. This is the child that is born within us when we make the commitment to rediscover ourselves in a more conscious way.

The shadow is often a Pandora's Box containing all the vices that everyone has and most of us deny. However, this shadow can also have virtues. In

Greek mythology, when Epimetheus (he who looks behind) opened the box, he let loose all the illnesses and suffering on humanity of that time. However, a virtue remained at the bottom of the box. That virtue was hope.

We need to reconnect with this and other virtues that are veiled by our vices. We can do this by observing our vices, uncovering our shadows, and seeing our stored hidden virtues. Then we have the opportunity to feel good about ourselves, feel worthy of our virtues, and be willing to take responsibility for expressing them to bring good into the world.

This is what is necessary for real change and growth. Without uncovering our shadows, we never get to benefit from our treasures. Instead, they remain imprisoned inside. We always know they are there, and it begins to eat at our subconscious that we have been unable to give birth to them. This deeply felt sorrow manifest as depression. Chronic fatigue syndrome is one way this depression manifests clinically, as we withdraw from life. The hidden toxins we have absorbed into our cells and tissues are what we have attracted in our veiled state. Integrating the shadow is the creative process of life.

We must be willing to acknowledge and share what we have to give. Then the inner wedding can occur, the integration of persona and shadow that is necessary for wholeness. This is the true marriage of masculine and feminine that needs to take place within every individual.

This book looks at the shadow from different perspectives—how it developed in our family upbringing, how it plays tricks on us all the time in order to be recognized, how it works in groups and institutions in the United States. Without recognizing our shadow, no advances of medicine will bring healing, and illnesses and diseases will continue to proliferate.

How do we do this work? Sometimes it entails going to therapy. Other times, we need to change our diet, exercise, and take substances and natural therapies that can help us change our chemistry and energies. Color, eye movement therapy, and sound frequency medicine can greatly assist our work here. Throughout, we need to develop daily objective and nonjudgmental capacities of self-observation. This means being willing to see and acknowledge a negative habit. At that moment, asking a question can be of great help. Why do I want to eat a chocolate bar right now? Why do I want to shop right now? Why did I get so angry at that person I work with? Asking the question opens the door to insight. Then, of course, there must be willingness to act on this insight, and change in that moment. Little changes gradually add up to the whole person we strive to become. Then we feel good about ourselves.

TRANSFORMATION OF THE FAMILY

To be fully human is to be contemporary, awake and conscious in the present, aware of how the effects of our past influence us in the present, not suppress them and yet not give in to them. This is not easy. It takes effort to build the strength to be able to behave consistently in this way. And it requires a circle of friends who share the same commitment to their own growth. This is community.

We are often hindered from becoming more human, more whole and healthy, by not having awakened an inner life that goes beyond a connection to our heritage. What does this mean? Humankind has progressed out of an original state of total identification with tribe and clan. It has incorporated race, religion, and family, as well as the present recognition of the interconnectedness of nations.

The family stands as a middle and stable ground between the isolated person and mass social groups. Yet the family in its present form is being assaulted from many directions. The pressures of the shadow forces of society, especially how they work through the economy and education, place undo pressures on the family structure.

What is family? The nuclear family is that form of group in which the trinity of father, mother, and children live together. This is the form of family most accepted in the United States, though single-parent families are becoming more common and perhaps changing that. However, everyone has a father and a mother. Everyone, from conception has that original trinity in his life.

Unfortunately, many people are not inwardly prepared and strong enough to begin a family. Social and economic forces often encourage people to marry too young and have families before they are ready. Stress from the responsibilities of children and debt, which force both parents to work, frustration, and nonintegrated shadow forces begin to manifest in various behaviors that do not contribute to health and healing. Both partners become overwhelmed and shut down authentic feelings and creativity.

Fear and a strong desire to conform to the norms of the family prevent real change. There is deep resistance to permitting hidden weaknesses and habits to be seen and discussed. These habits grow out of many years of denying our inner wounds, which derive from our families of origin.

In the first 21 years of life, we are normally very connected to family and heritage. When we do not acknowledge our uniqueness as we grow into adolescence and maturity, the effects of this accumulate and reveal themselves through such avenues as addictions, compulsive behavior, suicides, workaholism, rage, and psychopathic behavior. The family heritage often becomes stifling to us. Youthful and even middle-age rebellion is a cry to allow our inner selves to emerge and become active.

The two partners in a marriage often enter into an unwritten agreement to collude. This agreement states: "You tolerate and ignore my weaknesses and I'll do the same for you." To be clear, tolerance is a virtue. But collusion in order to deny each other's imbalances to keep an illusory peace is quite another matter. To compound this situation, members of the modern family are often tied together economically. Today both people often work outside the home to make ends meet. There is a shaky financial structure that both partners are fearful of upsetting if they start talking about deeper feelings.

When children are born into this kind of family arrangement, they are not greeted as the gifts they are. A child symbolizes the creative imagination of two people, the child's mother and father. Yet thinking this way is forgotten in the strains of daily living. If the marital relationship did not have a solid foundation to begin with, the child is not born out of creativity and wholeness, but out of the social drive and expectations to keep the family together.

The family is the focal point for all other elements of heritage: race, religion, creed, ethnicity, and nationality. Nevertheless, what at one time in our cultural development were appropriate and necessary structures to promote the development of family within each culture have now become blockages to growth. Multigenerational illnesses are surfacing all over the world, and especially in the United States, which has become the world's mixing bowl of cultures.

What has been hidden for centuries is now coming out in the open. All of this is very positive. Our roles, repressions, denials, and habitual ways of living are staring us in the face each day in our families, at work, and in other groups in which we are involved. This is the legacy of heritage that has a stranglehold on our creative lives.

Today something is emerging within and between us that is not heritage. This is the beginning of true community based on individuality. Simultaneously, the illnesses within families that for so long have been suppressed are now emerging. The hidden emotions and habits that went unquestioned for generations are now being called into the open. Something of a deeper and more nurturing nature is pushing to the surface in humanity today. The United States is the focus of this in the world, yet the effects are being felt in other countries and cultures, too.

Incest

An epidemic of physically and psychologically incestuous and abusive acts exists within families. Ignoring these realities is becoming more difficult. We lament these acts; we counsel so-called victims and perpetrators; and sometimes punish the victimizer. Yet this does not help us to resolve these difficult situations, because our solutions permit no new light and grace to emerge.

We need to understand abuse as part of stress and the breakdown of family that is occurring at this time and has been for the past 50-100 years. If we broaden our field of vision, conscious relationships based on recognition of the creative individuality of each of us can manifest in the family and the community at large. It is only when creating consciousness is incorporated within the family that the family can assume its rightful role as the safe place for another person to come into the world and grow into a fulfilled life.

What is incest? This is a very uncomfortable word. It implies that a great crime has been committed, often toward a child. Throughout history almost all cultures have had an incest taboo. This explicitly forbids incest, which is defined as sexual intercourse or other sexual activity between persons so closely related that marriage between them is prohibited. This taboo was designed to protect the blood lineage and to permit tribes and family lines to continue. Robert Stein provides an excellent understanding of this in his book *Incest and Human Love*.

When members of a family or culture observe this incest taboo, the child has space to grow up and learn the distinction between sex and love. Because sex is forbidden with the parents, love is free to grow. Likewise and necessarily parallel to this, a child's creative imagination flourishes in such a setting. The particular archetypal and unique qualities of the child's psyche gradually develop and take hold during the early years. This would occur well before the age of puberty and the flooding of life with the forces of sexuality and intellectuality.

When parents, teachers, health practitioners, and corporate businesses combine in encouraging these archetypal qualities to develop in children, these qualities serve as the children's protection and guide during the period of puberty, so that they do not lose themselves as they relate to peers and school. Today, children are not being given the support of an incest taboo.

Many children are exposed to one or more of a number of sexual and other abuses very early in life. This ranges from physical or overt sexual abuse to verbal language misuse by parent(s), to being shown acts that they are not psychologically developed enough to understand, magazines that give overt or subtle sexual messages, called subliminal suggestions, and television that overwhelms the senses with images the child cannot integrate. Or the child is pushed into being a surrogate spouse for one of the parents because the parental relationship is not present in a single-parent family or there is a strong degree of shame or denial between parents that is kept hidden.

With incest, the child's image of psychological wholeness is fractured. Our cultural obsession with mechanical laws and the rational mind have promoted and rewarded abstract intellectual development and suppressed healthy sexuality. The cost of banishing or suppressing both the instincts and the unconscious from which our life-giving archetypal natures spring is the loss of the qualities of creative imagination, inspiration, and intuition. Without these elements active in our lives, there is fear, resignation, boredom, and anxiety, and the shadow forces become overwhelming. These shadow forces are not only hidden in the psyche. They can be seen in the abusive, drug-infested, or shame-driven homes that habituate our nightly news events and daily talk shows and occur in all economic and social strata.

There is an abyss today between our divine and animal parts. We can see this in the manifestations of precocious clever intellectual development and in the many sexual diseases and aberrations. The incest wound that affects most people today is the disturbed relationship and split between sex and love. It is fed by a distrust of our animal-instinctual nature and a glorification of the rational mind. Our highly advanced mechanistic professional culture of sophisticated darkness has developed out of this split. So have most of the psychological and physical epidemics of today.

To return to the original question, what is incest? What does it mean today to be incestuous? Is this restricted to dictionary definitions and explicit examples of sexual molestation or rape? Incest is often the subject of talk shows on television. Incest is much broader than the sexual behavior we too conveniently want to restrict it to. Incest is in the multigenerational roles we continue to play out and that fracture us early in life.

We too often give ourselves permission to remain in driven lifestyles that are the shadow behind our persona, and we support each other in staying this way. We go to movies about heroes, yet most of us do not try to become a hero in our daily life. The hero in most cultural myths slays the dragon that lives in a hidden cave. This is where we hide the pain of what we have taken on early in life from the incestuous behavior of our original family. We act out the continuing effects of these wounds, and perpetuate them in the families we enter as fathers and mothers. In this way, we remain incestuously tied to the past through present patterns of behavior that are often self-destructive.

What are some of the contemporary results of incest wounds?

1. We too often have families that blindly follow certain precepts of religion, race, ethnicity, or national patriotism. In doing this, we often exclude or neglect others who are different and who may offer a real relationship outside the narrow confines of heritage. We become too comfortable with familiar settings that give us permission to go to sleep to our real selves. There is no awakening to who we really are beyond being a son or father, daughter or mother, or a lawyer stuck in a profession, or perhaps an Hispanic or white person with too much racial pride, to use several examples.

2. We are chained by mass emotional unconscious ties. Again in Greek mythology, Prometheus was chained to a rock. Each day, an eagle gnawed at his liver. Each night the liver healed. And the pattern repeated every day, until the hero Hercules released him from the rock. We are all chained to this rock. Each day our livers, which are the main metabolic

307

and detoxification organ in the body, are gnawed by the emotional drives and negative habits from our original incest wounds. Even worse, each night the liver tries to heal but often cannot. It is too overloaded.

When there is an accident or epidemic, we too often react in unconscious emotional hysterical patterns and lose focus. Our unconscious fear rises to the surface. Wounds of incest, denial, and shame linger in the unconscious, avoided at all costs in a society obsessed with comforts. These wounds manifest sometimes many years after the original event.

3. We too often are excessively attached to the physical body and its pleasures, pains, and comforts. Ancestry is rooted in the physical body through our genetic inheritance. Incest wounds grow and manifest today because of our excessive unconscious connection with these ancestral blood-lines that we maintain through our obsession with physical comfort.

4. There is an increased tendency to dissolve into a primordial unconsciousness and state of dependency characteristic of infancy. Elderly people with Alzheimer's disease as well as youths who seek death in drugs or suicide are two examples. John Bradshaw calls this patterned addictive behavior that comes when we are released from obsessive-compulsive behavior two sides of the same coin. We are either over-controlling, which is a compulsive state, or we have no control, as in addiction.

These two opposite sides of the incest problem feed off human nature and devour our lives. We are caught in the extremes, lacking a strong middle force of heartfelt feelings of trust and a rhythmic sense of life. When we are trapped in gravitating between these two extremes, we return to infancy, which is the time when the incest wound often began. We lack the courage and strength to meet and accept ourselves as we really are, wounds and all, and by doing this, become more human. Most people receive very little support, encouragement, or education to develop this courage and insight.

5. There is a loss of the imagination as the primary guide to growth and development.

FAIRY TALES AND INCEST

Throughout history, myths and fairy tales have portrayed many basic elements of the human psyche. They give a more imaginative and less intellectually hardened perspective on many of today's epidemics. In some of the more popular childhood fairy tales, such as "The Sleeping Beauty" and "The Frog Prince," the central character is under a spell. Often an evil witch has cast this spell. Frequently there is a drop of blood involved, and this is significant.

Children love to hear tales told over and over again. These stories speak to them in a language of images, and teach them in nonintellectual or abstract ways about deep truths of life. Most adults have lost the capacity to enter this imaginative world. Adults are under the spell of enchantment that is cast by an egocentric, intellectual-information culture of sophisticated darkness.

Children instinctively realize the truths in these fairy tales. Years pass. Childhood is followed by adolescence and then adulthood, with a growth in consciousness and abstract thinking that is often devoid of imagination.

How often do adults see or feel the deep wisdom in a fairy tale? More often than not we read the story to children to help them go to sleep, and then return to so-called important matters. In our adult state of mind, we view these tales as illusory, because we have lost the capacity to feel the depth of wisdom and simplicity. We have forgotten the words of the poet Wordsworth, "The child is father to the man, or what's a heaven for?"

Upon closer inspection, the composition of these stories reveals ways of understanding today's epidemic of incest. The witch is the clever intellect who focuses only on having more material possessions. She often lives in the forest of the subconscious. This is a subconscious that we in our rational sophistication have banished and continue to believe we can ignore. We do not realize that our creative possibilities derive in part from keeping a dynamic and living bridge between our conscious and subconscious. Our refusal to maintain this bridge leads to many of our contemporary incestuous problems. The subconscious habitual forces of family heritage become too strong, overpowering our childlike feelings of awe and wonder. They wreak havoc and chaos because we permit them to maintain a grip on us long after it was time for them to die.

Blood has been called our central spiritual fluid. Mephistopheles, the persona of the devil in Goethe's epic Faust, knew this when he asked for the blood of Faust in exchange for immortality. Sleeping Beauty pricked her finger and shed blood, and then went to sleep along with everyone else in the land because of the spell on her. That spell is the perpetuation of the bloodline as our primary way of relating to others. Rather than learning to relate to each other as conscious individuals, the blood relationship is often the path of least resistance. Many become parents before they have recognized and healed the wounds of incest from their own past. The flow of love becomes restricted in our blood-lines, and we pass the restriction on to our children.

The male-female relationship that is portrayed in fairy tales as prince and princess can give us insight into how we can break the spell of incest. The true masculine and feminine natures within each individual are reawakened and united again. These are the mysteries that are contained in many myths and fairy tales. They awaken within us an image of wholeness in what is called the Royal Marriage of masculine and feminine. We learn how to develop, as David Deida tells us, from immature to mature masculine and feminine. The archetype of union that children enter into with their mothers and fathers is often damaged or destroyed early in our lives.

Until parents themselves come to terms with their own weaknesses and wounds by being willing to observe and reflect honestly on a daily basis, there may be no healing of these multigenerational illnesses. Wounds are much more visible today than ever before.

What the child experiences is betrayal. The life-giving creative imagination and childlike nature that sustains growth in everyone begins to die early in many children. As the shadow forces take deeper hold, the faces and the behaviors of children change. As noted previously, this premature death of wholeness is encouraged by many social and medical practices we consider normal: devitalized foods early in life, vaccinations, and early intellectual education. The child grows up perceiving a fragmented partnership between our divine and animal parts. In *The Neverending Story,* a wolf threatens to devour the children. The wolf often symbolizes the cunning intellect and indiscriminate desire nature that devours everything.

Many of us correctly sense that incest taboos have broken down, and that it has become harder for our families to provide a healthy structure and protected safe space for children's growth. The family structure often remains as a shell of its potential. Today we see the results. Instead of being compassionate and imaginative in the face of this chaos, many call for more law and order, rigid discipline, and severe punishment. This is like looking in the mirror, not liking what we see, and then passing a law banning mirrors.

The power and respect of the creative imagination and of an open feeling nature are the true antidotes to these problems, as well as to cultural regeneration as a whole. Our creativity grows out of a redirection of the incest urge through participation in healthy cultural rituals and therapeutic dialogues. These rituals must be based on a true understanding and respect for life rhythms and the restrictions in the flow of love in our family constellations. Healthy rituals need to be part of our daily lives in our homes, schools, health care facilities, places of worship, and work. They provide the growing person with the guides to safe passage through major life changes. In other words, they give us glimpses of the divine in earthly life. We all need this.

The evolution of inherited blood lineage, from clan and tribe through ethnicity, and race to family, has been a necessary ingredient for our collective emergence from instinctual unconsciousness. A time arrives, as it has now, for us to move beyond the confines of heritage and into a true sense of brotherhood or sisterhood, of a shared humanity. Or, brotherhood and sisterhood that is based on individuality and community. The epidemics of incest and of chronic disease are signs that it is time to move on, to heal the wounds in our

310

families so that we may draw strength and love from those who have come before us. Chronic diseases reflect the decades of habitual lifestyles that have become comfortable because of our over-attachment to blood-lines.

When we become so wed to repeating past experiences that we do not perceive the inevitable passage from one cycle to another, then we risk being consumed by the forces of death that are released in this process, instead of learning to change these forces into constructive elements of regeneration. These death forces are the control, perfectionism, drive, shame, obsessions, compulsions, and codependency that are rampant today. The multigenerational wounds we act out in these and other ways produce a tomb that encases our creative capacities of soul and spirit. To reclaim our health and well-being, we need to transform the energies that are trapped in our lifelong habits. These energies will always seek expression. If we do not find ways to express them creatively, then these trapped energies will turn against us and weaken our cells, tissues, and organs.

CHAPTER 19

CYCLES AND RHYTHMS

What stops us from perceiving and acting on these insights we develop into the workings of our psyches. The answer is, in part, our lack of relationship with our unconscious. In addition, we do not acknowledge the significance of cycles and rhythms. In spite of well-documented research, our lives are becoming more chaotic and lacking in rhythms. Rites of passage through major life-changing events such as birth, puberty, marriage, or death are either ignored and denied, or are merely acknowledged and adorned in fantasy. We perceive one year as the next, one day as the next, and primarily see life in terms of how we are affected in our jobs and material well-being and comfort.

Because we focus too much on the physical and mechanistic, we do not observe the subtle changes in our lives through cycles. In the same way, we do not take account of the subtle changes in our health and well-being until these changes precipitate a more physical change that is often accompanied by pain or fatigue. We have become deficient in perceiving how participation in these cycles and rituals of life enhances our lives as beings of spirit and soul.

We need to develop faculties that are present but often underdeveloped. These faculties are of service to us as we learn to live more in the present. They help us by enhancing our capacities of observation, reflection, and honesty. Too often, our egotism and narcissistic self-absorption interfere with developing sensitivity to the more subtle aspects of life.

Nevertheless, cycles always occur, even when in our social and cultural arrogance, we choose not to recognize their reality and effects. Unfortunately, we are sometimes forced into this recognition by an accident or incapacitating illness, or by a major economic downturn or environmental disaster. Cycles have a life and death of their own. There is no life without rhythms and cycles.

At the end of every cycle there are usually aspects that are incomplete. For example, most of us have not fully lived our lives as children or adolescents. Due to emotional trauma, part of our essence or genius may have been repressed, as we took on roles in family dysfunctional environments. As a result, the forces of early life are not given freedom to play themselves out. These suppressed and distorted forces lead to organ weaknesses that manifest as psychological or physical illnesses later in life.

313

The nervous system develops in a healthy way when we are able to go through successive stages of development and meet the requirements of each stage. Dr. Gerard Gueniot, the French homeopath, describes how the nervous system that innervates all our organs does not fully myelinate until the age of four. However, when we are pushed to stand up before we are ready, or when we are exposed to emotional traumas early in life and change our posture as a result, or when we are vaccinated at birth, or fed animal milk before nine months old, these distortions change the body. They change the autonomic nervous system and alter the function of our internal organs.

This highlights again the importance of perceiving the whole of life as moving through interpenetrating cycles. When the cycles and rhythms of life are not honored, it is like completing a grade in school without being prepared for the next. Then what has not been learned and integrated weighs on us in the next grade and makes things more difficult. How often do we see children being passed into the next grade in school without being prepared? This is a reflection of what goes on in many of our lives. And we are burdening our children with our illnesses by continuing to do this.

Collectively Andromeda, the woman who is chained to the rock that symbolizes hardened intellect and fixed opinions and attitudes, symbolizes us in myth. This rock is next to the sea, our unconscious emotional ties. Out of this sea comes the dragon of our heritage of incestuous blood-lines that seeks once again to devour the enchanted captive. Andromeda is captive to cultural traditions that we continue to permit to possess our lives through attachment to the unconscious habitual patterns of contemporary family and social life.

The family is not the problem. The forces of inertia and hidden emotions, traumas, and secrets that possess people in many families are the problem. Many of today's physical and psychological epidemics strike directly at the perpetuation of these hereditary currents. They must be infused with new qualities of healing love. Our resistance to these changes and growth unnecessarily invokes the severity of our diseases.

To return to an earlier image, mother and father provide a nurturing environment for the child. This trinity is the physical embodiment of the underlying principle in the Christian tradition stated by the Christ: Where there are two or more gathered, there I am. The child in us symbolizes the rebirth and renewal of relationship and its creative capacities.

The children who are the physical reality of this inner symbol are being abused, neglected, and pushed too quickly. We are experiencing the fruits of our collective denials in the thousands of cocaine and alcohol addicted babies, those that are sexually, physically, or psychologically abused or neglected, and those that are pushed and accelerated in school to achieve before they are ready. The origins of many of the illnesses such as environmental illness, chronic fatigue, and autoimmune problems that are epidemic today can be traced to early life. Autism is the epidemic of childhood that has helped to make us aware. In autism, for a number of reasons, the young child withdraws from healthy contact with the world.

BREAKING THE SPELL OF ENCHANTMENT

We in our sophisticated darkness often disdain and frown on the feelings and imaginative faculties of childhood. Through the overwhelming realities of daily life, many of us have forgotten or have chosen to forget. We may recall Wordsworth, "Our birth is but a sleep and a forgetting." This forgetting of childhood serves an important purpose, up to a certain point in our development. To adapt as functioning adults we must forget parts of childhood. But the body stores the memory of traumas, even though we in our conscious minds forget. The time in life comes when the basic elements of childhood—trust, awe, wonder, and imagination—must be reawakened if our lives, both individual and collective, are to be renewed.

These childlike qualities are forces of the psyche that we keep imprisoned, like the witch, the clever manipulative intellect, who kept the little boy Hansel in a cell in Hansel and Gretel. He was imprisoned so that he could be fattened up. Look at the recent epidemic of overweight and grossly obese children. Do our children now reflect and suffer from our obsession with physical satiation and material comfort? After being fattened up, the witch eats the children. Does this not reflect how we in our advanced culture consume our childlike qualities by encouraging clever intellect and the competitiveness of sports?

In the story of Hansel and Gretel, the stepmother plotted to lose the children in the forest so that she could control her husband. He in turn was naive and too focused on his work, believing in the goodness of his wife. Though he was a heartful man, he was not sufficiently awakened within himself to see that there was a dark, controlling side to his wife. As a result of this relationship, the children were left abandoned in the forest. This abandonment is what many of us feel today and requires us to make fundamental changes in our relationships. We need to come to terms with the entrapments of heritage that are now deeply engrained in our individual, social, and cultural lives. Through a consistent process of honesty and feeling, detoxification, and a daily practice of meditation, mindfulness, and working with color and tapping exercises, we are able to gradually let go of these entrapments. We need to embody the true essence of family in our relationships: to awaken and give birth or rebirth to the sleeping power of love that exists, though often dormant, within every person.

In this way we break the spell of enchantment. We sever our unconscious ties with the destructive aspects of our original families by becoming aware of their effects on us today and being willing to make the necessary changes to allow our uniqueness to emerge. The love of our ancestors helps us grow and heal.

TURNING POINTS

We tend to look at past cultures with an attitude of superiority. Those cultures often knew of the vital importance of ceremony, ritual, and storytelling in helping people to transition through various phases of life. Key transitions such as birth, puberty, marriage, and death are the subject of many myths and fairy tales. This is no accident. Today there is little sense of childlike awe and wonder in passages through these portals, especially puberty and death. For others, such as birth or marriage, we do at least have ceremonies. Too often, young people reach puberty unprepared. Because of imbalanced diets, overexposure to television, zealous use of vaccinations too early in life, and schoolwork that is too intellectual, they reach puberty early.

Adolescence is often prolonged by college and even beyond. Many young people maintain too strong of an emotional connection to their mother or father. Bert Hellinger refers to this loyalty, this need to belong, as greater than the fear of death. Until the hero slays the dragon and emerges victorious, he is insecure, narcissistically self-centered, and self-absorbed. These qualities are age-appropriate to adolescence. But when they persist into adulthood because of what is not completed in adolescence, we are weakened and unprepared to mature in a healthy way. Insecurity is also expressed as a tendency toward self-destruction. Do these descriptions not accurately describe the growing epidemics in adolescence? The impulses of depressive self-destruction may take the form of eating disorders and other addictions, obsessive-compulsive behavior, psychopathic behavior, or even suicide.

Youths today are acting out in these ways partially because those who know better, namely the adults, have not matured. Many of us adults have not moved beyond our own adolescent attachments and comfort-seeking behaviors. How many of us have consistently striven to reawaken in ourselves the awe, wonder, and creative imagination of childhood? Most adults are still tethered to the cord, loyal to our incestuous family of origin connections, and cut off from the flow of love.

The family unit has become rigid. It is breaking down because of this rigidity, like a tree that breaks when the winds of change blow because it is not flexible enough to bend.

There is a difference between honoring our parents for what they have given us and remaining attached to them too long in psychological ways that harm us. There is a difference between honoring the sacred ceremonies and traditions of many traditional religions and races, and staying attached to them out of pride or fear of discovering our own uniqueness.

The purpose of relationship is to enhance each individual's creativity and trust in life and love, and awaken the sleeping imagination. It involves a return to childhood, but in a different way: consciously.

Like Hansel and Gretel, we must slay the witch who would keep us imprisoned and devour us in the forest of darkness that is our over-intellectualized culture of denial. We must return from exile to the land of our home, which is true human warmth. In doing so, however we will be changed. We will have left the womb of unconsciousness and have ventured out into the world of consciousness. This is a land where original light has been fragmented into the spectral differentiation of color, the rainbow, where the crystalline wholeness of being has fractured into multiple parts. In other words, we forget our feeling of wholeness and our feeling of being connected to a greater whole and come to identify with and see ourselves as separate. This reflects our current contemporary medical system of specialization. This world is pleasing to the senses. However, it may become a trap, a spell. We may lose direct contact with the sun, the center of our being and the source of all warmth. As this becomes our "normal" state of life, we then develop chronic illnesses like cancer, which involve lack of warmth. We are like the princess whose great orange ball fell into the depths of the water, the unconscious, and she awaits the Frog Prince to return it to her.

So often the hero and heroine in myths and fairy tales are prince and princess. The Frog Prince returns to his original human form by a kiss from the princess. The Sleeping Beauty is awakened from the witch's spell by the kiss of a prince who comes from a faraway land, which is the land of spiritual forces we have forgotten. He cuts a passage through the thicket of thorns, which are the sharp points of our attachments to possessions and achievements, the clever intellect on which we prick our fingers and shed our blood as we forget our life's true purpose or calling. After the spell is broken, the prince and princess are wed, as in The Frog Prince, Cinderella, The Sleeping Beauty, Snow White, and other stories of deep wisdom.

However, this healthy union of male and female is not the typical marriage of today. Through fantasy and illusion, marriages of today often unconsciously perpetuate the habitual patterns of incestuous behavior and hidden secrets from each person's family of origin. This habitual shame and denial limits the possibilities of each person's meaningful inner growth and development. In other words, each person is not guided, before marriage, to break the spells of family secrets so that the marriage can be lasting, and so that the offspring do not also have to bear these secrets in behavior and in organ development. Homeopathic treatment of both prospective parents can help greatly in preventing this passing on of hereditary tendencies to offspring.

Myths and fairy tales symbolize the marriage to our rich inner life. These stories appeal so much to children because they still feel the joy and exuberance of life's opportunities. Their connection with the inner world is very much alive.

We return from exile as separate adults and are reawakened to again discover the wonder of childhood. However, this return to childhood is not in the way of dim unconsciousness as it was many years earlier. At that time of life we were dependent on others for our growth and were not free-thinking people. Along the way we acquired an intimate relationship with the world and its sufferings. Too many of us, however, have gotten trapped in the dragon's cave of intellectual pride, experiencing the world only through physical senses. To be able to return from exile and enter into the future all the wiser, we must build a bridge to this former land, and cross over to the enriching land frequently. This is the bridge of transformation, and crossing that bridge is the hero's journey.

TRANSFORMATION

Transformation means to go beyond (trans) the form, to create new forms beyond those of the present. Transformation may be seen in three ways:

1. We often hold onto habitual patterns. They are comfortable and known, and so we feel more secure in them. But the trap is that by staying in this womb of false security, we stay separate from others and unknown to ourselves. Much of the chaos in the world is due to our denial of these realities. More people are choosing to deal with subconscious suppressed energies that intrude into our daily lives as they emerge. The violence and cruelty in some current events are misguided expressions of these energies.

2. From the opposite direction there is a precipitation of spiritual forces to which we are becoming more sensitive. The effect of these forces is to draw us closer together. We inwardly experience these spiritual forces as feelings born out of our suffering. Groups such as those that use the Twelve-Step program are good examples. The growing concern for the environment also reflects our increasing responsiveness to spiritual forces, because in caring for nature we forget our obsession with our own security issues

318

and raise ourselves to another level, one that includes the entire planet and all life. Another example of the influence of these spiritual forces is the growing fields of energy medicine and energy psychology.

3. Humanity stands in the middle between these opposite forces from above and below. We each need to create a living bridge within to connect the two, so that we may be strong enough to marry them in our daily lives. This living bridge is learning how to live in the present.

Past, present, and future are subconscious, conscious, and superconcious, respectively. Ken Wilbur provides excellent descriptions of these stages of human growth in his book *The Atman Project*. The past frequently intrudes from our subconscious habitual patterns into our present. And the future calls us through our superconcious intuitions.

Bringing these two forces together in the present is the process of transformation. These forces are not abstract concepts. They have a direct relationship to what occurs in our bodies. This trinity also expresses in our soul faculties of thinking, feeling, and willing. Our thinking is too often obsessed with past thoughts, or mental chatter. Our future is dormant, lacking purposeful movement that directs our limbs to create the future instead of to react as we often do.

We live in the present through our feelings, which as discussed previously are different from emotions. Feelings are of the heart. Emotions emerge when we react without thinking because our security seems threatened. Our reactions are often based on selfishness. Feelings usually arise when we selflessly respond in the moment to what is needed, whereas emotions are from the selfish side of life. The ancients expressed these emotions as the seven vices or the seven deadly sins: sloth, envy, lust, pride, anger, gluttony, and avarice. We need to be willing to observe which of these vices has taken hold. This gives us the power to transform our character weaknesses.

We can transform ourselves and regenerate our lives and our culture by creating the sacred space into which our souls can enter and become a reality in daily life. Each of the three aspects of the soul—thinking, feeling, and willing—requires a new impulse, as follows.

- The abstract thinking that is so predominant today is transformed into creative imagination that provides us with insight into truth.

- The indulgent personalization of emotions in often selfish and separate ways, which many of us stay in to keep us from experiencing depth of real feeling, gives way to a sense of inspiration that is accompanied by an appreciation of beauty.

- Finally, the will nature that in most of us is unconsciously and habitually driven is transformed into an active and conscious

- Intuitive will that guides us into right activities and a will to do good.

This means that we gradually learn to trust our intuition instead of fearing our shadow. First, however, we must be willing to acknowledge the existence of that shadow, the banished side of our nature, the part of us that is predominant when we do not care about others. By doing this, we develop the spiritual strength to acknowledge the presence of our shadow side and yet not feed it or let it run our lives.

Doing this conscious work reawakens childlike qualities within us. We feel worthy to return to the innocent trust that we see in the eyes of a young child, the feeling of inspiration, and the imaginative and creative qualities of our being. We return again to childhood but in a different way, now consciously awakened to the suffering in the world and within ourselves. We complete the circle in this return, yet always on the next upturn of the spiral rather than at the initial level.

The circle of the whole is always greater than the sum of its parts. This principle embraces both our positive and negative sides. It is much more difficult to relate to other family members when all are gathered together, as opposed to communicating on a one-to-one basis with individual family members. The difficulty that we encounter is the entire family entity. It comes out especially at holidays and birthdays, and stifles real relationship between people.

To transform is to change completely in composition or structure, so that the new composition may better embody what we are integrating on deeper levels. But how do we do this? How do we create a living bridge within ourselves between the part of us that is still tethered to the limitations of heritage through our drive and unconscious habits, and the opportunity of a greater life that we are being called upon to live in these times?

We cannot create this bridge simply by repeating the same rehashed past experiences with new window dressing. Doing things in this way is taking the path of least resistance. It is being a slacker, like the character played by Michael J. Fox in the movie *Back to the Future*. It is doing just enough to get by. This is the path that many of us still choose to take because it is the most comfortable, as if that is the main goal of human life. Our social and cultural institutions often support us in this laziness.

320

The parts of ourselves that are unresolved remnants from our continue to obsess us in the present are the narcissistic and sel complacencies of our consumption-oriented culture. We have become the destructive and all-absorbing Nothing that was portrayed in the movie *The Neverending Story*. The Nothing consumes the world's resources and our own life's dreams for the sake of comfort and gratification of the senses. In this imaginative movie, it is the wolf who is the spokesman for the Nothing. The wolf is the guardian of darkness and clever intellect. Our wolf lives in the halls and streets of Wall Street, and enchants us with get-rich schemes steeped in selfish individualism that slowly eats away our true humanity.

We are now being confronted by the cultural arrogance of these attitudes, as evidenced by the following:

- The growth in self-destructive occurrences and activities such as suicide, drug abuse, eating disorders, and other psychological epidemics

- The rise in health care costs, which in part reflects our obsession with the physical and keeping many people alive and hooked up to machines long after they need to be let go.

- The decay and breakdown of the transportation infrastructure (planes, bridges, roads, railways).

- An epidemic of diseases—AIDS and other viruses, cancer, heart disease, and other chronic degenerative conditions.

Viruses serve us in a positive way. These microorganisms often have no cell wall of their own. They get into our cells and change the DNA structure. They do this to serve their own growth rather than ours. The activity of viruses, which we so fear, mirrors many aspects of our culture. There are numerous social and cultural examples of how we penetrate boundaries in order to serve our own ends, or the ends of our business, without concern for the other.

The pervasiveness of subtle manipulative advertising penetrates our minds, disturbing our capacity to think clearly and stimulating our most base and narcissistic emotions, so we will buy products that others want us to buy rather than those we need. Our thinking becomes distorted subtly so that we believe we need the item. Many of us do not pay attention to whether a product will harm us. And children do not have the discriminating capacity to know whether an object they are attracted to will harm them. So perhaps there is a relationship between the epidemic of parasitic viruses and the epidemic of license to penetrate the boundaries of others without conscience.

Perhaps the crystalline forms of viruses resonate with the crystallized habits in our lives, which lead to toxins and imbalances in our bodies and infection by the viruses and the microorganisms they change into that feed on these toxic bodies.

It is unfortunate that many people develop chronic viral problems. In integrative medicine there are many therapeutic approaches that are effective in helping people to heal these problems. Yet these viral problems remain with us as epidemics, because our health care system is trapped in old patterns of financing and thinking.

These problems are interrelated, and they represent the symptoms of both personal and collective illnesses. Yet we are dealing with them in piecemeal and mechanistic ways. We continue to let our behavior be run by emotional patterns formed in our past. We believe what we are told, that problems are solved primarily by more money or more technology and that discovering the genetic blueprint will lead to the cure for cancer, Alzheimer's, and many other diseases. We believe because these problems are increasing, permeating our lives and health, and disturbing our comforting slumber.

The obvious solution is to be more honest and observant, so that we can transform and regenerate our lives. When we do this, illness is no longer necessary, because we have taken up the mantle, the lessons of life that were trying to be revealed to us in the illness.

We need to recreate and reform the bridge of the living present each day out of our creative endeavors and honesty. Groups such as Alcoholics Anonymous know this. Their motto is "One day at a time." The substance of the bridge that we build comes from our past experiences. We continue to reform the bridge when we embrace this past substance as our own, rather than deny it and find scapegoats to blame. Then through the enhanced capacities of perception and observation that we have striven to develop, we gradually transform our old patterns and liberate their trapped energies for more constructive endeavors.

Many of today's problems originate in our headstrong arrogant, intellectual assumptions that the future can be built in the same way as the past was. And the past, with its unconscious emotional undercurrents, rises up to constantly create problems. Our capacities of observation have become weakened, especially when it comes to seeing the whole picture instead of the parts.

We often lack these capacities because we become absorbed in our own thinking, which is self-centered and emotionally reactive. Or, we are constantly being over-stimulated through the five physical senses, always craving more. These two poles—narcissistic thinking and the desire for more things and experiences—are twin curses in this culture. Under their spell, we slowly die because we have forgotten our truth.

Often these two polarities combine. The capacity to embrace the full spectrum of relationship is fractured in this chaos, and manifests in the imbalances in our biochemistry of organs and tissues, which in turn provides opportunities for microorganisms to multiply within us. As noted repeatedly, through the illnesses we develop, we are given the opportunity to become more conscious of our illness-generating lifestyles. This is the positive role of illness, one that we too often ignore.

We often engage the day unconsciously, habitually, still possessed by our past experiences and our obsessive unfulfilled desires. This hinders us from being able to observe and feel each moment the presence of something, someone, or some idea that is new. To be able to do this requires a willingness to respond in the moment to subtle changes in our daily environment. As long as we are possessed by our pasts and obsessions, we will continue to create a future out of past molds that are rapidly decaying. We must create the bridge to a regenerated future out of an enhanced capacity and willingness to be in the present.

SYNTHESIS

There is no transformation without observation. We engage in the art of observation by taking notice. Through observation we are able to perceive correctly how the parts have come together to form the whole. By keeping alive this perception of the whole, we are able to see the right relationship of every part to the other.

Synthesis is the opposite of analysis, the prevailing scientific approach today. In analysis, something is broken down into its constituent parts in order to learn how the whole functions. But in our contemporary obsession with analysis, which dominates education, health care, and the workplace, we lose our vision and imaginative capacity, our capacity to sense the needs of the whole, which is synthesis.

Synthesis requires us to develop the capacity to objectify and detach. We loosen our attachments to observing the world in our past habitual ways, which means through our subjective emotional and self-absorbed experiences. These attachments are the spell of forgetting that encourages us to continue to live in the old but comfortable ways. Under this spell, we are often deluded into thinking that there are no consequences.

The process of loosening our attachments is learning how to die. We die in a small way each night when we let go of being awake and of experiencing the world through our thinking and five physical senses. By letting go of control, we enter the realm of sleep and dreams. Unless we learn to do this consciously, to prepare for sleep and our experiences at night, we are not able to get the rest we need. And so we have a growing epidemic of insomnia and other sleep-related disorders.

To objectify is a process of learning to view and feel our experiences as if we are watching a play. This is not an easy process, because it means we have to see ourselves without judgment, without likes or dislikes, as we are. Yet

ess is vital if we are to fulfill the purpose of transformation and re-
therwise we stay stuck in doing battle as the hero, and we never
yond this into a greater and more conscious wholeness.

This is the central task of the second half of our lives—moving into
wholeness. Few of us learn to master this task. We remain stuck in the habitual behavior of trying to fulfill our unfulfilled desires from incomplete tasks
in earlier cycles of our lives.

We see the tremendous growth in premature degenerative tendencies
and diseases of aging after age 35 or 40. These diseases occur at the time of
life when our forces of regeneration and rejuvenation atrophy, and include
physical diseases such as arthritis, arteriosclerosis, and cancer, as well as
Alzheimer's disease and other forms of senility. As discussed previously,
during the years when our vitality is stronger, many of us do not embrace
the principles of wellness. We choose to continue living primarily through
our fixed habitual patterns and stay too much in the past. As a result, when
the body begins to decay and degenerate, we fall into the trap of too closely
identifying with these organic processes. This is because our more detached
inner childlike nature, our capacity to be present, has not been sufficiently
awakened.

This is true in both old and young people. We become too subjectively
attached to our own life experiences and physical bodily comforts, and
believe these are what it means to be healthy. Many people identify too
much with decaying forces in their body as they age. The elderly return to
the dim unconsciousness of childhood, a time of life that they may never
have left. They become childishly demanding and dependent on others.
This often occurs after a lifetime of being too independent, which is not
the same as being individualized or individuated in Jungian terms. The
term independent has come to mean separate, not inclusive. As the population ages, we are confronted with the economics and unnecessary human
suffering of these denials.

THE SHADOW KNOWS

As we begin to invoke an active process of transformation in our daily
lives, opposite forces hidden within us make their presence felt. This is the
force of certain authorities within us that have long obsessed and possessed our thoughts and activities. These authorities are often unknown to
us consciously until something such as an illness or an accident occurs.
These unwelcome problems frequently happen when these forces act according to their own will and are not under our purposeful conscious
direction. These authorities will often come to the opening of the cave like
dragons that have held the princess captive and will not surrender her
without a fight.

One of these authorities is the shadow, discussed earlier. The shadow is nothing more than the forces of our imprisoned psyche that we must embrace if we are to grow.

A second authority is our opposite inner nature. A man's inner nature is feminine. A woman's inner nature is masculine. Each man is composed of masculine and feminine qualities. Each woman likewise has both a masculine and feminine nature. Men often do not acknowledge their feminine, receptive, nurturing side, called the anima by psychiatrist Carl Jung. Men often perceive femininity as weakness, although this is changing. Or they may suppress hints of this inner feminine nature if they think it conflicts with their strongly masculine self-image or persona. Likewise, a woman may so identify with her feminine nature that she denies her masculine side, the animus. When she does this, of course, this denied masculine will possess her life and cause problems. What we deny often emerges to consume us and cause us to interact with the people around us in ways that are not helpful.

Myths and fairy tales that told stories of marriage were really addressing the reunion or healing of the separated duality within each of us. This is the true significance of the Royal Wedding of the prince and princess. The two have been freed from the spell of incest that chains men and women to one aspect of their nature at the expense of being undermined by the other more hidden aspects.

BREAKING THE SPELL OF FORGETFULNESS

When the evil fairy enters uninvited into the party and casts the spell of death on the princess in The Sleeping Beauty, the good fairy who brought gifts for the princess after the evil fairy knew that she could not undo the spell. She did not fight the evil spell, as we cannot directly fight the dark side of our nature without giving it more control over our life. The good fairy was able to find a way to redirect the negative effects of the evil one's spell so that it would be temporary and would be able to be broken. She cast a spell that put the princess and all others in the castle to sleep. This was the spell of forgetfulness that comes over many families.

Breaking this spell is possible only with conscious effort. It has become more difficult to break the spell today. We collude with each other so that we can be comfortable with our habits and have every modern convenience.

Many often escape from the work of consciousness by pursuing abstract intellectual and professionally narrow pursuits. This is part of the immature masculine nature of our culture (discussed in Chapter 4). It infects both men and women. In our striving to dominate the earth, to have all knowledge and

power, and to control without risks, we have been under a spell of unconsciousness or forgetfulness. We have been acting as if what we do not know
does not matter and will not affect us. To awaken from this spell, we must do
the following:

- Engage in the true spiritual or royal marriage portrayed in
  fairy tales and myths. This is the marriage of masculine and
  feminine natures within each of us, the healing of incest
  wounds.

- Embrace unconscious shadow forces, and be responsible
  for the results, external and internal, of our denial of these
  forces. To be responsible means to be willing to respond,
  in the present, to what is needed in order to bring healing
  in any particular situation. We need to ask for help from
  superconcious guiding forces that are always present and
  ready to guide (for many, this is God, Allah, angels, ancestors, the goddess, and others). And we can also use
  Hellinger's family constellation work to help us.

Just as in The Sleeping Beauty, the good fairy did not fight the spell directly but acknowledged its strength, we must be honest about the strength
that our habits have over us. The principle is that fighting negative forces directly only empowers them. For example, we cannot fight the power of an
unconsciously driven addictive behavior, but we can learn to reflect, observe,
and be honest in the moment, each moment. We can ask ourselves: Why am I
doing this? How am I? How do I feel? Instead of being obsessed by past experiences and unfulfilled desires that continue to possess our behavior, we
learn to live in the present and therefore have the tools to create a regenerative
future instead of a future that perpetuates addictive illnesses. This requires an
effort of the conscious will and the willingness to take risks. Simple exercises,
like those in Rudolf Steiner's booklet entitled *Overcoming Nervousness*, can
be of great help.

We awaken the conscious will in part by asking questions of ourselves
when we feel stuck. Also, doing little things daily gradually awakens our will.
Watering a particular plant at the same time of day helps, or writing in an observation notebook, or changing a habit in the moment, as in choosing to eat
slowly if we tend to eat fast. We can take a deep breath and pause, and be present in the silence. We can pay attention to the subtle colors in nature. The
effect of these efforts is cumulative.

THE THREE GIFTS

How do we initiate and maintain the process of transformation? The myth of Perseus and Andromeda suggests an answer. When Perseus set out to slay the Gorgon Medusa and free the princess Andromeda from the chained rock, he was provided with guidance in the form of three gifts. With these gifts he would be able to do the work himself, and not have the gods do the work for him. This guidance took the form of a shield to protect and reflect, a helmet of invisibility, and winged shoes.

The three gifts symbolize three human qualities that are necessary on the road of transformation. Respectively, these are reflection, observation, and honesty. The shield gave Perseus the possibility to reflect, the helmet to enable clear observation, and the winged shoes to be strong enough to be honest.

The three gifts were worn on three major areas of the human body.

- The shield that is worn next to the chest is the gift of being able to reflect on life. We can accurately reflect only by being vulnerable, willing to feel, and not judging our experiences as good or bad.

- The helmet of invisibility on the head is the gift of being able to observe clearly. This only becomes possible as we clear the mind of attachment to abstract and crystallized intellectual thoughts, and begin thinking imaginatively. Then we become invisible. In other words, we can then do the work of our transformation without having this precious work exposed to those who would destroy our efforts. It is like protecting an infant by wrapping him up in our arms.

- The winged shoes are obviously worn on the feet. Our feet permit us to move through the fog of unfulfilled desires and ascend toward becoming who we really are only if there is a willingness to be honest with ourselves.

These three together—reflection, observation, and honesty—help us create and maintain the living bridge between past and future, to touch the divine on earth, as Sir Walsingham said to Elizabeth I, Queen of England, in the movie Elizabeth. We enhance our capacities to reflect and observe with clarity and honesty, meaning that we stop filtering our perceptions because we do not like them. Our perceptions are not clouded by the fog of past experiences, or what Aldous Huxley called seeing through a glass darkly. Our perceptions can be guided by the creative imagination that is ever-present within us, though too often dormant. At the same time, we become more honest with both others and ourselves about our reflections and observations. We are especially more aware of our observations about the habitual patterns of behavior that continue to obscure the light of day and keep us in darkness.

Reflection

The Gorgon Medusa is an image of the hideous appearance that we assume when we choose to remain too connected to our past through the habits we use to shield ourselves in the present. Perseus killed Medusa with a shield. This shield permitted him not to look directly into the Gorgon's eyes, an act that would have turned him to stone. How does this relate to our daily lives?

When we compulsively and longingly gaze into the past, we turn to stone—we become rigid. Our hardening habitual patterns, which the Medusa personifies, have become so strong that if we (like Perseus) try to confront them directly, without the shield of reflection, they will overcome us. Perseus is the personification of that quality in ourselves that enables us to reflect on our past habitual patterns. We can do this in silence in therapeutic dialogue, and in other ways. Fighting our habits directly often empowers those habits, which can harm us, rather than disarm them.

Perseus waited, observed the Gorgon's movements, which were the movements of our heritage-ingrained habits. Then he cut off her head, which was covered with writhing snakes in place of hair. The snakes symbolize the uncontrolled and unregulated desires that rule our heads too much when we are trapped in habitual behavior.

Reflection is the capacity to look at ourselves objectively, to see ourselves as others see us, to see how our habits set us up for illness. Then we more clearly perceive the subtleties of any situation because our perceptions are less distorted by driven emotions or habitual thoughts. Only by doing this do we really get the job done right and feel we have fulfilled our purpose.

Perseus used the reflection in the shield to see where the Medusa was hiding. He reflected to see where the shadow (Medusa) was hiding. This is what we need to be doing—reflecting, not analyzing. Only in this way could he slay her and the writhing serpents. We often must reflect on the difficult parts of ourselves in order to gain insight and choose the right course of action. To stare at the Medusa directly would have turned Perseus to stone. To look directly at our dark side requires preparation and inner strength. If done prematurely, we may become more rigid, because of the fear this premature direct gaze generates.

We need to develop the willingness to receive reflections from other people, especially from those we trust. This helps us to break the spell of too strongly identifying with our often narrowly structured personas or masks.

The moon is not a source of light. It is the reflection of light. The moon itself is dry, cold, and barren—in short, lifeless. It is the reflection of the past. This is like what occurs during life when we perpetuate our past experiences and the personas we have built. We forget to seek the source of true light and warmth, the sun, the center of our being. In sum, we expand into a deeper conscious awareness and purposefulness of life by learning to reflect on ourselves. This helps us to emerge from patterns of self-obsession that, as with Narcissus who got stuck admiring his own reflection in the pond, will lead to death even while we are still alive.

The wicked queen in Snow White asks the question, "Mirror, mirror on the wall, who in this land is the fairest of all?" She vainly expects and indeed demands to hear that it is she who is the fairest. She is the Narcissus in each of us, in love with her reflection, cold and distant like the reflective moon, without the sun-generated warmth of human heart and feeling. Like the self-obsessed person of today, she is intolerant of any answer other than the one she wants to hear. We do not want to hear that there is a problem with the persona or mask we have developed as our appearance in the world.

The path of allowing ourselves to become open and sensitive to others and to ourselves requires willingness to give and receive reflections without judgment. As we are able to become more detached from our emotions and passive self-absorption, we may offer and receive reflections in more artful and imaginative ways. In the quality of compassion that develops through appreciation of our shortcomings rather than denial of them, we are able to offer reflections as discernment without crossing the line into personal judgment.

It is not easy to offer reflections or to receive them from others. Often, we hear them through our shame-based and narcissistic natures. Then we reject, deny, or ignore the reflection, or use it against others or ourselves. This especially occurs in those who were shamed early in life and prevented from working through their weaknesses.

Additional ingredients of self-observation and honesty are required in order to become inwardly strong enough to receive these reflections and embrace them as one's opportunity for growth. And all of these are critical ingredients in a healthy transformation of the workplace and of our illness-generating health care.

Observation

There is no transformation without observation. When we learn to observe without thinking and without fantasizing, the doors open. Through observation we perceive the whole picture composed of its constituent parts. We remain centered in the present and prepared for what in the Buddhist eight-fold path is called right action. Through observation, we enter into a more direct and intimate relationship with the world. In this way, all things become visible. Little children do this all the time.

When Perseus wore the helmet of invisibility, he could clearly observe what was occurring around him. He had become invisible. We become invisible by being in a constant state of observation. We stop reacting emotionally. In so doing, shadow forces from our suppressed unconscious do not rise up without awareness and lead to reactions. Such reactions often make us unnecessarily visible by the circumstances they attract. In the process of transformation, shadow forces must come to the surface, to the light of day, so that we can see and embrace them, and guide them in positive directions.

This quality of observation is vital to the process of healing. It gives us the fuel we need to build the living bridge between our conscious and subconscious. This bridge enables us to unfold our creative capacities. We learn to observe not only the obvious, but also the subtle. In this way, we stir the imaginative faculty into activity. Only through the creative imagination do we develop as beings of wholeness.

The mechanistic and materialistic world as it currently is steals the creative imagination. It does so daily in many ways, including the following.

- Education that stifles and rigidifies

- Television that manipulates through the mind control of advertising

- Entertainment that emphasizes "formulas for success"

- A social environment that promotes work which is often mechanistic and suppressive to human creativity

- Health care that promotes fear, dependency, and suppression of symptoms

The list goes on. We are either chained to past experiences through our fixation with abstract thinking and reactive emotionalism, or rushed into the future driven by an overly fantasizing mind before we are inwardly prepared to meet the future without destroying it. This is like the sailors on Odysseus's ships who, upon hearing the voices of the sirens, lost their heads and hurled themselves on the rocks in self-destruction. We succumb to the spell of Rumpelstiltskin, arrogantly thinking we can easily weave straw into gold and find contentment without doing the necessary required inner work. Hence the rush to buy lottery tickets and gamble.

Our educational system is obsessed by a spell known as analytical deduction. We break things and people down into their parts in order to learn why they work. We are like the tailor in Grimm's story, The Tailor in Heaven, cutting all the fabric to pieces with our mechanistic intellect in order to sew it back in a different way without imaginative creativity or life-renewing wholeness or understanding. Our schools increasingly stress intellectual abstract thinking while robbing the other aspects of a child's sense of wholeness—the arts that strengthen feelings and physical education that strengthens the will. Medical schools also thrive on this type of thinking.

A child who emerges from this narrow system becomes a kleptomaniac. This means that his strongly built head-thinking nature, mechanically trained and separated from the whole of life, has an attitude of theft toward all of life. We are raising children with an arrogant cleverness of excessive egocentricity and megalomania. These are infantile feelings of omnipotence and grandiosity, especially when retained later in life. Can I make my first million dollars before I'm 28?

To remain in this state is to be more like the blinded Oedipus than like St. George. Oedipus conquers the sphinx, the dragon of the abyss that is the devouring unconsciousness, which keeps us in a primeval state of dependency and hinders our development. But after slaying the dragon-sphinx, Oedipus commits incest with his mother and slays his father. These two represent respectively the unconscious (mother) and the conscious ego (father). Oedipus fails because he does not observe. He loses his sense of direction and returns unknowingly to his town of original birth. He marries his mother, who represents his past unconscious patterns and habitual patterns of heritage, thus committing incest. After discovering what he has done, he does what so many people who are caught up in narcissistic behavior do. He becomes self-destructive, in his case, by blinding himself. He refuses either to accept what he has done and not judge it, or to develop an imaginative antidote to his illness.

Does this myth not speak directly about our present situation? As we perpetuate an intellectually clever egocentricity we are in turn being increasingly devoured by what in our self-absorbed complacency we do not care to observe or act on. The devouring is evidenced by the increase in child abuse and neglect, depression, and self-destructive behavior occurring in our times. These destructive tendencies are typically not observed until circumstances force us to see. Even then we judge and condemn these tendencies and their consequences, and find scapegoats to blame. In reality, these destructive behaviors and tendencies are the objective manifestations of a cultural outpouring of decay.

How do we counter this outpouring of decay in ourselves? The answer lies in seeing. Who comes along in Little Red Riding Hood to slay the wolf and rescue her? None other than the hunter. And what are the qualities of the hunter that bring success? They are:

- Attentiveness to what is around (keen observation)

- Receptivity and readiness to accept and respond to what comes next (embracing without judgment)

It is interesting that Dr. Joseph Mercola, in his book *The No Grain Diet*, and other authors are encouraging us to return at this time to the hunter-gatherer diet. Perhaps this means we need to be more attentive and prepared. There is a balance to strive for by being prepared and alert yet not being hypervigilant.

Little Red Riding Hood, who personifies the childlike nature in all of us, is about to be devoured by the big bad wolf. This means we are devoured by what we have denied. Then we are cast into the abyss of the unconscious until we are rescued by the hunter, or until we become the observer of our subconscious patterns. If we don't become our own observers, these patterns will continue to haunt us through environmental toxicity, terrorism, and illness.

Honesty

St. Michael slays the dragon and is vigilantly observant of the dragon's nature so he is not consumed by its offspring. So is Hercules in destroying the Hydra. This brings us to the third quality that is necessary for transformation: honesty. By enhancing our capacities to reflect and observe, we come face to face with ourselves and with the world as it really is. We increasingly take note of how our habitual patterns keep us tethered to the past. They are the fog that obscures the light of day in our sophisticated darkness. Without a developed sense of self-honesty, the enhanced faculties of reflection and observation are minimized. This is dangerous when we are facing a devouring wolf. Let's return to The Frog Prince. The princess mistreated the frog who she had agreed to take as her companion because the frog had rescued her large ball, symbolizing the sun, from under the water, representing the subconscious realms of life. In being honest and true about the results of her actions, she kissed the frog.

This released the frog from his spell and returned him to his original form as a prince. The princess in turn was also released from her bonds to her father and was able to enter freely into marriage. Her lesson was to stop running from commitment and embrace what she had attracted. She had wanted the frog that had done her a great service simply to go away. Both frog-prince and princess were liberated from the spell of the past, the old ways of looking at the world unconsciously and intolerantly. What freed them from these chains of habitual behavior was the spirit of service of the frog-prince and the princess's willingness to look at herself honestly, to see herself as she is.

THE TASK

The task at hand is to transform our culture by not permitting the forces of decay and destruction to act in uncontrolled and unbalanced ways. If we do not make the necessary changes, these forces will lead to chaos without regeneration. For real transformation with regeneration to occur, we must be willing to enter into the new forms of relationship found in the subtext of fairy tales and myths. We then construct a living bridge between our past habitual patterns and comfortable lifestyles that have provided the substance for our culture until now, and a future of true community committed to drawing out the talents and creative genius of every individual in the fulfillment of life's purpose. This is what healing illness is all about.

As we build and maintain this bridge, we are showing that we have the capacity to be an integral part of everyday life in work, family, and other social involvement, while at the same time maintaining an active connection with our inner self and purpose. We are then flexible enough to pull back when we become over-involved in daily matters and give ourselves the space to observe and reflect on our experiences and what is occurring in the world, so we can more clearly perceive the next step that is called for in our development. We are able to feel the objective and subjective of the two polarities of life's drama, masculine and feminine, day and night. We gradually learn to identify exclusively with neither, and we move purposefully as needed between both. This is the living bridge of healing.

In practicing these principles we take note of how much our fixed behavior patterns and rigid attitudes have maintained a hold on our lives. We enter into new forms of relationship by viewing others beyond the confines of persona or heritage as individuals with dreams and destinies to fulfill, and with weaknesses and wounds that will prevent growth when ignored. Until we do this daily, the negative forces will grow stronger and eat away at the foundations of our lives. All the drugs, surgeries, vitamins, economic patch-ups, and educational quick fixes will not prevent the negative focus from becoming stronger.

CHAPTER 20

THE CREATIVE ARTS AND HEALING

O ur feeling nature is being starved today in this land of plenty with its growing percentage of the population who are overweight. True feelings, in contrast with emotional reactivity, are often suppressed in our culture. What encourages the growth and active expression of the feeling nature? The answer is the arts.

The true role of the arts is to reawaken within each of us a sense of artfulness and rhythm in life by consistently applying the principles of art to each day's process of unfolding. For example, consider rising each morning and playing a musical instrument for 15 to 20 minutes or doing artful movement such as tai chi, yoga, or eurythmy. This is a valuable tool in growth and development.

Through activities such as these, we begin to notice that the particular rhythm or sense of the music varies from day to day. We are drawn today to move differently or to play the music differently from yesterday—different chords, different rhythm, and so on. This brings us into the moment. It helps us to understand experientially rather than intellectually that today is different from yesterday, even though the routines of the day may have us believe otherwise.

We are apt to believe that one day is like the next, that days vary only in externals, such as how the weather changes or who may be ill and not at work or school. However, each day is inwardly different and we are different each day. We die each night upon sleeping and are reborn each morning upon rising. If we do not put forth the effort to observe the differences, which engaging in artistic activity can help us do, then we are more prone to go to sleep during the day and miss opportunities, creative inspirations, or new possibilities in relationships.

Beginning a day with music or another creative art brings us into a creative stream. This sets up a resonance that provides a matrix for all events and interactions of the day. We generate this matrix out of our inner being. It gives us strength to deal with the mechanization and habitual patterns of the day. Otherwise, we are gradually overwhelmed and lose ourselves, and then retire at night with a vague sense of uneasiness and resignation.

We take note of the subtle overtones in a piece of music, or of the ways that our hands move with assurance. Each day has a different pattern on the keyboards or in sculpting with clay or in painting with colors. In the same way, we begin to become more aware of subtle variations throughout the day. The essence of who we are lives and breathes in these subtle areas. To be more aware of these subtleties requires an enhanced quality of receptivity and a willingness to wait.

Each of us must again become like a child with a feeling of awe and wonder, learning how to trust all aspects of our being so that no parts of ourselves are banished from the kingdom of light into the world of shadows.

Even after all these years, I myself still resist this trust in myself, in being childlike without feeling self-conscious, I still am somewhat driven to place informative reading above artfulness. Healing is a lifelong process.

FEELINGS AND THE CREATIVE ARTS

The creative imagination is under assault beginning very early in life. This comes from all sides, including the following:

- Family disharmonies

- Hidden shame and dishonesties

- Toys that do the work for the child and leave nothing for the imagination

- Television that encourages passivity and stereotyped thinking

- Drugs taken early in life that have hindered or overexcited the development of the nervous system, so that the higher faculties such as imagination do not develop in healthy ways

Without our creative faculties, we are weakened and more susceptible to taking the path of least resistance. We live subconsciously and habitually through comfortable and socially encouraged behavior that keeps us too tethered to our heritage. The song of the childlike imagination recedes—as Wordsworth wrote, "Our birth is but a sleep and a forgetting."

As the strength to become whole fades within us, the always-present death instinct is unleashed and becomes destructive. This is what we face today. And this is why new forms of relationship, such as the consciousness communities described in this book, must be developed and must permeate all human interactions. They are the living antidotes to the rampant death forces of the wolf that threaten to devour our culture.

In these new forms of relationship, we learn to assist each other in drawing the negative forces away from another person until that person's creative forces can become strong enough to provide a balancing force. This is the true process of healing.

336

The arts are vehicles of inspiration. Any of the arts, such as architecture, sculpture, painting, music, poetry, drama, and movement, can be vehicles for creative expression. One certainly need not be an "artist" to create art. Without knowing how to read music, we can sit at a keyboard and create beauty that inspires us to enter with greater feeling and vulnerability into life's mysteries. Without knowing any of the so-called rules of poetry, we can write spontaneously in a rhythmic fashion. These exercises become the vehicles of self-transformation.

Furthermore, they serve as a living process to take the undigested knowledge in our lives—knowledge that can otherwise create more chaos—into a process of creative assimilation and expression. Often when we are playing music, writing poetry, or sculpting, events of the day or contemporary life situations come onto the screen of our conscious minds. These are the often-unnoticed fragments of knowledge and life that yearn to be integrated into the whole.

Beyond any of the specific creative arts, we need to develop a sense of the artfulness of everyday life so that we do not get trapped in the constant drum of daily duties, projects, habits, and readings. And the cornerstone of the art of living is a lifestyle of observing our process and seeing it as an artful development that is unfolding. This requires and teaches us to develop an artful ritual to everyday life. In this way, we can transform the senses, so that not only do they help us in our daily life, but they also are inner receiving points for our soul/spiritual natures. As painting teaches us to see the subtle changes in hue, so we are training ourselves to see the subtle changes in our relationships and work. As we teach ourselves with sculpture about the life of forms, we train ourselves to see our relationships and lives as more mobile and less fixed. With music, we teach ourselves to be able to hear what people and events are really saying to us, beyond the words. With poetry, we learn that words have a beauty that we hardly ever express in daily life. When we engage in movement or dance, we develop an inner sense of movement, of where we are going with our lives, of "knowing" our next actions.

Living out of a sense of being is what Edward Whitmont refers to in *Return of the Goddess* as the transformed feminine nature that we greatly need in our illness-generating culture of predominant masculine and paternalistic values. This sense of being that lives in an active feeling nature puts us in touch with the mysteries of transformation and acts as a guide through the abyss of the death forces of our contemporary world.

Without art there can be no healing, and the death forces will become rampant. Only with a renewed artfulness to life will there be positive and constructive movement in the economy, education, or health care.

Through practicing the art of living as a lifestyle of observation, we can again return to what is termed the Sophia, or wisdom in action.

There is no life without art.

337

The arts are gifts from God. This is why much of the great art of history was done in the service of religion. But we are all artists. Art can help us greatly in the process of personal and collective transformation.

Many in the medical and psychology fields see art as therapy for the handicapped or mentally ill. This prevalent attitude is slanderous to the human soul and spirit. This slander originates in our predominantly mechanistic ways of processing, and in the economic priorities of medicine.

There are other reasons that arts such as painting or sculpture are not generally embraced as therapies for all illnesses and all wellness programs. Many of us are afflicted with a general lack of creative participation in life and work. And our educational system rewards abstract intellectual thinking rather than the development of cognitive faculties. The country as a whole denies death, and our major institutions support this denial. An artful process that enhances a life of feeling and helps us to go through a living process of healing and self-renewal brings up this resistance in many of us.

ARCHITECTURE

Architecture is the first in a sevenfold classical procession of the arts: architecture, sculpture, painting, music, poetry, movement, and drama.

Architecture is form and structure. In architecture, we use the mineral kingdom (calcium and other minerals) to build. The central characteristics of mineral forms are rigidity, immobility, and stillness. Buildings have a certain structure that provides grounding and space. Because of its connection to the mineral kingdom, the art of architecture corresponds to our physical body, which is our vehicle for growth and development. The mineral content of our physical bodies provides strength to this form, if we have enough of the right minerals, and if they are in the right relationship with each other.

Though minerals exist throughout the body, they are most densely concentrated in the skeleton. The human skeleton is that form within a human being that corresponds to an architectural structure in the world. The same is true for each art form. When we begin to perceive the world and our lives in artful ways, by seeing the interrelationship between our own form and the architectural forms we build, life begins to have more meaning. Then we will build structures that are alive with human creativity, rather than the predominant forms of building today, which are merely functional and mechanistic.

SCULPTURE

Sculpture is the force that gives life to form. A sculptured form often appears more alive than a building. Why is that? After all, human effort has

338

gone into creating both. One obvious answer is that many buildings are mass-produced whereas sculpture is more individual. However, even mass-produced sculpture seems to have more life to it.

In sculpture, we perceive movement and flow. Life is movement; only in death is there stillness. This is not a mere abstract statement. When a person stands still in life and tries to stay the same, to stop time and keep things the way they are, this person ceases to permit life to become alive within him and to be inspired by life.

Sculpture is one antidote or remedy that we can apply to help heal the overemphasis on head-oriented abstract intellect. To begin with, what is to be sculpted must be wet in order to be molded and shaped by the hands. Thus the life-giving forces inherent in water give life and movement to what is dry and lifeless: earth. An image of sculpture in the human body is the muscles that contain more water than almost any other organ in the body. In contrast to the relative dryness of the bones, muscles give the body a sculptured and living image, a flow of movement.

In order to sculpt creatively, we must permit the spontaneous and nonintellectual intelligence that lives in our arms and hands to give shape and movement to the clay. The head must remain empty of thinking. This is the same principle as in spontaneous therapeutic writing for 20 minutes per day. Our hands are guided to create living textures within the form.

In essence, the sculptor feels the inner vital sculpturing forces that reside within a human being, forces that live and weave in constant movement throughout life. This is experiential understanding, rather than what we read in a book and do not grasp with our whole being. Sculpting is a being-centered knowingness rather than a head-centered abstract fact. It is as if in the process of sculpture the head empties out into the arms and hands. The head, empty of the constant chatter of thinking in which we engage all day, can now reflect on what is being created and silently observe what is coming into outer expression from within, by way of our hands.

Working with sculpture is not easy. For many people a noncreative life has become the norm. Unconscious habitual patterns kill creative spirit. We live primarily through the physical senses, which exist for the most part in the head (sight, hearing, taste, smell). Because of an excessive and artificial stimulation of our senses from early in life, which often begins early in each day of our lives through food or television, we become trapped in the head. We experience the world primarily through our senses, which no longer reflect spirit. There is a negative wedding between abstract, dry intellectual thinking and excessive physical sense stimulation. Life becomes like a prison, and the head is the jail. We live from thought to thought, book to book, meal to delicious meal, billboard to billboard. Our creative will and sense of well-being atrophy. Epidemics of drug addiction, eating disorders, and other obsessive/compulsive disorders have developed from this social and cultural soil. This is the depleted soil of family dysfunctional illnesses and decaying cultural institutions that do not enrich the living spirit.

The principle of wholeness is shattered in these very common American situations. When our creative individuality is deadened, our daily behavior is wed to an abstract clever intellect that thinks it knows more than it does, and our physical senses are over-stimulated, we become ill. Rationalizing and lying to ourselves becomes the norm and slanders the spirit. We promote and continue bad laws and social measures, as well as intolerance and prejudice.

Our more human parts will always try to reassert themselves. The urge to wholeness is a basic soul urge. The soul and spirit parts of us, which we too often have banished into dormancy, but which others may notice in our eyes, will make their presence known, whether through accident, physical illness, or compulsive addictive behavior. This will continue until we acknowledge the suffering born of their denial.

We do not have to permit things to go to this extreme. We can emerge from our separate lifestyles and cognitively appreciate what is occurring.

We can invoke living forces into our daily lives, and learn to let go of the controlling self that is trapped in the head. A major way to do this is by enlivening our senses through the arts.

When we sculpt, we live our way into form. This helps us to feel more at ease with our own physical form. Each day, we increasingly express the living movement of sculpting forces, rather than the dead images we absorb through television advertising. We gradually emerge from a lifestyle of being trapped in the head, so that our lives can be filled by images that move us and guide our activity. This is why the image of Mother Mary holding the baby Jesus, or the statue of David, or the Buddha, is so appealing. They remind us of what our lives are really about, why we are here.

Family-centered dysfunctional behavior that has produced millions of people with compulsive behavior disorders originates in a lack of trust in our sense of self. The process of sculpture helps us to trust in life, in our individual uniqueness and our creative capacities, in our abilities to perceive and respond to change. This art is a living antidote to the illnesses of our time.

Memories and feelings from early in life often come to the surface when sculpting. This occurs because the process of sculpting brings us back into the flow of time, out of which we have stepped at some point in our lives. It will remind us of our true birthright, our creativity that we have repressed or denied. The separation of past, present, and future dissolves. The sculpting forces enliven our sense of movement and flow as qualities of time. It places us into what Dr. Klinghardt calls the "intuitive body." This is the same place we can do family constellation work.

By entering into a process of sculpture we permit ourselves to be involved in a creative process as both a participant and an observer simultaneously. We engage in an active creative process through spontaneous movement of the hands. At the same time, we observe what we are creating. This awakens our dormant capacities to observe, so that we can exercise this capacity every day.

340

With sculpture we are creating a breathing process with our soul. The artfulness of sculpture may remind us of an unlived life. The irritation that may result may be the anger of our over-controlled personality that does not want to surrender its position of control in our life, so that the soul's urges toward wholeness and development may be fulfilled and bring a true sense of self and well-being.

Participation in the art of sculpture gives us a sense of knowingness and trust in the creative movement of all of life. This trust deepens when we also engage in other arts such as painting or photography that awaken an awareness of the subtleties of light and color, or music that provides an inner experience of tone, or the inspiration of poetry and drama. These give us strength to meet each day with a deepened sense of self.

We need to see the gift and grace of sculpture and the other arts as means of growth and transformation, and place them at the center of healing. Then the phantoms, the spectres, and the demons that arise out of the hidden recesses of our psyches and undermine our lives can be consciously and artfully reintegrated into a more honest and life-sustaining culture of individuality and community.

PHOTOGRAPHY

While writing this book, I rediscovered photography. I would buy film, load the camera, go out and shoot pictures, and have them developed. But I became discouraged as the slides that were developed from one roll of film after another were mediocre and did not reflect the beauty that I had seen through the lens.

In the past, at this point of frustration I would have set aside photography as I had done with music, painting, and other art forms. This time, however, I began to pay attention to the weaknesses in my character that were being revealed in this process. I observed how these weaknesses were reflections of certain illnesses in my life. I avoided paying attention to details, to persistently strive to stay with and master something.

A professional like myself is often trapped in his head, thinking too much. After a number of years at my work, I discovered certain formulas of success, and learned how to apply these formulas by the rules of the social economy in order to keep my status and money. Then I bought a camera, arrogantly thinking that if I take pictures they will turn out well.

However, when the pictures do not turn out as expected, I became irritated. This irritation is a reminder that the professional like myself is indeed trapped in a certain lifestyle. I was being reminded of my illness. Before developing sufficient inner strength, I would turn away from this in anger, or find a scapegoat for this apparent failure, or buy an automatic camera to do all the work, or move on to something else. And so, I would come to terms with the weaknesses of my character. This behavior is common to many more people than just professionals. Unless we dissolve hardening habitual behavior patterns, our egotism continues to be fed. And this character weakness, if I allow it to continue, leads to accidents or illnesses. The effort in comprehensive medicine is to perceive what organ needs support so that this weakness can be lessened. In this situation the organ is the kidney. This can be treated with herbs, or homeopathics, or color, for example.

What the art of photography offers is the opportunity to become involved in life. I began to become knowledgeable in the various facets of photography—film, lighting, lenses, and so forth. I learned to observe. There are subtle changes in light and dark, and shades of colors, as they move through the times of the day. I became familiar with how different types of substances absorb or reflect light.

Also, I learned how to wait. Often, I would sit somewhere and wait for the light to be just right for a picture. In the movie *The Natural*, there was a scene in which the main female character, played by Glenn Close, stood up in the stadium, and the light of the sun appeared to radiate from her. The director explained in an interview that they had waited for the right time of day for this to occur at that exact spot. We all need to learn to observe and wait for the right time. This is the art of healing.

After a while, I began to sense and feel what was right. When looking through a camera lens and focusing at different levels, we see things in ways that our normal intellectual brain-connected eye rarely sees. It becomes obvious how things that seem to our everyday sight to be separate and unmoving are in fact in movement and in relationship with everything else around.

One day, I attempted to take pictures. The feeling of right timing and lighting was not there. Several hours later, while writing at my desk, I looked out the window and noticed the light on a small bush. I jumped up, grabbed the camera, and shot a roll of slide film. This would not have happened unless I had come out of my thinking head, observed the light, and then acted on this perception. In the short period of time it took to shoot the pictures, my whole being became active. I went from thinking about writing to feeling the colors and light of the day to the conscious activity of taking photographs. This is healing.

When these three aspects of our selves—thinking, feeling, and activity—work more closely together, their corresponding inner soul qualities of imagination, inspiration, and intuition also become stronger. Thinking becomes more imaginative. Destructive emotions give way to feelings of inspiration, which grow out of a childlike feeling of awe and wonder that the art of photography enhances. Activity becomes more consciously and intuitively directed. This describes the awakening of the feminine nature, the capacity to wait and be actively receptive to what comes toward us, and then to respond through intuitively guided activity.

In these ways, photography becomes an artful antidote to and to many others in our professionally controlled soc' trapped in intellectual and habitual thinking, cut off from tl tion. For several days after shooting these pictures, I often c perceived colors in movement, remembering what happeneu went in and out of focus through various distances. I began to perceive not just space but also time. I started to perceive emotional and physical ailments differently, not as still events from the past, but as energies whose movement is restricted but which may be redirected if I observe and wait for the right timing.

It is important to notice that, once again, we do not fight against the weaknesses in our character or punish ourselves for having acted out of an imbalanced or one-sided temperament. Through participating in this artful way of living, we invoke inner soul qualities in daily life. These give strength, so that while the weaknesses of character and temperament may still be present in the shadows, they do not attract our attention, as they used to before. In this way, they gradually die of attrition. This process often requires years.

We need to build gradually a new structure of thinking, feeling, and activity that continually draws the inner essence of our being into daily life. The creative arts help us do this. They become agents of healing in which everyone can participate. In this way, we take the arts far beyond where they are today—another exhibit we pay 20 dollars to see or a painting we purchase to hang on the living room wall.

The arts lead us toward living an artful life. This enlivens our feeling nature. Our feeling nature then becomes the living bridge between past and future, intellect and activity. It provides an opportunity to heal inner weaknesses by drawing out latent strengths. In these ways, the illnesses we incur by living in a professionally sanctioned society of specialization are observed, taken account of, and transformed.

CREATIVE WRITING

In the willful act of spontaneous writing we open a dialogue within ourselves. We create a bridge between subjective and objective, unseen and seen, inner self and outer persona. Daily writing and other positive daily disciplines are a vital part of the biographical process. Through writing, our inner subjective awareness becomes objectified or visible on paper. This is a powerful way to observe, reflect, and develop an honest sense of our selves. It's like looking into a mirror and reflecting on what has come out from within us and is now in front of us on paper to read and to work with. By writing, we define the day. We draw from the worlds of our subjective experiences, and bring these experiences into present time.

By writing spontaneously, we create a bridge between the two poles of our being: thinking and activity, head and hands. Writing is an act of will in which we give ourselves permission to express objectively what we have experienced. We then reflect on what has been written. This completes the circle, which then becomes a circle of protection in which we feel safe to open our feeling nature a little bit more.

Why is it important to our process of healing to create a living bridge between our two poles? Today the value of feeling is greatly denied. Results of denying our feelings range from mild neuroses and obsessive-compulsive disorders to depression. The feeling pole is the middle ground, the bridge that connects the thinking and willing faculties of the soul. It is the living present that connects our past and future. Our feelings are our sensitivity. When this sensitivity is traumatized early in life, we contract to defend ourselves. We then become too headstrong or too habitually driven in our actions, and lack trust in our feelings and sensitivities.

Our circle of protection is being invaded today from many directions. The result of this weakness of boundaries can be seen in epidemics of environmental illness, autism, and autoimmune diseases, along with anxiety disorders and insomnia. The common thread among all of these seemingly separate illnesses is a loss of protection that is continually infused into our lives when the thinking, feeling, and activity parts of ourselves are connected instead of separate.

Our culture promotes two avenues of escape from being in the present, from a life of feelings.

- One is through the intellect, which in our society often culminates in becoming a professional. A professional is someone who is rewarded with stature and financial reimbursements for being clever and holding a storehouse of information. It matters not whether this knowledge is used wisely or in the service of others. We forget the line that Scrooge's dead partner said as he wailed from the afterlife, "Mankind was my business."

- The other avenue is through the will. The soul forces of the will are engaged through activity. This activity becomes socially acceptable in the multimillion dollar industry of sports. But there is a large reservoir of unconscious will forces in each of us and in society as a whole that become destructive to life. We see this in the increase in drug abuse, child abuse, psychopathic and compulsive behavior, and violent crime.

Without awakening the living middle ground of feeling, there can be no real healing, regardless of whatever drug, operation, herb, or structural manipulation we undertake.

Spontaneous writing is one significant way to enliven the bridge connecting the poles of thinking and willing (activity). Writing is the bridge that connects will through the hands with thinking through the eyes and brain. In a very positive way, the process of thinking that awakens through spontaneous writing is not mechanistic, information-based abstract thinking. Instead, it is a perceptive and aware genre of thinking in which we consciously practice the art of synthesis, or putting things together into a whole picture. More typically we think through analysis, where we break things apart to understand how the whole works. The danger with analysis is that we assume in our egotism that we can operate or irradiate the part and the cancer will be gone. Cancer and all other diseases are diseases of the whole person, and can only be healed by applying the art of synthesis. Spontaneous writing, creating a bridge between thinking and willing, objective and subjective, day and night, encourages us to develop a rhythm of breathing and a living dialogue between opposite poles of the human constitution. This is therapeutic in any illness.

Writing with spontaneity and honesty means being willing and vulnerable to permit ourselves to see what our inner self needs to express in that moment. This has great practical significance. It enables us to gradually begin depersonalizing things that we have been taking too personally. We educate ourselves in the art of detachment. Creative writing is self-education. We have an opportunity to reveal that which is often churning within us and buried in a sea of chaos below the diaphragm after we have swallowed and stuffed our feelings. We release and give expression to our trapped parts in a rhythmic and orderly fashion according to the way and timing by which it needs to be expressed. In this way we create a free space for real relationship with others and ourselves . Out of this space we can deepen our qualities of imagination, inspiration, and intuition.

This has relevance to illness and healing. Churning emotions do not remain buried. They upset the delicate balance and rhythmic functions within the metabolic and reproductive spheres of our constitution. By writing in a regular and willfully spontaneous fashion, we superimpose a self-generated rhythm on this chaos of suppressed feelings. This is the process of healing we invoke each day by engaging in this process of creative writing.

Of what does this writing consist? Is it merely the mechanical description of what we do during the day, as in a diary? No. During the day, when a recollection of a particular event or feeling enters, that is the moment to write. Something is coming to the surface in order to be seen. When written, it is seen, and not hidden anymore. There are many things that occur during the day to which we remain blind and unaware because we do not discipline ourselves to observe and reflect in the moment. At the end of the day, sit in a quiet place that you have dedicated to this work, at a time that provides you some leeway for freedom of expression. Bring together what you have written earlier that day. It is like making a necklace every day with the stones, the written observations and feelings that have been gathered during the day. They are gathered from your soul as it speaks to you through the events of the day.

Writing creates a picture, a field of time in which you can begin to see how seemingly separate events of the day are in reality parts of a common thread, a pattern of relationship. Writing creates a painting. You begin by painting the picture of a particular event. As you continue to write, other aspects of the day, other thoughts, words, or deeds, portray varying shades of the painting. Writing about one aspect of the whole leads to writing about another aspect, and this in turn leads to a third, if you give yourself permission to do this. The events you write about will often come out in a different order from the way they occurred in actual life. Just as suppressed feelings from early in life may surface years later, so an event in the morning has a particular relationship with another event later in the day, or earlier in the week. Until you permit this stream of time to open within you, these relationships may not be apparent. Permitting this stream of time to open helps you become less rigid and more adaptable. These are the hallmarks of healing on mental, emotional, and physical levels.

For this to be effective, you have to be honestly forthcoming in your writing. Just write it down. Become a scientist in the true sense of the word, willing to observe and understand without trying to control or judge. This is the difference between the artistic scientist and the intellectual mechanistic scientist of today.

Why is this exercise so vital a tool for self-healing? To answer this, let's look at the direction the economy is moving today. In the context of writing by hand, and its role in healing, Alvin Toffler's book *Powershift* talks about how the time interval it takes for ideas to manifest, from when a person has an idea, to when that idea manifests in the physical world in the marketplace is much shorter now than it was even five years ago. He indicates that knowledge is power. Other books and articles say much the same.

What is going to happen to us as the economy moves more in this direction of the present and near future? As time speeds up, how does this affect the rhythm of our lives as well as the rhythmic function of internal organs? Our internal rhythms are often greatly upset because they are still based on the time rhythms of tradition over thousands of years. These rhythms are much slower and are measured in terms of generations rather than hours, weeks, and months. The slower rhythms of generations are built into our physical constitutions. Our chaotic dysfunctional emotional lives grow out of the stress and lack of rhythm that accompany the breaking down of the old rhythms of tradition in our bodies without an accompanying discovery of how to regenerate with new rhythms. As a result of our arrhythmic lifestyle, we have epidemics of addiction, obsessive-compulsive disorders, depression, immune system weaknesses, and other chronic illnesses.

346

We are inventing computers that can run faster and require smaller spaces. Because we have benefited materially from this, we have blindly permitted our lives to be run by the rhythms of computers. Many people do not write by hand anymore. They sit at a computer and compose, and think this is advanced because the writing is accomplished more quickly.

Writing at a computer and writing with a pen and paper are quite different experiences. It is crucial that this difference be appreciated. Writing with the hand awakens the conscious human will forces that are often asleep. Writing with the hand, if we do not rush ahead as fast as we can, is like sculpting words on paper. It becomes an artful process of connecting head and hand. The setting for illness in many people is a combination of will that is asleep, with feelings that are suppressed or muted, leaving the head and intellectual, mechanistic thinking as the only awake part of a person's soul life. This state of affairs is the cause of much illness. No bottle of pills, whether pharmaceutical or homeopathic, is going to correct this.

By engaging in active creative writing, the conscious, self-directed human will is awakened. The stream of inner life is given the opportunity to flow forth and be seen. Creativity does not come from the head, but rather from the union of imaginative thinking with real feelings and conscious guiding will. We then become able to meet the forces of technology as master and not as slave. Then we can work on computers without becoming one.

This process is portrayed in the mythology of the centaur. The first stage is horse-man, the centaur. Next the man rides the horse. The human aspect is now distinct but still wedded to the animal soul nature. Finally, the man or woman walks the horse, with a focused mind that is not possessed or driven by the animal psyche of instinctual drives, mechanistic thinking, and selfish egotism.

It is the will to power and control, which is really the desire of our mask personas, that drives our activities and distorts life rhythms and organ functions. Technological marvels may put money into our hands in seconds or clothes at our doorsteps within hours. Without developing an active inner human rhythm, however, we will become even more driven and anxious than we are today as the forces that are constantly being over-stimulated become even more predominant in our lives.

To be able to work with new technology in a constructive fashion guided by human soul faculties, we need to be able to channel and redirect into human creative activities our animal will to power. This creates a positive rhythm for the chemistry of the body. Creative spontaneous writing is one way to build this positive self-image. If one is willing to look, then such writing gives insight into the denials that many of us live. It also offers a sense of having communicated with our selves. This living process of growth does not occur when we write at the computer.

This book was initially written in longhand. I observed whether or not my handwriting was legible. When it was not, I knew that rushing had entered my creative work. I felt the inspiration enter my psyche, and I became too impatient to see how it would manifest, or too fearful that it would disappear, instead of trusting that with my conscious efforts this higher guidance would show me how to create sentences.

You may recall stories of driven artists who hurriedly rushed to complete a painting. This is the classic picture of the artists—eccentric and hurried, off in their own worlds. Their works may have been great, but they were often one-sided individuals who had difficulty with groups. What we need today is not one-sided artistic drive, but rather an artfulness of everyday life that connects all parts of the whole in synthesis and supports us in developing a rhythmic life guided by the principles of the soul.

When we write creatively, we are choosing to be in the present. When we commit to such a decision and consistently act on it, the wholeness of a given situation opens up to our vision. We then see what we need to see. The act of surrendering to the process of spontaneous writing is a willingness to see what is needed at the moment.

If we do not like what we have written and judge it or ourselves, then we remain stuck in a particular pattern of rigidity in our personal nature. We too often become driven by what we think we want in the future. We narrow-mindedly demand that things be done in a certain way and done immediately. Yet the result is never good enough for us. It never measures up. We are obsessed by the acceleration of time and the material things we want in such a world. This reality applies up and down the socioeconomic ladder, from savings and loans executives to 14-year-old car thieves to teachers and doctors. Yet because we do not learn to honestly observe, reflect, and respond in the moment to what is needed, there is no spark of insight. And we remain driven.

Exercises such as creative writing create bridges that help us to connect the separate parts of our lives. The pieces of the broken mirror are slowly put back together again so that we can see who we really are, instead of who an accelerated and technology-driven culture and educational system wants us to be. We actively participate in our own healing, instead of trying to find the magic drug or surgery or vitamin or herb. By doing creative writing, we create new positive rituals that awaken a self-generated rhythm of education and healing.

WRITING IN TRAUMA

Another form of writing, similar to but distinct from creative writing, is writing in trauma. Research has shown that engaging in a certain type of writing can help us heal the emotional traumas that are often buried within. This is different from the creative writing just discussed. The technique is as follows:

- Find a quiet, safe space.
- Begin writing about a particular experience of trauma.

348

- Keep your pen on the paper.
- If you get stuck, keep writing. Do not stop writing.

Writing in this way helps the brain move the emotional content of trauma away from areas that can cause problems in your autonomic nervous system, and toward areas that are safer for memory storage. Such writing also accesses the part of your autonomic or unconscious nervous system that supports healing and regeneration of body cells and tissues.

Upon finishing, feel free to discard what you have written. What is important is the process, not the product.

PART V

COMPREHENSIVE MEDICINE: HEALTH CARE THAT WORKS

CONCLUSION

W e are at a threshold in medical care today. The hardened encasement held in place for over a hundred years by our primarily mechanistic, materialistic field of allopathic modern medicine is beginning to crack. In spite of an onslaught of pharmaceutical advertising, hospital promotions, insurance company plans, and governmental restrictions in care, millions of people are seeking alternative care. While there is no doubt that the timely use of drugs and surgery can be beneficial, the virtually exclusive reign of these two pillars of modern medicine has not improved the quality or financing of health care. The touting of the American health care system as the best in the world is a delusion. An increasing number of major university hospital medical researchers, FDA employees, and company managers are disclosing the truth at the risk of losing their jobs or tenure. Yet the amount of media misinformation and pharmaceutical advertising continues to rise even as the shell is cracking more.

What we need at this time are inclusive, sweeping changes in health care. Continued jockeying for position and control is immature and harmful. It is time for those in positions of authority to cooperate in pulling back the tight reins that modern medicine holds on our health care and health finances. This book is written to offer a panoramic and wide-ranging perspective and groundwork for how we can make the necessary changes.

The public needs to become aware that much has already been put into place to create the kind of health care system I write about in this book. Fear-mongering special interest groups who have much to lose if we make the necessary changes would like us to believe differently. We are by no means beginning from scratch. Many thoughtful and intelligent people in fields of health care that are outside the modern medical model have been laboring and refining their skills and observations for decades. And so have an increasing number of conventional medical doctors and nurses, under the rubric of integrative medicine. These practitioners, often derisively dismissed as being part of what has been called alternative or complementary medicine, have had to build practices based on effective outcomes in order to survive. Patients have kept coming and paying out of pocket because they have been getting results.

In conventional medicine, patients return for years even though they know the medicines are not working, because the care is being financed by their employers or government-based insurance plans. Integrative and alternative practitioners have led the way in evidence-based and outcome-based medicine. They are not the quacks that media bias would lead us to conclude. While there are undoubtedly those in these fields who make unsubstantiated claims, this pales in comparison to what is happening in conventional medicine. Even the AMA admits that adverse reactions to drugs are a leading cause of death in the United States. And even though the forces of materialistic greed have also become part of integrative and alternative medicine, nevertheless, there are far more such practitioners who have developed effective ways of helping people heal.

This last sentence is significant. Changing health care is at its core not a financial issue. It is a deep spiritual and personal issue. Otherwise many people without financial wherewithal would not seek care outside their insurance plans. These people are not being duped. Rather, they have researched the options, especially with the explosion of the Internet, and have concluded that integrative and alternative approaches are their best chance of healing.

The floodgates are ready to open, because all of us sense at a deep level the need for this to happen.

Imagine a room filled with all the sick people in the United States, which, if we are honest, are many more of us than our statistics show. These sick people are crowded into this small room, and fearful. The walls of the room are covered with notices and advertisements from pharmaceutical companies, insurance companies, hospitals, and physician organizations. This room, however, is in the middle of a much larger building, the rest of which is only sparsely being used. This space is taken up by the growing number of integrative and alternative diagnostic and therapeutic modalities. Some people inside the small room have been successful in walking through the doors and into this greater space, have improved in health, and have come back to tell the others.

Someone inside the crowded room asks, as did Dr. Jay Cohen of the School of Medicine at the University of California at San Diego, "Why isn't integrative medicine our primary form of medicine?" The doors into this greater space are open to walk through, yet most people inside are unaware of what lies outside or fearful of the unknown or of the cost of taking such a step. There are many who work in conventional medicine that know that the doors of the room need to be swung open.

Studies reveal that "Perhaps a third of medical spending is now devoted to services that don't appear to improve health or the quality of care—and may make things worse." (Elliott S. Fisher, professor of medicine at Dartmouth, 2003) Yet critical mass for change has not yet been reached. The drive toward the needed changes must come from the general public which is growing increasingly distrustful of the drug companies and knows that politics, mostly bereft of moral integrity, is rife with hidden selfish economic incentives.

How can we reach critical mass to bring about the necessary changes in our health care system?

Owners of large and small businesses who have insurance plans for employees need to come together and demand that insurance policies begin to give workers more freedom to explore other options. The frontiers of these options can be gradually expanded in phases.

354

Hospital executives and boards of directors need to lay down the law to the medical staff that the gates must be opened. It is obvious that to leave things as they are is more risky to financial survival than to open the gates. Practitioners representative of many integrative and alternative modalities in their communities need to be invited into hospitals to begin serious dialogue. It is time to open doors and trust in people's common sense to determine what they need and what works. The principles outlined in this book can be foundational starting points. Hospitals and medical centers at all levels need to begin by establishing departments of integrative medicine, followed by departments of energy medicine. In the latter, physicists, acupuncturists, homeopaths, light and color therapists, sound frequency therapists, microcurrent therapists, and many others who work with frequency would actively participate. Even though allopathic physicians have stiff resistance to these changes, they will benefit greatly from them, and when the changes do occur, will breathe a big sigh of relief and begin to embrace much that they opposed.

Government health care planners at all levels, including those who manage Medicare and Medicaid, must stop blindly reimbursing the tremendous overuse of cardiac surgeries and cancer chemotherapies, and demand to review much of the evidence-based integrative and alternative medicine. If a homeopathic practitioner, for example, can provide a certain number of therapeutic successes that show the effectiveness of his therapies, then he should receive better reimbursement for patient care. For example, a homeopathic medical doctor in Virginia treated a patient with Lupus with homeopathy. Not only did the patient symptomatically improve without pharmaceuticals, but her objective laboratory measurements of the disease improved.

Hospitals must overhaul current dietary policies that still serve devitalized food to patients and employees. Every hospital and clinic needs to provide nutritious food as part of a new mainstream medicine.

Hospitals and clinics must regularly employ practitioners of effective forms of trauma release such as EMDR (eye movement desensitization and reprocessing) as an integral part of care for people with chronic disease. These labor-intensive therapies will become much more common than surgery.

Medical boards must immediately stop any further prosecuting of non-allopathic practitioners, unless they have been shown to cause harm. Furthermore, the rules and regulations must be fundamentally changed. All practitioners, whether lay homeopaths, integrative physicians, allopathic physicians, or color and sound therapists, have the right to practice free of persecution if they have shown evidence of sufficient training and certification in their field. This will permit the public to gravitate to therapies that work, which will happen if legal and economic barriers are removed. And these therapies by certified practitioners must be reimbursed by insurance plans which are not restricted to conventional medical doctors, and which exist to help people heal.

The media must cover all of these developments so the public can learn from what is presented and make their own decisions and so no secrets are kept from the common man and woman.

All of this requires that we take a risk; that we have the courage to make needed changes. There is no effective change without risk. The Founding Fathers risked their lives by signing the Declaration of Independence. There will continue to be significant resistance to these changes from those who have benefited the most from the status quo, and they will continue to convince most of us, out of fear, to stay crowded together in the tiny room.

There will also be significant structural and financial shifts as part of these changes, and there will be important questions to ask. For example, the present health care industry, which is highly allopathic and drug and surgery driven, is a major employer in many communities across the country. Communities depend on tax revenues from health care employees in order to meet basic municipal needs.

Many governmental agencies are overstretched in meeting needs, which involves maintaining a needed social safety net. The major reason that certain epidemic illnesses declined historically was not because of the introduction of vaccinations, but rather due to the improvement in social and personal hygiene that was often financed by governments cooperating on many levels.

Most of the health care employees work in laboratories, X-ray departments, surgical suites, and other specialized and highly technical diagnostic and therapeutic areas in allopathic specialty medicine. Most medical school graduates still gravitate to these fields for prestige and income.

Hospitals, insurance companies, physician organizations, and pharmaceutical companies will use the media to spread the fear that if the necessary changes are implemented, many people will be out of work, local governments will have even less tax revenue, and people's health care will worsen. The latter will not happen, and with good planning that is inclusive of all parties, health care employment can remain high. It will grow even more because it will become more interesting and meaningful.

Laboratories are very helpful in comprehensive medicine. Regular lab testing in hospitals and labs can be greatly expanded and more effective, with proper training. Nationally recognized laboratories such as the Great Smokies Diagnostic Laboratory in Asheville, North Carolina, and Doctor's Data Labs in Chicago have been doing good work for years and can step up to train many other labs.

The same is true in radiology. Instead of so many X rays and mammographies, technicians will also do thermographies and other noninvasive testing and imaging that help practitioners diagnose and treat people before symptoms get too advanced.

Nurses will play a big role in coming changes. They will gradually be more liberated from their compressed role as dispensers of drugs with limited patient contact. Their work will become much more interesting. They will be trained more in patient care that includes therapeutic baths and compresses, psychological therapies, and nutritional IVs. And their participation in therapeutic teams with doctors, psychotherapists, energy medicine therapists, nutritionists, and others will be a key to therapeutic success.

Surgical departments are often the most powerful in the hospital because they bring in the most money from insurance and government reimbursement. This connection must be broken for the sake of our personal and economic health. Surgery is undoubtedly sometimes needed and good surgeons are necessary in every community. However, the emphasis must now be on the myriad of therapies that, when employed properly, can and often do prevent unnecessary surgeries.

Before any surgery, assuming that the patient is in no immediate danger from a delay in surgery, all non-surgical approaches to a particular illness that have evidence of success will be explored. For example, the ongoing increase in the number of hospitals that provide cardiovascular surgeries would be directly threatened if well-proven integrative medicine therapies were applied on a large scale. Chronic infections and heavy metal toxicities in the coronary arteries are often at the root of these diseases. Of course, people who wish to have surgery or any other procedure would have the right to pay for this out of pocket. But no governmental agency or insurance company would fund these unless they were they only alternative.

This brings up the often-used argument of the sacredness of the doctor-patient relationship. Allopathic medical doctors claim that a main reason they are fighting against insurance companies and government agencies for their patient's good care is the sacredness of the doctor-patient relationship. However, the medical profession is misusing this mantle of sacredness as a smokescreen to maintain control. In reality, any form of therapy that would take away their business and professional standing threatens most physicians. Physicians obtain most of their continuing education from educational programs that are pharmaceutically funded. They know very little about the integrative medical programs that they try to convince their patients not to follow. So the doctor fears loss of income and prestige and the patient fears his doctor's disapproval. This way of doing things must end.

How will the hospital stay in business if it is not receiving money from surgeries, special procedures, lab tests, and drugs that it currently uses? The answer is that if creative, honest, and clear-thinking people come together with no hidden agendas, these concerns can be worked through positively. The courage to take risks that are involved with these changes is paramount.

As I mentioned at the beginning of the book, for many years of my professional life, I worked simultaneously as an emergency physician and a practitioner of integrative medicine. Emergency medicine was my main source of income. I then became medical director of a holistic clinic and received a good salary. After two years I left the clinic and took the risk of living as a comprehensive medical doctor. I was full of doubt. Going back to emergency medicine would have been the easy way out, but not the best way for my future development.

In many respects I was still on level one of the three levels of the masculine (as described by David Deida in *Intimate Communion*): over-concerned with acquisition and being in control, and fearful of not having enough. Out of a desire for security, I had wanted to work in a medical institution and receive a paycheck. During those years, after leaving the holistic clinic, I was also doing what Deida calls level two work: facing my demons, doing self-improvement, facing fears.

Yet the time came in my life to take a risk, to step into unknown territory, and to have the courage to discover who I was beyond an employee. Some people have done this much earlier in life than I did; others never do it at all. This risk taking is level three: becoming open and relaxed in one's real self, letting go, giving freely, and trusting, even if it is painful. Or, in the words of one of my guiding mentors, Rob Robb, being abundantly myself. Part of my move to live as a comprehensive medical doctor was to accept a reduction in my finances. I was willing to accept this because I wanted to see only 6-7 patients a day in order to deliver what I felt was quality care, and to have a healthy quality of life myself. I had to let go of believing that only money allowed me to be safe, secure, have fun and trust.

My purpose for telling this story is that when I consistently practiced facing my fear, opening up to life even though I have fear, my linear fear-based thinking shifts into thinking in terms of patterns, relationships, trust, and letting go. Answers not apparent to me before emerged. This is what Karl Maret, M.D. calls "Awakening the Dialogue of the Heart" (www.heartmindcommunications.com).

The same thing will happen in hospitals, for example, with such issues as where funds will come from if surgery and procedures are decreased. The demand for effective care will grow so much as the word spreads about these changes that new creative solutions will have to be found to deal with the demand. It also likely will happen that many who are able will come forth with philanthropic funds to support these transitions. The reason why philanthropic gifts are not approaching the level at which we need them is that health care is still trapped in old forms, structures, and arrangements that are fear based.

These risky steps must be taken if we are to open up our closed system and let it breathe in new energies. There is no rational alternative. It will take time, and it will not be easy. But it will bring great joy and health to many. It is the soulful thing to do.

Our health care system, and the state of our general health and well-being, will get much better once the medical establishment is no longer an enabler, needing patients who are dependent and who therefore must remain in states of chronic illness that require drugs. This codependent-enabler mentality between patient and medical establishment must end for our general health and well-being to improve. Patients will open up and respond by seeking care that helps them heal rather than stay dependent. For those who have difficulty with this transition and resist changes, the solution is loving, firm attention and encouragement to make the slow, incremental changes needed. The time it will take will vary from person to person, from city to city.

All of this is still only the first step in where we need to go in the future. There are already those who have been working for years on steps that are two or three or more ahead of where we are now. These are the sound therapists, the shamanic healers, and anthroposophical professional-community arrangements. The idea of health associations is something to be explored.

The next step we need to take, however, will only become visible once these initial steps are taken. The problem with what we call innovative thinking today is that programs based on this thinking (and these are the programs that investors are willing to fund) know in advance what steps two, three, and four will be as a safeguard against risk. Remember how Kevin Costner's character in the movie *Field of Dreams* asked the character played by James Earl Jones, "What do we do next?" Jones's character responded in his wonderful, deep voice, "How the hell do I know?" Costner's character immediately said, "Of course." He knew instantly that the next step would only be obvious after they completed the current step. This is trust. It is not blind faith. Rather, it is based on sound principles and capabilities and a willingness to take reasonable risks.

We can imagine future steps. Once we begin to break down the rigid shells of modern medicine, these movements will lead to other movements. The energies released in these activities will liberate funds from many directions for this Common Good. We may see different arrangements of professionals, like those at the anthroposophical community in Spring Valley, New York, where physicians are not paid according to conventional standards, but according to what they, as part of a community, say that they require for the coming years. The market in efficient and relatively inexpensive forms of energy medicine, many of which have been banned by the FDA, will open up and make the home and local community much more effective in actively participating in healing. We may see more communities with local currency, as in Ithaca, New York—dollars that re-circulate in communities and become forms of barter for those whose regular incomes do not sufficiently meet their current health care needs.

We will need regional and national comprehensive medical health centers that can serve as teaching facilities and places where chronically ill people can come for extended periods of time for deep help and support, like Paracelsus Foxhollow Clinic near Louisville, Kentucky. Such centers will increase in number as the economic arrangements I've outlined come into existence on a greater scale in our health care system.

All of this will occur if we:

- Hold true to the vision of what we need

- Stay mindful of what it will take to manifest this vision

- Are willing to take the necessary risks to open up the system

- Remain devoted to the principles of service and healing that are the true calling of the healing professions

A sense of dignity and meaning will return to the healing professions. Creativity will blossom in many sick people, so that we can only begin to imagine what they will offer to the greater society as gifts of genius for the betterment of all.

WHAT TO DO NEXT

PERSONALLY

- Make the changes in your own life that promote health and healing and prevent or help heal illness. If you are not striving to walk the talk, other efforts at healing will be less meaningful.

- Follow the Basics, implement lifestyle changes, and make changes to establish a new foundation of wellness in your life. Develop ways of dialoguing with your subconscious and changing habitual patterns. Such methods as tapping (mental field therapy) and David Deida's work may be very helpful. Let yourself become more creative. It will open new worlds for you and help you to change habitual patterns.

- Act with courage and conviction on your principles toward what you feel, regardless of obstacles.

- Read and study magazines and web sites, and attend lectures.

IN CHOOSING A DOCTOR

- Seek physicians who understand the need for integrative/comprehensive medicine and are practicing it daily, and who are willing to listen and be open. Work with them on deeper psycho-emotional issues, and with toxicities and deficiencies.

- Don't stay loyal to a doctor who cannot support you with integrative/comprehensive medicine. Many of us have strong feelings of loyalty. These are deep patterns and sometimes need to be broken. Doctors or dentists can be very nice and have good intentions, and still do harm. Our health needs to come before loyalty to our doctors.

- Think twice about taking drugs that are prescribed for you and try to find effective alternatives, which is often possible.

361

ECONOMICALLY

- Learn more about health associations, how you can form one in your area, and hire good integrative/comprehensive practitioners.

- Educate yourself in new forms of economy in health care.

- If your employer's health insurance limits availability to integrative/comprehensive health care, and health insurance is necessary, make every attempt to ask the employer to add an option, if possible. Ask the integrative/comprehensive practitioner about reduced rates.

- It may be necessary to pay more out-of-pocket expenses for integrative medicine for a while in order to turn your health around. Do not let insurance coverage dictate the tests and treatments that offer the greatest opportunity for healing.

LOCALLY

- Press for your local hospital to hire integrative/ comprehensive medical doctors and other health practitioners.

- Start or sponsor organic or biodynamic gardens as a source of healthy food. This is a way to build community.

POLITICALLY

- Support efforts to eliminate state medical boards. They do not really protect the public, and largely exist to protect the allopathic medical profession from legitimate competition.

- Sign up for Dr. Mercola's new nonprofit health association (www.mercola.com).

SOCIALLY

- Make investments in health care companies that support these changes. If stock portfolios have pharmaceutical investments, this is actually supporting old forms of medicine. Look into green investments.

- Don't base your hopes of a retirement nest egg on the success of pharmaceutical, tobacco, and chemical companies. This does not support a healthy environment for our children.

- Find like-minded individuals in your community and workplace who understand the need for these changes.

BIBLIOGRAPHY

Achterberg, Jeanne; Dossey, Barbara; and Kolkmeier, Lesley, *Rituals of Healing*, New York: Bantam Books, 1994.

Benson, Herbert, MD, *Timeless Healing*, New York: Scribner, 1996.

Berman, Phillip, *The Search for Meaning*, New York: Ballantine Books, 1990.

Black, Dean, *Health at the Crossroads*, Springville, UT: Tapestry Press, 1988.

Blair, Justice, *Who Gets Sick*, LA: Jeremy Tarcher, 1987.

Bly, Robert, *Iron John*, New York: Addison Wesley Publishing Company, 1990.

Botmanghelidj, F. MD, *Your Body's Many Cries for Water*, Falls Church, VA: Global Health Solutions, 1997.

Bott, Victor, MD, *Spiritual Science and the Art of Healing*, Rochester, VT: Healing Arts Press, 1984.

Bradshaw, John, *On the Family*, Deerfield Beach, FL: Health Communications, 1988.

Breggin, Peter, MD Toxic Psychiatry, New York: St. Martin's Press, 1991.

Breiling, Brian J, ed., *Light Years Ahead*, Tiburon, CA: Light Years Ahead Productions, 1996.

Callahan, Roger, *Tapping the Healer Within*, Chicago: Contemporary Books, 2001.

Campbell, Joseph, *Transformations of Myth Through Time*, New York: Harper & Rowe, 1990.

Carnes, Patrick, *Out of the Shadows,* Minneapolis, MN: Compcare Publications, 1983.

Carter, James P., *Racketeering in Medicine*, Norfolk, VA: Hampton Roads Publishing Company, 1993.

Casdorph, H. Richard, MD and Walker Morton, MD, *Toxic Metal Syndrome*, Garden City Park, NY: Avery Publishing Group, 1995.

Choprak, Deeprak, *Quantum Healing*, New York: Bantam, 1989.

Cohen, Jay, MD, *Overdose*, New York: Penguin USA, 2001.

Coyle, Michael, *The Four Underlying Causes of Illness*, Petaluma, CA: Elbow Room Publishing, 1999.

Cummings, Stephen and Ullman, Dana, *Everybody's Guide to Homeopathic Medicines*, Los Angeles: Jeremy Tarcher, 1984.

Deida, David, *Intimate Communion*, Deerfield Beach, FL: Health Communications, 1995.

Dethlefsen Thorwald, *The Healing Power of Illness*, Rockport, MA: Element Inc., 1990.

Dosch, Peter, MD, *Manual of Neural Therapy*, Heidelberg, Germany: Karl Haug Publishers, 1984.

Dossey, Larry, MD, *Healing Words*, New York: Harper Collins, 1993.

Dossey, Larry, MD, *Prayer is Good Medicine*, New York: HarperCollins, 1996.

Edwards, David A. MD, HMD, *Theory and Practice of Biological Medicine,* Reno, Nevada: BioMedical Research Institute, 1995.

Eknath, Easwaren, *Dialogue with Death*, Petaluma, CA: Nilgiri Press, 1981.

Erasmus, Udo, *Fats That Heal, Fats that Kill*, Burnaby, BC Canada: Alive Books, 1986, 1993.

Ewald, Paul, *Plague Time*, New York: The Free Press, 2000,

Gerber, Richard, MD, *Vibrational Medicine*, 3rd ed. Rochester, VT: Bear and Company, 2001.

Glas, Norbert, MD, *The Fulfillment of Old Age*, Hudson, New York: Anthroposophic Press, 1970.

Glockler, Michaela, MD, *Medicine at the Threshold*, London: Temple Lodge Publishing, 1997.

Goldberg, Burton, Editor, *Alternative Medicine: The Definitive Guide*, Berkeley: Celestial Arts Press, 2002.

Gordon, James, MD, *Manifesto for a New Medicine*, Reading, MA: Addison-Wesley Publishing Company, 1996.

Hamer, MD, *Summary of The New Medicine*, E-Fuengirola, Spain: Amici di Dirk, 2000.

Harrison, John, MD, *Love Your Disease: It's Keeping You Healthy*, Santa Monica, CA: Hay House, 1989.

Hawkins, David, MD, *Power vs. Force*, Sedona: Veritas Publishing, 1998.

Hay, Louise, *You Can Heal Your Life*, Santa Monica: Hay House, 1984.

Hellinger, Bert, *Love's Hidden Symmetry*, Phoenix, AZ:.Zeig Tucker and Company, 1998.

Huggins, Hal, DDS, *It's All in Your Head*, Garden City Park, NY: Avery Publishing Group, 1993.

Illich, Ivan, *Medical Nemesis*, New York: Pantheon Books, 1976.

Janiger, Oscar, MD, and Goldberg, Phillip, *A Different Kind of Healing*, Los Angeles: Jeremy Tarcher, 1993.

Janov, Arthur, MD, *The Biology of Love*, Amherst, New York: Prometheus Books, 2000.

Johnson, Robert A., *Owning Your Own Shadow*, San Francisco:.Harper San Francisco, 1991.

Khalsa, Darma Singh, MD, *Brain Longevity*, New York: Warner Books, 1997.

Kimbrell, Andrew, *The Human Body Shop*, New York: HarperCollins, 1993.

Kirchner-Bockholt, Margarete, MD, *Fundamental Principles of Curative Eurythmy*, London, England: Rudolf Steiner Press, 1977.

Klatz, Ronald MD and Goldman, Robert, MD, *Stopping the Clock*, New Canaan, CT: Keats Publishing, 1996.

Kleinman, Arthur, MD, *The Illness Narratives*, New York: Basic Books, 1998.

Kurtz, Ron & Prestera, Hector, *The Body Reveals*, New York: Harper Howe, 1976.

Lappe, Mark, *When Antibiotics Fail*, Berkeley, CA: North Atlantic Books, 1986.

Lievegoed, Bernard, MD, *Man on The Threshold*, Stroud, UK: Hawthorn Press, 1985.

Lievegood, Bernard, MD, *Phases: The Spiritual Rhythms of Adult Life,* London: Rudolf Steiner Press, 1997.

Lindorff, Dave, Marketplace Medicine, New York: Bantam Books, 1992.

Mander, Gerry, *Four Arguments for the Elimination of Television*, New York: Quill Press, 1978.

Mattman, Lida, *Cell Wall Deficient Forms*, New York: CRC Press, 2001.

McAllen, Audrey, *Sleep,* Gloucestershire, England: Hawthorne Press, 1981.

McGarey, William MD, *Edgar Casey and the Palma Christi*, Virginia Beach, VA: Edgar Casey Foundation, 1975.

McTaggert, Lynne, *The Field: The Quest for the Secret Force of the Universe*, New York: Quill, 2003.

Mees, L., MD, *Blessed by Illness*, Spring Valley, NY: Anthroposophic Press, 1983.

Meineg, George, DDS, *The Root Canal Cover-Up*, Ohai, CA: Bion Publishing, 1994.

Mercola, Joseph, DO, *The No Grain Diet,* New York: Plume, rev. 2004.

Moore, Robert & Gillette, Doug, *King, Warrior, Magician, Lover*, San Francisco: Harper San Francisco, 1990.

Moyers, Bill, *Healing and the Mind*, New York: Doubleday, 1993.

Murphy, Christine, *The Vaccination Dilemma*, New York: Lantern Books, 2002.

Myss, Caroline, *Anatomy of the Spirit*, New York: Crown Publishers, 1996.

Myss, Caroline, *Why People Don't Heal and How They Can*, New York: Harmony Books, 1997.

Nelson, Dawn, *Making Friends with Cancer*, Tallahassee, FL: Findhorn Press, 2000.

Ornish, Dean, MD, *Love and Survival*, New York: HarperCollins, 1998.

Oschman, James, MD, *Energy Medicine: The Scientific Basis*, New York: Harcourt Publishers, 2000.

Oski, Frank, MD, *Don't Drink Your Milk*, Brushton, NY: Teach Services, Inc. 1996.

Peck, M Scott, MD, *The Road Less Traveled*, New York: Simon & Schuster, 1978.

Pert, Candace, *Molecules of Emotion*, New York: Scribner, 1997.

Pizzorno, Joseph, ND, *Total Wellness*, Rocklin, CA: Prima Publishing, 1996.

367

Rechtschaffen, Stephan, MD, *Timeshifting: Creating More Time to Enjoy Your Life,* New York: Doubleday Books, 1996.

Rechtschaffen, Stephan, MD and Cohen, Marc, *Vitality and Wellness*, New York: Bantam Dell, 1999.

Rogers, Sherry, MD, *Tired or Toxic*, Syracuse, NY: Prestige Publishers, 1990.

Ross, Julia, *The Mood Cure*, New York: Penguin USA, 2003.

Rossman, Martin, MD, *Healing Yourself*, New York: Simon & Schuster, 1987.

Rossi, Ernest, *The Psychobiology of Mind/Body Healing,* New York: W.W. Norton & Company, 1993.

Rubin, Jordan, Patient, *Heal Thyself*, Topanga, CA: Freedom Press, 2003.

Ruiz, Don Miguel, *The Four Agreements*, San Rafael, CA: Amber-Allen Publishing, 1997.

Sanford, John. *What Men Are Like*, Paulist Press: New York, 1988.

Schmidt, Gerhard, MD, *The Dynamics of Nutrition,* St. Gallen, Switzerland: Proteus-Verlag, 1980.

Schmidt, Michael, MD, Smith, Lyndon, MD and Sehnert, Keith, MD, *Beyond Antibiotics*, Berkeley, CA: North Atlantic Books, 1993.

Shealy, C. Norman, MD and Myss, Caroline, *The Creation of Health*, Walpole, New Hampshire: Stillpoint Publishing, 1993.

Sheldrake, Rupert, *Seven Experiments That Could Change the World: A Do It Yourself Guide to Revolutionary Science*, Rochester, VT: Park Street Press, 2002.

Sheldrake, Rupert, *The Presence of The Past: Morphic Resonance and the Habits of Nature*, Rochester, VT: Inner Traditions, Intl., 1995.

Siegel, Bernie, MD, *Love, Medicine and Miracles*, New York: Harper Rowe, 1986.

Siegel, Bernie, MD, *Peace, Love, and Healing*, New York: Harper & Rowe, 1989.

Small, Jacqueline, *Becoming Naturally Therapeutic*, Bantam Press: New York, 1990.

Stein, Robert, *Incest and Human Love*, New York: Viking Press, 1974.

Steiner, Rudolf, *Spiritual Science and Medicine*, Great Barrington, MA: Steiner Books, 1989.

Stevens, Rosemary, *In Sickness and in Wealth*, New York: Harper Collins, 1989.

Stockton, Susan, *The Terrain is Everything*, Aurora, CO: Power of One Publishing, 2000.

Strauss, Anselm, Ed., *Where Medicine Fails*, New Brunswick, New Jersey: Transaction Books, 1984.

Toffler, Alvin, *Powershift*, New York: Bantam, 1990.

Valone, Thomas, Bioelectromagnetic Healing - A Rationale for its Use, Washington, DC: Integrity Research Institute, 2000.

Walcott, William, *The Metabolic Typing Diet*, New York: Doubleday, 2000.

Walker, Martin, *Dirty Medicine*, London: Slingshot Publications, 1993.

Weil Andrew, MD, *Health and Healing*, Boston, MA: Houghton, Mifflin, 1983.

Weil, Andrew, MD, *Spontaneous Healing*, New York: Alfred Knopf, 1995.

Whitmont, Edward S., *Return of the Goddess*, New York: Continuum, 1997.

Whitmont, Edward, *The Symbolic Quest*, Princeton: Princeton University Press, 1969.

Wilbur, Ken, *The Atman Project*, Wheaton, IL: Theosophical Publishing House, 1980.

Wilder, Barbara, *Money is Love: Reconnecting to the Sacred Origins of Money*, Wild Ox Press, 1999.

Wilson, Lawrence, *Nutritional Balancing and Hair Mineral Analysis*, Prescott, Arizona: L.D. Wilson Consultants, Inc., 1998.

Wilson, Lawrence, *Sauna Therapy*, L.D. Prescott, AZ: Wilson Consultants, Inc, 2003.

Williams, Donald Lee, *Border Crossings*, Toronto, Canada: Inner City Books, 1981.

Wiley, T. S., *Lights Out*, New York: Simon & Schuster, 2000.

Zavik, Jeffrey, *Toxic Food Syndrome*, Ft. Lauderdale, FL: Fun Publishing, 2002.

Ziegler, Alfred, *Archetypal Medicine*, Dallas, TX: Spring Publications, 1983.

Zieve, Robert, MD, *Rhythms in Time: The Homeopathic Future*, Chadds Ford, PA: Robert J. Zieve, MD, 1993.

ABOUT THE AUTHOR

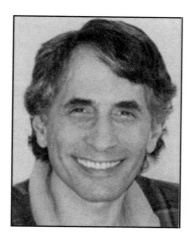

Robert J. Zieve, M.D., is an author, lecturer, and practitioner of Comprehensive Medicine. His practice includes homeopathy, European biological medicine, anthroposophical medicine, neural therapy and nutrition. He has also worked as a Board-Certified specialist in Emergency Medicine for over twenty years, and has served as a past emergency department director.

Dr. Zieve has extensive experience in the general practice of integrative medicine. This includes helping patients with illnesses that include autism, Lyme disease, and other chronic infections, neurodegenerative disorders, hormonal imbalances, cancer, chronic fatigue syndrome, fibromyalgia, auto-immune disorders, and depression.

He combines and integrates a synergistic approach to healing that includes homeopathy (both classical and drainage), biological medicine, neural therapy, homeopathic, and color treatment through acupuncture meridian points, nutrition and intravenous therapies, oxygen therapies, and heavy metal detoxification. He is also trained and experienced in the use of Insulin Potentiation Therapy in the treatment of cancer. In addition, Dr. Zieve applies an anthroposophical approach that includes anthroposophical remedies, therapeutic eurythmy (a movement therapy), as well as biographical therapy and topical therapies.

His work also includes many applications of energy medicine. These include microcurrent therapies, color and eye movement therapies, and emotional freedom techniques with tapping. On deeper levels, Dr. Zieve works with the psychodynamics of a patient's illness in the context of family history, employing Dr. Bert Hellinger's work in order to determine both the relationship of illness to unresolved family dynamics and the effective therapeutic dialogues that will help a patient heal.

Dr. Zieve is a graduate of the Ohio State University College of Medicine. During his training, he was instrumental in setting up one of the first community programs in the nation for evaluating children for lead poisoning. After completing his medical training, he took instruction in homeopathic medicine under the auspices of the National Center for Homeopathy, as well as studying with several well-known homeopathic medical doctors in Ohio. Dr. Zieve has also completed the two-year training course for physicians in anthroposophical medicine. In addition, he has studied for five years with Dietrich Klinghardt, M.D. of the American Academy of Neural Therapy in Seattle, Washington. Dr. Zieve has also completed a two-year training course with The Biological Medicine Foundation under the auspices of Thomas Rau, M.D., and has studied with Dr. Rau at Paracelsus Klinik near Zurich, Switzerland.

Dr. Zieve has lectured to groups in both clinical orthodox medicine and holistic medicine for more than twenty years, both locally and nationally. He was an instructor in university courses in clinical anatomy and physiology as well as body-mind dynamics for three years in San Diego. Dr. Zieve has taught at the Southwest College of Naturopathic Medicine, and has given lectures in integrative medicine to hospital medical residents. He has also spoken at educational forums for psychologists and parents, in such areas as community development, homeopathy, wellness, and holistic home care throughout the United States. For three years, Dr. Zieve was a participating lecturer and organizer in a national educational program for physicians training in European biological medicine.

The Arizona Homeopathic and Integrative Medical Association elected Dr. Zieve as their President for the 1998-99 year, and then re-elected him in 1999 for another term. Dr. Zieve practiced integrative medicine in Prescott, Arizona from 1991-99. In November of 1999, he accepted a position as Medical Director of Paracelsus Foxhollow Clinic near Louisville, Kentucky for two years. He is trained in European Biological Medicine as it is practiced at the Paracelsus Klinik in Switzerland, with which Foxhollow is affiliated. Dr. Zieve also practiced for two years in Chadds Ford, Pennsylvania, near Philadelphia. During this time, he was invited to be a guest physician at two major hospitals in the Philadelphia, PA area.

Dr. Zieve returned to Prescott, Arizona, in April 2004, to practice, write, and teach.

372

An updated version of his first book, *Rhythms in Time: The Homeopathic Future,* first published in 1987, may be ordered at his web site: www.pinetreeclinic.com. The office telephone number is 928-778-3500. The office address is Pine Tree Clinic for Comprehensive Medicine, 1000 Ainsworth Drive, Suite A-220, Prescott, AZ 86305. Send e-mail to: drzieve@pinetreeclinic.com.